THE
ULTIMATE WOMEN'S GUIDE TO BEATING DISEASE

AND LIVING A HAPPY, ACTIVE LIFE

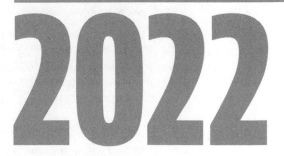

2022

FROM THE EDITORS OF BOTTOM LINE

**The Ultimate Women's Guide to Beating Disease
and Living a Happy, Active Life**

10 9 8 7 6 5 4 3 2 1

ISBN 978-0-88723-000-4

Bottom Line Books® publishes the advice of expert authorities in many fields. These opinions may
at times conflict as there are often different approaches to solving problems. The use of this material
is no substitute for health, legal, accounting or other professional services. Consult competent
professionals for answers to your specific questions.

Telephone numbers, addresses, prices, offers and websites listed in this book are accurate at the time
of publication, but they are subject to frequent change.

Bottom Line Books® is a registered trademark of Belvoir Media Group, LLC.
535 Connecticut Avenue, Norwalk, CT 06854-1713

Belvoir.com || BottomLineInc.com

Bottom Line Books® is an imprint of Belvoir Media Group, LLC, publisher of print and
digital periodicals, books and online training programs. We are dedicated to bringing you
the best information from the most knowledgeable sources in the world. Our goal is to help
you gain greater wealth, better health, more wisdom, extra time and increased happiness.

Printed in the United States of America

CONTENTS

Preface xi

1 • AGING WELL

The Secret to Successful Aging 1
Five Things That Are Surprisingly
    Better After 70 3
Reassuring News About Vaginal Estrogen
    for Menopause 5
Resveratrol Supplements Improve
    Menopause Symptoms 6
Earlier Menopause Linked to Man-Made
    Chemicals 7
DIY Honey-and-Lemon Face Mask 8
Tired of Looking Tired? How to Erase
    Undereye Dark Circles and Bags 8
Feel Better, Live Longer: Sitting 101 9
Feeling Dizzy? Get the Correct Diagnosis 10
Vertigo: Not Just Dizziness 11
Stay Safe and Secure When You Live Alone 13
Sugar Shortens Lives—but Not Necessarily
    Through Obesity 15
You're Never Too Old for Cavities 15
Surprising Danger of Earwax 16
Heart-Healthy Diet May Save Hearing 17
Poor Vision Linked to Dementia Risk 17
Coping With Eye Floaters 17
Don't Miss Your Eye Appointment 18
This Eye Surgery Improves Driving Safety 19
Will I Ever See My Feet Again? My
    Flat-Belly Quest 19
Intermittent Fasting and Older Adults 20

2 • BRAIN HEALTH

Train Your Brain for Better Memory
    and Greater Joy 21
Headaches? Memory Loss?
    Blame Menopause! 23
The 3 Steps to Worry Less…and
    Enjoy More 24
Strength Training Starts With the Brain 27
How to Remember Names… 27
Alcohol and the Brain 28
What's in a Drink? 30
A Makeover for Your Mind 30
Case Study: What to Do About That
    Failing Memory 32
Treating Hypertension Could Reduce
    Dementia Risk 32
4 Natural Ways to Prevent Dementia 33
Danger for Women: Dehydration and
    Dementia 35
Promising News About Dementia Risk
    from Parkinson's Treatment 35
Dementia Alerts 36
Parkinson's Patients Are Given Drugs
    That Work Against Each Other 37
A Blood Test for Alzheimer's 38
Dementia Patients Often Get
    Ineffective Drugs 38
A Novel Way to Identify Alzheimer's
    and Predict Its Progression 38
Multiple Sclerosis Symptoms Improve
    With Mindfulness Meditation 39

Contents

Strenuous Physical Workouts Tire the
Brain Too 40
More TV Viewing, Greater Cognitive Decline... 40

3 • CANCER CARE FOR WOMEN

3-D Mammography Is Best for Breast
Cancer Screening 41
Earlier Breast Cancer Screening Saves Lives 42
A Fasting Diet May Boost Breast
Cancer Treatment 43
Menopause Help for Breast Cancer Survivors.. 43
Breast-feeding Reduces Ovarian Cancer Risk .. 46
Honeybee Venom Kills Hard-to-Treat
Breast Cancer Cells 46
New Treatments Are Increasing Lung
Cancer Survival 47
How to Protect Your Colon: The 5 Essentials... 47
A Chinese Herb May Reduce the Risk of
Colon Polyps 49
Colorectal-Cancer Screening Should Start
Sooner Than You Think................................ 50
Gum Disease Raises Cancer Risk 50
Severe Sunburn Can Make You Sick.................. 50
Routine CT Scan Predicts Heart Disease
in Breast Cancer Survivors.......................... 50
Cutting-Edge Cancer Care 51
A Psychedelic Drug Offers Years of Benefits
to Cancer Patients.. 53
Cognitive Issues Linger in Breast Cancer
Survivors on PPIs... 53
If You Had One HPV Cancer, You're
More Likely to Get Others 53
Seaweed May Treat Skin Cancer and MRSA..... 54
An Aspirin a Day May Make Cancer
More Dangerous for Older Adults................ 55
Combining Cancer Drugs Improves
Leukemia Survival 56
Beware of Cancer Treatment Side Effects........ 56

4 • DIABETES AND BLOOD SUGAR CONTROL

The Hot Flash/Diabetes Connection 57
Probiotics Help People With Type 2
Diabetes... 58
New Option for Preventing Diabetes................ 58
The Gut Bug That Protects Against Diabetes... 59
Acid Reflux Drugs May Increase
Diabetes Risk 60
The Hidden Risks of Normal-Weight Obesity.... 61
Flax and Pumpkin Seeds May
Fight Diabetes 62

COVID-19 Causes Dangerous Spikes
in Blood Sugar.. 63
Diabetes Makes COVID-19 Worse and
Possibly Vice Versa 63
Statins Raise Diabetes Risk 64
Stem-Cell Treatment May Cure Diabetes 64
Weak Grip Strength Can Predict Type 2
Diabetes Risk 64
Diabetes Vaccine Under Investigation 64

5 • EMOTIONAL RESCUE

Surprising Cause of Anxiety…and
How to Heal It.. 65
Ways to Keep Anxiety from Spiraling............... 67
The Narcissistic Partner..................................... 68
Are Your Clothes Ruining Your Mood?
How to Dress to Feel Your Best.................... 70
Art Relieves the Stress of Caregiving................. 72
Adults With ADHD Are More Likely
to Get into Car Crashes 72
A Faux Commute Could Be Good
for You.. 72
Social Anxiety May Affect Your Memory.......... 73
Remember in a New Way 73
Time and Money Traps That Can Rob
You of Happiness 73
A "Gratitude Jar" Can Help Lift
Your Spirits 75
"Doomscrolling" Makes a Bad Time
Span Worse 75
Depression After Surgery 76
Use Instagram to Lift Your Spirits 76
Make a Big Change in Small Increments........... 76
Finding Meaning After the Death of
a Loved One... 76
"Mind Over Matter" Can Reduce
Inflammation.. 78
Are You a Precrastinator?.................................. 79
How to Prevent Problems Before
They Erupt.. 79
Happiness Lies in Change.................................. 81
Playing Hard-to-Get Pays Off............................ 81
Four Hidden Marriage Killers 81
Full House: How to Make It Work..................... 83
Boost Your Spirits by Helping Others 86
Spread the Love! 86
Myths Many Older Women Believe
About Alcohol Consumption 86
Solve a Recurring Sleep Problem
With a Sleep Journal..................................... 86
Alcohol-Related Deaths Have Doubled 87

Why Some People Feel Stress More
Intensely Than Others.....................87
7 Tools to Help You Through the
Rough Patches 88
Change Your Mind About How to
Change Minds 90
The Right Way to Help People Who
Ask for Your Help 92
Best Ways to Regulate Your Emotions 94
How to Get Beyond Small Talk......................94
How Not to Be Annoyed by People
Who Annoy You.........................95
How to Tell If You're the Toxic Person
in Your Workplace—and How
to Be Better 96
Beat Loneliness With the Grandkids.................97
Steps to Forgiveness 97
When You Fear You're Not Good Enough......97
Better Ways to Avoid Loneliness....................99
Detox Your Relationships 99
Magic Mushrooms Can Relieve Depression ...101
Calming "Monkey Mind"..................102

6 • FOOD, DIET AND FITNESS

5 Ways to Change Your Attitude and
Get Healthy 103
Small Wins With Big Payoffs 104
Shared Success Stories Help Young
Moms Lose Weight, Get Healthier 105
Lose Your Quarantine Weight Gain...............106
Alpha Lipoic Acid Lowers Body Fat
and Weight..............................106
Trick to Eat Less...........................106
Taste Bud Rehab: Stop Craving Bad Food 106
Guilt-Free Snacks from Top Food Bloggers ...107
Satisfy a Sugar Craving: Choco-Banana
"Nice Cream" 108
Beat the Afternoon Slump: Matcha
Cupcakes...........................108
Postworkout Hunger: Avocado Sweet
Potato "Toast" With Hummus 108
When Dinner Isn't Ready: Creamy Curried
Red Lentil Dip With Raw Veggies and
Tortilla Chips 109
Movie Night: "Cheesy" Popcorn With
Nutritional Yeast......................109
Coffee: Drink Up for Less Body Fat 110
Healthier Coffee Drinking............................111
Beware the Keto Diet for Weight Loss 111
3 Food Myths That Could Hurt You.............111
Going Meatless Without Going Hungry.........113

Lentil Cassoulet With Lots of Vegetables.....113
Artichokes and Shell Beans Braised in
White Wine 114
Tamarind Tempeh Kebabs...............115
Lab-Grown Meat Is Coming.....................115
Some Foods May Contain Unlisted
Ingredients 115
Spices May Reduce Risks of a High-Fat,
High-Carb Meal.........................116
Extraordinary Olives.............................117
Hummus and Beans Often Are
Contaminated.........................117
Hidden Dangers in Food from China 118
Beyond the Cucumber: Pickled Vegetables
Are a Tangy Treat 118
Lemon Dill Kraut 120
Spicy Carrot and Lime Salad....................120
Prebiotic Foods May Improve Sleep and
Reduce Stress 121
Organic Apples Are Better for Gut Health 121
Fatty Foods Can Hamper Concentration.........122
Using Only Sea Salt or Gourmet Salt
Can Lead to Iodine Deficiency 122
Don't Throw Away Expired Milk 122
How to Cook Safely With Nonstick Pans 122
Switch to Sourdough Bread........................123
Easy Gluten-free Sourdough Bread Recipe 123
Immune-Boosting Recipes That Are
Bursting With Flavor 124
Chicken Almond Satay Wraps 124
Roasted Sweet Potato and Kale
Quinoa Bowl 125
Roast Cod with Fennel and Tomatoes.........125
Zesty Papaya Salsa.........................126
Super Spinach Hummus 126
Unsweetened Dried Fruit..........................126
Homemade Fruit Leather 126
Skip the Soda 127
Foods to Wash—and Not Wash.....................127
The Sweetener Stevia Could Disrupt
Your Gut..............................127
Calcium: The Rest of the Story 127
The Vitamin Deficiency You Don't
Know You Have..........................130
You Can Have Confidence in Vitamin C
Supplements............................132
Vitamin C Is Associated With Higher
Muscle Mass 132
Strength Training After 50...........................132
Beat the Heat: Five Surprising Ways to
Keep Cool 134
The Beauty of Winter Hiking.........................136

Contents

Make Money When You Walk........................ 138
Build Muscle With This "Rubber Band"
    Workout.. 138
Free Ways to Do Workouts at Home............. 140
Cutting-Edge Athletic Shoes to Up Your
    Performance 141
Exercise Outside 141
Too Busy to Exercise? "Fidget-cisers"
    Can Help Anytime, Anywhere..................... 142
It's Time to Get Back on a Bike 144
Bicycles That Won't Break the Bank 145
Create a "Peloton" Experience for Less 146
How to Spot-Train Your Butt 147
Raising the Barre 148

7 • GET THE CARE YOU NEED

Women Need More Attention in Medical
    Research 149
Don't Let Medical Care Take Over
    Your Life.. 150
The Best Way to Advocate for Your
    Health: Ask the Right Questions 152
What a Health Coach Can Do for You........... 154
E-Coaching: Your Virtual Guide 156
Banish Physician Phobia.............................. 156
How to Survive the Hospital Now 158
Don't Be Misdiagnosed 160
Lead Shielding Does Not Protect
    During X-rays.. 161
Before You Say "Yes" to Outpatient Surgery... 162
Virtual Post-Op Visits Work 162
Make the Most of Video Visits with
    Your Doctor 163
Best Health-Monitoring Devices to
    Have at Home 164
Owning a Pulse Oximeter............................. 165
Trusted Health Resources 166
The Right Way to Measure Your
    Blood Oxygen....................................... 166
Cannabis Use Before Surgery 167
Many Medicines Can Trigger Tinnitus 167
Reduce Delirium Risk After Surgery 167
Beware Websites Offering Online
    Prescriptions.. 167
Managing Medication Side Effects................. 168
Drugs That Alter Your Gut Microbiome 170
Popular Drugs That Can Lead to
    Eye Problems 171
Problems After Gastric Bypass Surgery 173
Key to Treating Chronic Digestive
    Conditions 174

Are PPIs OK?.. 174
NSAIDs Do Not Make COVID-19 Worse 175
A Natural Medicine Advocate at the
    Hospital Emergency Department 175
The Pros and Cons of Chiropractic Care 176

8 • HEART AND STROKE HEALTH FOR WOMEN

Heart Disease in Women: A New
    Paradigm for Prevention & Treatment......... 179
Heart Failure is Deadlier for Women.............. 181
Heart Attack or Passing Panic? 181
Mediterranean Diet Beats Low-Fat Diet
    for Heart Attack Patients 182
Omega-3 Supplements Really Do Help
    Prevent Heart Disease 183
New Way to Help Treat Heart Failure 184
Hot Flashes and Night Sweats Are
    Linked to Heart Attack 184
How Hard Are You Exercising?...................... 184
Silent Heart Attacks 185
A Novel Way to Predict Heart Failure
    Prognosis 187
Carpal Tunnel Syndrome: A Harbinger
    of Heart Failure?................................... 188
Busting the Cholesterol Myth 189
3 Questions to Ask Before You Start
    Statins: Personalizing Your
    Risk Profile 192
Most People Don't Benefit from
    Low-Dose Aspirin 194
Nocebo-Effect May Explain Many Side
    Effects of Statins................................... 195
"Broken-Heart Syndrome" and COVID-19 195
Sudden Cardiac Arrest May Not Be
    So Sudden 195
Blood Pressure Mistakes 196
Blood Pressure Meds at Night 198
Long Work Hours Are Linked to
    High Blood Pressure 198
Low Blood Pressure: No Symptoms?
    No Problem 198
All About Resting Heart Rate........................ 199
Training for a First-Time Marathon................. 200
Mealtime Linked to Heart Health 201
When It Seems Like You're Wearing a
    Heart Monitor Too Long… 201
A Flavanol-Rich Diet Lowers Blood
    Pressure.. 201
The Truth About Life After Heart Failure 201
LVAD for Heart Failure................................ 204

Beware of Atrial Fibrillation After
Any Surgery......................................205
Say Goodbye to A-Fib 206
Positive Thinking Could Help Prevent
a Stroke...208
Protein Helps Fight A-Fib.....................209
Speech Therapy After Stroke Does Not
Have to Be Rushed...........................210
Restore Mobility and Sense of Touch
After a Stroke 210
Heavy Drinking Increases Waistline—
and Stroke Risk................................210

9 • INFECTIOUS DISEASES

Put an End to UTIs 211
Better Probiotics Could Lead to Better
Vaginal Health 213
COVID-19 Symptoms Can Linger
for Months 213
Once Exposed, the Immune System
"Remembers" COVID Well 216
What We've Learned About Treating
COVID-19 216
Fever: To Treat or Not to Treat? 218
Is It a Cold or COVID-19? 218
MMR Vaccine Booster Could Improve
COVID Outcomes 219
Better Cleaning to Kill Germs..............220
Be Careful When Using Potting Mix ...220
Disinfect Your Home After a Virus 220
5 Natural Ways to Repel Mosquitoes ...220
Too Much Salt Lowers Your Immune
Defenses 221
Fecal Transplant Better Than Antibiotics
for C. diff Diarrhea 221
Can You Be Immune to Lyme Disease?...222
Eyeglasses Can Protect Against
Viral Infection 222
Best Humidifiers to Fight Viruses........223
Six Ways You May Be Showering
Wrong..224
Help for Fever Blisters 224
Alcohol-Free Hand Sanitizers Protect
Against COVID-19 225
Rescue Dry, Chapped Hands................225
Humans vs. Virus: Curing Hepatitis 226
Another Strange Sign of COVID-19.......226

10 • NATURAL HEALING REMEDIES

Super Immune-Boosters Your Doctor
Doesn't Know About..........................227

If You Catch a Cold...Pelargonium.................229
After a COVID-19 Infection: Healing
Your Brain and Body 229
Restorative Yoga Is the New Power Yoga......232
Morning Light May Speed Healing After
Mild Concussion 235
Natural Cure for an Abnormal Pap Smear......235
Natural Therapies That Ease Parkinson's
Symptoms..236
Let Nature Be Your Medicine 237
Irritable Bowel Syndrome Eased
by Walking..238
Stopping Inflammation Is More Important
Than Ever: 9 Ways to Reverse Chronic
Illness, Prevent Infection and More 238
Chronic Indigestion Relieved With
Acupuncture.....................................240
Curcumin Effective for Ulcerative Colitis........240
Charcoal: A Versatile Treatment 241
Face Rash Cured from the Inside Out............242
Finding Natural Relief for SIBO.........243
Acupuncture Before Surgery Lessens Pain.....245
No-Hassle Natural Therapies for
Varicose Veins..................................246
Bye, Bye Baker's Cyst: No Cortisone,
Drugs or Knee Surgery 247
Calming the Pain of Chronic Tendonitis.........247
Excellent Health Benefits of Chamomile........248

11 • PAIN RELIEF FOR WOMEN

When Menopause Causes Arthritis...How
to Ease the Pain and Get Back to Life 251
Got Painful Hand Arthritis? Get Relief
Without Drugs....................................253
Arthritis Drugs Linked to Depression 254
Ease Your Pain With These Soothing
Self-Massage Tools............................255
How to Relieve Muscular Pain Points 257
Relieve Your Neck Pain 258
Breakthroughs in Migraine Relief 259
Beware Uncommon Symptoms of Jaw
Problems That Lead to a Temporo-
mandibular Joint Disorder (TMJ).................259
Yoga Improves Migraine Treatment...............261
What to Take for a Tension Headache—
No Drugs Needed..............................262
High-Tech Help for Migraine Pain 263
Green Light Reduces Migraines.......................263
Surprising Migraine—Dry Eye Connection.....263
The Role of Cannabis in Pain Management
Is Unclear 264

Contents

Sit Smarter and Prevent Pain 264
For Knee Arthritis, PT Beats
    Steroid Injections 264
Prevent Gas, Pain and Intestinal Bloat 265
8 Stretches That Ease Your Aches and Pains ... 265
The Four-Step Plantar Fasciitis Plan 267
Suffering from Sciatica? 269
Debilitating Sciatica Relieved in 10 Minutes ... 269
Counting Down Can Keep Pain in Check 270
To Live Pain-Free, Take Care of Your
    Fascia: Here's How 270
3D Technology Makes Knee Replacement
    Better Than Ever 273
Fight the Rise of Autoimmune Disease 275
Bee Venom Injections Relieve Knee
    Osteoarthritis 277
Tryptophan Shows Potential to Relieve
    Celiac Disease 277
Thriving When There Is No Cure 278

12 • PHYSICAL INJURY AND BONE HEALTH

Physical and Emotional Trauma Linger in
    Your Body: How to Free Yourself 281
4 Common Moves That Lead to Injury…
    And How to Do Them the Right Way 283
3 Easy Ways to Relieve Your Pain
    from an Injury 285
Danger of Plant-Based Diets:
    Bone Fractures 286
Can the "Love Hormone" Prevent
    Osteoporosis? 287
Steroids for Asthma Linked to Osteoporosis .. 287
After an Accident: Healing Lasting Anxiety
    and Insomnia Naturally 288
Beware of This Hidden Cause of Falls 288
Balancing Act 289
How to Do Computer Work With
    Thumb Pain 290
Why Does Dizziness Linger After a
    Bad Fall? 291
Is Whiplash More Dangerous If It
    Happens Again? 292
Is Shoulder Pain a Rotator Cuff Tear?
    Don't Trust Your MRI 293

13 • PREGNANCY AND REPRODUCTION ISSUES

IVF Offers Clues to Future Health Problems .. 295
New Microbiome Therapy Fights Recurrent
    Vaginal Infections 296
Drinking and Miscarriages 297
If You're Having Trouble Getting Pregnant,
    Check Your Thyroid 297
Typical Drug Doses May Be Harmful
    for Some Pregnancies 297
Which Antidepressant Is Linked to the
    Most Birth Defects? 298
Postpartum Depression (PPD) Alert 299
"Vascular Storm" Blamed for Severe Flu
    During Pregnancy 299
Natural Birth May Reduce Infants'
    Health Problems 300
Is Your Daughter or Daughter-in-Law
    Pregnant? For Family Harmony,
    Follow These Five Rules! 300
"Mommy Brain" Is Largely a Myth 301
Late Pregnancy and NSAIDs Alert 301
Surgery for Benign Breast Disease Does
    Not Affect Breastfeeding 301

14 • RESPIRATORY CONDITIONS

Why You Can't Catch Your Breath. 303
Know the Symptoms of a Lung Emergency ... 305
Danger of Using Petroleum Jelly in the
    Nose to Moisturize Nostrils 305
Breathe Better: Four Easy Exercises
    to Strengthen Your Lungs and
    Restore Good Health 306
Pulmonary Rehabilitation for COPD
    Saves Lives 307
Why We Sigh: The
    Biology and Psychology of Those
    Deep, Audible Breaths 308
Air Pollution Damages Gut Bacteria 310
A Healthier Home 310
Dangers in Dust 311
Secondhand e-Cigarette Exposure Is
    Dangerous 311
Cleaning Products Linked to Childhood
    Asthma 312
Teas That Relieve Asthma 312
Milk Allergy in Babies May Be
    Overdiagnosed 312
A Simple Pill Could Block Severe Allergic
    Reactions 312
Your Heartburn Could Be Caused
    by an Allergy 313
Surprising Solution to Recurrent Nasal
    Infections 314
Thirdhand Smoke Can Affect People
    Even in Nonsmoking Environments 314

15 • VERY PERSONAL

Demystifying Incontinence 315
Less Sex Linked to Earlier Menopause............ 317
Talking Testosterone 317
Pornography Doesn't Affect Relationship
   Satisfaction—at Least Not in the
   Short Term 318
Clean Your Bottom Better............................... 318
Beware This Smell When You Pass Gas......... 320
How to Sweat Less and Stop the Stink 320
Bad Breath Despite Good Dental Hygiene?.... 322
Treat and Prevent "Maskne" 323

Drug-free Constipation Cure: A
   Vibrating Pill 323
Floating Poop Could Be a Sign of Trouble..... 324
New Treatment for Heavy Bleeding
   from Fibroids 324
Swelling in the Legs: Consider
   May-Thurner Syndrome 325
Drooping Eyelids: Aging Isn't Always
   the Cause.. 326
Women Fall Asleep Faster After
   Intercourse....................................... 328

Index 329

PREFACE

We are proud to bring to you *The Ultimate Women's Guide to Beating Disease and Living a Happy, Active Life 2022*. This essential volume features trustworthy and actionable life-saving information from the best health experts in the world—information that will help women beat the most deadly conditions.* In the following chapters, you'll find the latest discoveries, best treatments and scientifically proven remedies to keep you living a long, happy and active life.

Whether it's heart care, the latest on breast cancer prevention and treatment, breakthrough treatments for hot flashes or cutting-edge nutritional advice, the editors at Bottom Line Books talk to the experts—from top women's health doctors to research scientists to leading alternative care practitioners—who are creating the true innovations in health care.

Over the past four decades, we have built a network of literally thousands of leading physicians in both alternative and conventional medicine. They are affiliated with the premier medical and research institutions throughout the world. We read the important medical journals and follow the latest research that is reported at medical conferences. And we regularly talk to our advisors in major teaching hospitals, private practices and government health agencies for their insider perspective.

*"Leading Causes of Death in Females," Centers for Disease Control and Prevention (*http://www.cdc.gov/women/lcod/2017/index.html*).

In this 2022 edition, we've gone beyond diseases and have included several chapters of life-enhancing health information on pregnancy, pain, depression, fitness, nutrition, quality medical care, digestive health and aging...all of which are essential to living a happy, active life. And it's all backed by breaking studies and top health experts. Also note that respiratory diseases, according to the Centers for Disease Control and Prevention, are now considered one of the top three causes of death in women of all ages (same percentage as stroke).

The Ultimate Women's Guide to Beating Disease and Living a Happy, Active Life 2022 is a result of our ongoing research and connection with these experts, and is a distillation of their latest findings and advice. We trust that you will glean new, helpful and affordable information about the health topics that concern you most...and find vital topics of interest to family and friends as well.

As a reader of a Bottom Line book, be assured that you are receiving well-researched information from a trusted source. But please use prudence in health matters. Always speak to your physician before taking vitamins, supplements or over-the-counter medication...stopping a medication...changing your diet...or beginning an exercise program. If you experience side effects from any regimen, contact your doctor immediately.

Be well,
The Editors, Bottom Line Books
Norwalk, Connecticut

Chapter 1

AGING WELL

The Secret to Successful Aging

Successful aging is the ability to take pleasure from things that you enjoy, to discover new things, and to live your life in a way that is meaningful—at any age. It requires discipline and commitment throughout your lifetime. Although it is never too late to begin, the earlier you commit to the habits that promote successful aging the better.

In my book *Successful Aging: A Neuroscientist Explores the Power and Potential of Our Lives*, I use the acronym COACH to describe the key habits necessary to age successfully and lead a happier life: Conscientiousness, Openness, Associations, Curiosity and Healthy lifestyle.

Conscientious people are dependable, reliable and proactive. They seek medical attention when they are sick. They listen to a doctor's advice and take their medications. They live within their means and put money aside for future needs and retirement.

Being open to new experiences is crucial to successful aging and can even help prevent cognitive decline. Try a new sport, join a book club or take piano lessons. You will feel better physically and mentally.

Associations with others, through friendships and hobbies, keep you engaged and not isolated. Maintaining these associations and adding new ones gives you new perspectives and can lead to new relationships as well as shared interests.

Curiosity should never wane. People who are curious are more apt to challenge themselves intellectually and socially. They are also more likely to be interested and engaged. Curiosity helps to make us mentally agile and alert and helps to boost the immune system.

Follow a healthy lifestyle. Exercise is key to both physical and emotional health, but there is too much emphasis on aerobic exercise and lifting weights. Although going to the gym is helpful, being in nature is better. Taking walks in natural surroundings, going on hikes or riding a bike keep our minds active. An extra 20 minutes on an elliptical machine is good for the heart, but it does not stimulate your mind.

I have learned that there is no one right diet for everyone. Maintaining a healthy

Daniel L. Levitin, PhD, an award-winning neuroscientist, musician, and best-selling author. Dr. Levitin is the founding dean of Arts & Humanities at the Minerva Schools at the Keck Graduate Institute, San Francisco, and James McGill Professor Emeritus of Psychology, Neuroscience and Music at McGill University in Montreal, Quebec, Canada.

weight is key to successful aging, but it's fine to eat dessert occasionally.

A good night's sleep is essential for health and cognitive function. Restorative sleep allows the body to engage in cellular repair processes and for the brain to digest all of the experiences of the previous day. Disruptions in sleep can lead to depression and anxiety and raises your risk of high blood pressure, cardiovascular disease, diabetes and obesity. It also weakens your immune system. The National Sleep Foundation recommends seven to nine hours of sleep each night for adults ages 26 to 64, and older adults (65+) should get seven to eight hours.

It's not always easy to sleep, and it gets harder as we age. I recommend that you have a ritual before you go to bed. Take a bath or read or listen to relaxing music. Go to bed at the same time each night, and get up at the same time each day. Don't drink alcohol before bedtime. Sleep in a darkened room, and use earplugs if necessary. I don't recommend sleeping pills such as *zolpidem* (Ambien) or *eszopiclone* (Lunesta), especially for seniors, as they can cause confusion and double the risk of falls and hip fractures. Additionally, they disrupt the normal rhythms of sleep. I do not generally recommend natural sleep aids such as melatonin either. Supplements are not regulated by the U.S. Food & Drug Administation, so their quality is not guaranteed.

Keep Working

Working keeps your mind engaged. It gives you a routine and keeps you from being isolated. If you must retire, retire to something else: Volunteer, teach a class, tutor or become a mentor.

The easiest way to be happy is to help others. Helping others gives our lives purpose. It even helps with the minor aches and pains we have, as they recede when we are focused on others.

Be Grateful

Being grateful allows you to feel more positive emotions and to deal with adversity. There is also evidence that it can lower stress levels and give people an optimistic approach to life. Studies have shown that genes can make some people more grateful and others less so. To help boost your gratitude, try making a list of even simple things that you are thankful for, such as "I'm grateful I can still read," or "I'm happy my friend called me today."

Other Factors

High blood pressure, diabetes, cancer and Alzheimer's disease often run in families, but genes are not destiny. Research has shown that diet, exercise and sleep can lessen the risk or delay the onset of chronic illnesses.

Many studies show that (happily) married people live longer, but a bad relationship can actually shorten your life. Many single people live long, happy lives. The key is to connect with people in other ways.

We Get Happier as We Age

Numerous studies have shown that after age 50 people tend to get happier. A study by the Office for National Statistics in England found that 65 to 79 is the happiest age group for adults. A different study found that happiness peaks in the 80s. Older people have fewer arguments and come up with better solutions to conflict. They are also better at controlling their emotions, accepting misfortune and coping with the ups and downs of life.

While we tend to grow happier, depression can still strike at any age. If you lose interest in things you previously enjoyed or feel sad, hopeless, or empty over an extended period, talk to your doctor.

Busting Brain Myths

Your body and brain age. This is natural. We cannot run as fast as we could in our 20s at age 60. But when it comes to brain health, decline is not inevitable. Failing memory is one of the biggest misconceptions about aging. If you are over 60 and forgot where you put your keys or glasses, you might fear that it is the beginning of dementia, but teenagers forget their cell phones, and middle-aged people lose their car keys all the time. No one suggests that those lapses are a sign of Alzheimer's disease. While people are quick to draw that conclusion for seniors, those little memory lapses are normal at every age.

The more we use our brain, the better we will succeed both mentally and physically. Being mentally engaged, whether it's through work or play, keeps us interested, present and sharp. These habits are the foundation of successful aging.

Five Things That Are Surprisingly Better After 70

Adriane Berg, Esq., founder of Adriane Berg & Associates, a firm that helps companies market to the boomer and mature generations. She author of 14 books including *How Not to Go Broke at 102: Finding Everlasting Wealth* and *The Totally Awesome Money Book for Kids*. She is also an attorney and helped found the National Academy of Elder Law Attorneys. Listen to Adriane's *Generation Bold Radio Show* at AdrianeBerg.com.

Certainly, there are a variety of good things that older age brings, many of them discussed and explained by developmental scientists. For example, we are supposed to become more transcendent of the world around us, less ego-driven and more focused on our legacy. At least so said sociologist Lars Tornstam in his theory of gerotranscendence. So, too, we are supposedly on the cusp of greater wisdom as we pass 70.

Frankly speaking, so far at least, I have enjoyed none of these boons as I glided past 70 into 71 and soon 72.

Hats

What did happen, however, was I began to look exceptionally good in hats. *Here is the humble proof…*

Now, when I was a slip of a girl of only 65, I had not yet acquired that magnificent Queen Mother look that gives one the impression of aging royalty. A hat might cover a wrinkle or bring me into better light, but it did not serve to make me seem enigmatic, as it does now. I have become a romantic figure in a hat. Hats are head turners on older women, but sadly merely ornamental and a touch silly on the young.

I recently saw on the website Sixty and Me an interview with Judith Boyd, aka the "Style Crone" and a former psychiatric nurse, on the subject of women's passion for hats as we age. She mentioned cancer, hair loss and hats that cover baldness. Indeed, many years ago, I accompanied a friend who was getting Reiki at Beth Israel Hospital in Manhattan as part of her cancer treatments. One of the fascinating features of the cancer-recovery floor was the retail establishment that was a hat shop. It sold both men's and women's hats.

Hats are therapeutic, outgoing and anti-ageist. Why? Because they overtly say, *I am here*. Not invisible. Try to make me disappear, and I'll spite you with a hat that cannot be ignored.

Travel

I have visited 82 countries so far. Despite COVID-19, I plan to travel as soon as allowed by law. But as I age, I become more and more a traveler rather than merely a tourist. I enter the bones of a place…I become an inhabitant. I am not alone on this. Airbnb —embodying that ultimate ideal of living in a place, not merely visiting—is an elder-boomer phenomenon. So much so that President Obama invited Airbnb, along with Uber, to attend the 2015 White House Conference on Aging to emphasize the growth of the sharing economy as a purely boomer-driven market sector.

Then, too, intergenerational family travel takes on greater meaning when you yourself represent the oldest generation in the group. That continuity of life, which goes far to assuage the fear of its ending, is most sweetly pronounced during family vacations. Memories are as deep as your first kiss or your first look at the Eiffel Tower.

For boomers, even the family vacation must be accompanied by "an experience." In fact, the concepts of experiential travel is part of the travel industry's lexicon when describing trends of older boomers, who, like me, were born from 1946 to 1950. Lately a new term, "authentic travel" or "immersion travel"—the desire to meld and be part of the culture, cuisine and life of the area—is associated with adult travel.

Sex

Now this gets a bit edgy. Remember the great line purportedly expressed by Oscar Wilde and many wise others—"Do what you like only don't scare the horses"? Well, after 70, sex becomes another thing that one can enjoy without taking one's temperature and wondering if the drugstore test kit will turn red or blue. No concerns any longer that "we've lost it," as we often had in our postmenopausal years.

By 70, we are reconciled and fully understand which ships have sailed and which remain afloat and are seaworthy. Moreover, sexual tolerance is the peculiar bailiwick of elders, as we understand any port in a storm, to maintain the nautical allusions. Plus, there is not much by now we either have not tried, pledged to never try or planned to try before the final curtain.

As nothing is much of a surprise, we can vicariously and tolerantly take extreme joy in the loving of others, whether on screen, on the stage, in a book or in bed. We wear a perpetual broad smile when we see any type of love, having lived long enough to understand its rarity.

So how come sex and 70 seem contraindicated? Because of ageism, you silly billy. Loren Stein in her article "The 70-Year Itch," opines: "Horny old broads, dirty old men. These commonly used terms speak volumes about how society views older people who are interested in sex." Why talk when we are ridiculed? "The silence, say experts, allows misconceptions to flourish—including the widespread assumption that seniors lose interest in sex and are or should be asexual."

Interior Design

We know by now whether we are a minimalist or a maximalist. And our surroundings suit us as never before. Although downscaling isn't easy, your home and your closet do look better afterward.

But there is a lot more to "senior design," now called "universal design." Why? Because what started as a concept for design that is accessible to seniors is now understood to be beneficial for all ages.

Yes, over 70, we are saving the planet one bathroom at a time, insisting on going green and conserving water with every flush. Toilets are now created for conservation (Check out Architizer.com/blog/practice/details/water-saving-toilets/) I have worked with water conservationist, Gunnar Baldwin, to show architects the demand for saving water.

Health-care design and hospitality design have merged for that luxurious bathroom and bedroom that feels like heaven. Even down to the mattress for better sleep, an essential for healthy aging, interior design is simply better when it's all about us.

Your Finances

You are likely to be richer after 70 than before—for two good reasons. First, 70 is the age when the highest Social Security is attainable, and many workers wait until that age to collect. Second, 70 is the usual age that a pension is maxed out, following the Social Security model.

So, at age 69, you may not have those two basic sources of passive income. By 70, you do. In fact, between 2013 to 2016, there was a large surge in wealth mostly to folks over 75. *According to Forbes, citing the Fed-*

eral Reserve Board's Survey of Consumer Finances...

"The relative affluence of today's elderly is historically unprecedented. Never before have the 75+ had the highest median household net worth of any age bracket. Today, the typical 80-year-old household has twice the net worth of the typical 50-year-old household. As recently as 1995, they were about equal."

What's more, people older than 70 are still working. If that sounds unrealistic, it's not. And because of this, the US government passed the Secure Act to allow for IRA contributions at any age so long as you are working. There are a whole host of new regulations, mostly tax-oriented, that were passed in recognition that many boomers will be collecting Social Security, pensions and working well after 70, making their incomes much higher than that of younger folks.

A Final Word Here

Certainly, there are have-nots at all ages, and we must not be sanguine about the future of aging and wealth in a society where retirement could last 40 years. Ageism often prevents healthy elders from working. But know this—since the 1980s, poverty rates among seniors have consistently been much lower than those among the young. "In 1966, 28.5 percent of Americans age 65 and older were poor; by 2012, just 9.1 percent were," according to the Pew Research Center.

So if you are wise, you will save when younger and plan to rejoice when you reach 70.

Here's the punchline—live so you want to reach your 70th birthday.

Do you want to make your life better right now whatever your age? Remember how long life is. Don't sweat the calendar. Take care of yourself, your pocketbook and, above all, your hat rack. Make sure you get to 70... it's mostly in your control.

So why not live like the best is truly yet to come?

Reassuring News About Vaginal Estrogen for Menopause

Carolyn J. Crandall, MD, MS, professor of medicine, David Geffen School of Medicine at the University of California at Los Angeles, and lead author of a study titled "Breast Cancer, Endometrial Cancer, and Cardiovascular Events in Participants Who Used Vaginal Estrogen in the Women's Health Initiative Observational Study" by researchers at University of California, Los Angeles, published in *Menopause*.

Let's say you're a woman going through the menopausal transition. You're experiencing burning and itching in your vagina...you often feel an urgent need to pee... and sex is uncomfortable.

So your physician recommends that you try vaginal estrogen. It's effective for these issues, and it's available as a cream, an insert or a ring. Unlike oral hormone therapy, it won't help with hot flashes, but you're not particularly bothered by them.

So far, so good. But when you get home and open the package, you see a "black box" warning that you're at slightly increased risk for heart attacks, strokes, blood clots and breast cancer. Whoa!

Relax. There's growing evidence that these claims are unwarranted. The latest and largest study to date has found no increased health risk—and even possible benefits— from this form of hormone therapy.

Background: "Genitourinary syndrome of menopause" can include symptoms such as dryness, burning and itching in the genitals...pain while urinating...a feel of urgency when it comes to urination...lack of lubrication (and sometimes pain) during sex... and frequent urinary tract infections. These issues affect as many as 45 percent of women in the menopausal transition and can last into postmenopause.

One established treatment is low-dose estrogen delivered directly to the problem area via vaginal inserts or ointments—that is, vaginal estrogen. Even though the majority of the estrogen stays where it is needed to do its job, a small amount of estrogen enters the bloodstream and can travel throughout the body. While all the evidence to date has suggested that it's safe, there hasn't been a comprehensive study that answered the question—until now.

Study: The Women's Health Initiative Observational Study began in 1993 and enrolled nearly 100,000 women who were between the ages of 50 to 79 at the start of the study. During the course of the study, questionnaires were sent to the participants every few years to collect information about risk factors and various health conditions, including cancer, blood clots and heart disease.

For this particular analysis, researchers looked at women who used vaginal estrogen and compared them to women who didn't use any form of hormone therapy. In the end, there were 45,663 women in this analysis—and about 4,200 had used vaginal estrogen. They were followed for an average of 6.4 years.

Results: After adjusting for various risk factors for heart disease, clots and cancer, women who had used vaginal estrogen were not at any higher risk for invasive breast cancer, colorectal cancer, stroke, blood clot or premature death.

Surprising finding: Women who went through "natural" menopause—that is, women who didn't have a hysterectomy—who used vaginal estrogens were actually at reduced risk for both heart disease and hip fracture compared with those who did not use vaginal estrogens. Whether this is due to low levels of systemic estrogen as a result of the vaginal estrogen therapy or simply a healthy lifestyle in women who choose this method isn't known.

Bottom line: Vaginal estrogen is effective in treating the genitourinary symptoms of menopause, and this study adds evidence to support its safety.

Most forms of vaginal estrogen won't help with hot flashes, however. If hot flashes are your issue, talk to your doctor about hormonal and nonhormonal approaches.

Nor is vaginal estrogen the only effective resource for genitourinary issues. Recently, the FDA approved Intrarosa, a DHEA vaginal suppository that helps the body create estrogen in vaginal tissues. There are also many nonhormonal ways to manage vaginal dryness, including natural lubricants. And Kegel exercises are key to treating urinary urgency and overactive bladder.

But if you decide that vaginal estrogen is right for you, rest assured—there's growing evidence that it's safe. According to the American College of Obstetricians and Gynecologists, vaginal estrogen is safe even for breast cancer survivors, who are often advised to avoid systemic estrogen.

There's one exception—Femring, a vaginal ring that has high levels of estrogen. Unlike other vaginal estrogen products, it actually is approved to treat hot flashes. But because of the high levels of estrogen, it likely has systemic effects and is not recommended for women who are breast cancer survivors.

Resveratrol Supplements Improve Menopause Symptoms

The study titled "Long-term Resveratrol Supplementation Improves Pain Perception, Menopausal Symptoms, and Overall Well-being in Postmenopausal Women," University of Newcastle's Clinical Nutrition Research Centre, Australia, *Menopause*, August 2020.

A new study from researchers at the University of Newcastle's Clinical Nutrition Research Centre in Australia finds that resveratrol supplements in postmenopausal women may reduce symptoms of menopause and improve quality of life.

Resveratrol is a naturally occurring compound found in the skin of red grapes. Some studies have found that resveratrol has anti-inflammatory and antioxidant properties. Studies suggest that resveratrol may relieve symptoms of type 2 diabetes and arthritis. It has also been linked to protection against the thickening of arteries that causes heart disease.

The Resveratrol Supporting Healthy Aging in Women (RESHAW) study is published in the journal of the North American Menopause Society, *Menopause*. This was a two-year study that included 125 healthy, postmenopausal women. The women were randomly assigned to receive resveratrol supplements (75 mg twice each day) or a placebo. Neither the women nor researchers knew which group was getting a placebo or the supplement (double-blind study).

The women answered questions about their menopause symptoms, including pain perception, mood, depression, sleep quality, quality of life and other menopausal symptoms, such as hot flashes.

As the study ended, the researchers concluded that the resveratrol group had significant improvements compared to the placebo group. These included less aches and pains, less hot flashes, better sleep, better quality of life, and better cerebrovascular function (as measured by blood flow in the brain).

Menopause symptoms are caused by the loss of the female hormone estrogen that occurs with age. Resveratrol is a phytoestrogen—an estrogen-like compound that occurs naturally in foods. The other treatment for menopause symptoms is hormone replacement estrogen. Hormone replacement therapy has been linked to a higher risk for heart disease and breast cancer.

Earlier Menopause Linked to Man-Made Chemicals

Study titled "Associations of Perfluoroalkyl Substances with Incident Natural Menopause: The Study of Women's Health Across the Nation," led by researchers at University of Michigan School of Public Health, Ann Arbor, published in *The Journal of Clinical Endocrinology & Metabolism*.

It's become increasingly well-known that a variety of consumer products, including nonstick cookware, pizza boxes and stain repellents, have long been manufactured with a class of potentially harmful man-made chemicals known as PFAS (short for the tongue-twister per- and polyfluoroalkyl substances). These chemicals also have been found in contaminated drinking water.

Even though word has spread about PFAS' potential dangers and their use in manufacturing has declined, they are "forever chemicals" that do not break down over time. Most people in the US have been exposed to PFAS. These chemicals have been linked to a range of health problems, including elevated cholesterol levels, negative effects on the immune system, liver damage, high blood pressure and increased risk for certain types of cancer, such as kidney and testicular.

Now: Research has revealed yet another concern about PFAS. High levels of these chemicals can accumulate in women's bodies and may cause menopause to occur earlier than usual. This can be significant because earlier menopause may affect women's heart and bone health and possibly lead to quality-of-life issues that are more common after menopause. The median age of menopause of women living in industrialized countries is 50 to 52.

Study details: To investigate PFAS levels in women, researchers from the University of Michigan School of Public Health used data from 1,120 midlife, premenopausal women who were enrolled in a 17-year study called the Study of Women's Health Across the Nation.

After blood samples were taken, the study participants were divided into four groups based on their PFAS levels—low, low-medium, medium-high and high. Women with high levels of PFAS had a 63 percent greater risk of earlier menopause compared with those who had low levels of the chemicals in their blood.

For women with high PFAS levels, menopause occurred two years earlier, on average, than in women with low levels, according to the study, which was published in the Endocrine Society's *Journal of Clinical Endocrinology & Metabolism*.

DIY Honey-and-Lemon Face Mask

To prevent acne and slow aging, make this simple concoction. Mix one tablespoon organic honey with the juice from one-half small lemon. Apply the mask to your face and neck, avoiding your eyes. Leave it on for 20 minutes. Rinse with warm water, then cold. Honey is antibacterial and full of antioxidants, while the vitamin C in lemon juice helps form collagen, the protein that gives skin its elasticity.

Sejal Shah, MD, dermatologist in New York City, quoted on TheHealthy.com.

Takeaway: While efforts have been made to reduce the use of PFAS in manufacturing, it is virtually impossible to completely avoid it. Exposure to PFAS most often occurs through contaminated drinking water. Eating fish that live in contaminated water is another way that people can be exposed to PFAS. To avoid these possible sources of exposure, check with your local or state health and environmental quality departments for PFAS water contamination or fish advisories in your area.

Tired of Looking Tired? How to Erase Undereye Dark Circles and Bags

Doris Day, MD, cosmetic dermatologist in New York City and clinical associate professor of dermatology at NYU Langone Health. She is a member of the medical advisory board for the Dr. Oz Show and coauthor of *Beyond Beautiful: Using the Power of Your Mind and Aesthetic Breakthroughs to Look Naturally Young and Radiant.* DorisDayMD.com

D o you long to have smooth skin around your eyes—no puffiness or hollows, no dark circles, no lines or wrinkles? *Getting more sleep and drinking more water*

are important, but there are some less obvious causes and do-it-yourself solutions…

•**Drinking too much alcohol.** Alcohol depletes your skin of water, and the sugar increases skin inflammation. Also, when people drink, they typically eat foods high in salt and low in nutritional value, further increasing dehydration and inflammation. Cut back on alcohol, and you'll see the difference within a day. Alcohol also can disrupt sleep. An occasional drink is fine, but always have extra water when drinking alcohol.

•**Allergies cause increased redness,** and rubbing will further darken and irritate the skin under your eyes. If you have seasonal allergies, start taking allergy medication a week before they tend to start. Speak with an allergist if over-the-counter treatments are not enough.

Rubbing can create a response in the skin, which leads to inflammation, wrinkling and dark circles. When you're tired from staring at your computer or phone screen, suffer from sleep deprivation or are having an allergy attack, resist the urge to rub out your discomfort. Instead, gently pat on eye cream or try the home remedies below.

•**Vascular inflammation.** Blood vessels under the skin can be prominent if there is irritation in the area, causing dark circles. Use a firming eye cream or one that reduces inflammation such as ISDIN K-Ox Eyes. Products that have white and green tea extracts also work well. My product, CE HPR Eye Cream, has a high-potency retinol and vitamins C and E to firm and reduce puffiness, redness and dark circles.

Fast Home Remedies

•**Tea-and-honey-soaked raw cucumbers ease eye bags and lighten dark circles within minutes.** Cucumbers are cooling and astringent, honey is anti-inflammatory, and tea has antioxidant properties. Green tea has the most healing benefits, but black or white tea also will work. This brew can last up to a week in the refrigerator. The best time to do this is morning and evening.

Brew four cups of strong tea. Add three tablespoons of honey. Let the tea cool to room temperature. Add one cucumber, cut into about 16 thin slices. Refrigerate for at least four hours.

To use, lie down, close your eyes and put one cucumber slice on each eye for about two minutes.

If you don't want to wait hours for a remedy, you can simply place moist tea bags on your eyes. Again, green tea has the most benefits, but black and white tea also will work.

Dip two tea bags in a cup of room-temperature water for 60 seconds. Take them out, and squeeze out the water. Lie down and close your eyes. Place a damp tea bag on each eye for three to five minutes.

Feel Better, Live Longer: Sitting 101

Carol Krucoff, C-IAYT, E-RYT, a yoga therapist at Duke Integrative Medicine, a member of the *Bottom Line Health* advisory board, and author of the book *Yoga Sparks*.

Our bodies are made to stand. Not only does sitting increase pressure on the spine, but doing it too much has been linked to reduced life expectancy. When you add poor posture to excessive sitting, it can lead to chronic back and neck pain, headaches, shoulder pain, and even carpal tunnel syndrome. It can contribute to digestive, respiratory, and circulatory problems.

Sitting less and improving your posture when you do sit can reduce pain and boost your health.

Assess Your Posture

First, pay attention to your posture right now.

• **Is your head thrust forward from your shoulders?** Does your chin poke up? Are you looking down?

• **Does your spine have its natural "S" curves or is it more like a "C"?**

• **Are you sitting on the two hard knobs at the base of your pelvis** (the ischial tuberosities or, colloquially, the sit bones) or on your sacrum?

• **Are you holding tension in your shoulders?** Your brow? Jaw?

Improve Your Alignment

Now take a moment to adjust your alignment with a yoga move called Seated Mountain Pose. First, make sure you're sitting on the sit bones. To find them, you may need to reach your hands under your bottom to feel for these knobs, then gently move the flesh of your buttocks aside so you can feel your sit bones releasing down onto the surface on which you're sitting. Next, put both feet on the floor or, if they don't reach, on a flat or slightly angled footstool. Make sure the stool does not push your knees higher than your hips. Your thighs should be parallel to the floor. If you are tall and your knees are too high, elevate your chair or add a cushion to get into proper alignment.

Once you feel grounded, extend the top of your head upward and lengthen your spine. Stack your joints so that if someone were looking at you from the side, they'd see your ear over your shoulder and your shoulder over your hip. Keep your chin parallel to the floor. Don't tilt it up or tuck it in.

When working on a computer, make sure the screen is at a height at which you can look straight ahead or just slightly down. Set up your keyboard so your forearms are parallel to the floor. Because it can be hard to have good alignment when working on a laptop, try plugging your laptop into an external monitor and keyboard.

Relax your shoulders away from your ears. Holding the shoulders in a tightened, raised position over time can lead to fatigue and pain.

Take an easy, full breath in so that your abdomen expands; then as you exhale release any tension in your face, jaw, and throat. Imagine a light shining out from your breastbone and direct it forward, not down at the ground.

If your chair doesn't support this good posture, consider placing a support (such as a rolled towel) at your lower back.

Keep It Up

Once you're in proper alignment, try to stay there, but recognize that it's common to fall back into a slump for a variety of reasons, including eye strain, fatigue, and old habits. If you find yourself straining to see a computer screen, invest in a pair of computer glasses to reduce the temptation to lean forward to see the screen. If you're slumping due to fatigue, take a brief walk or stand up and stretch frequently, preferably for a few minutes every hour. If possible, use a headset so you can stand up and move around whenever you're on the phone.

If you must remain seated, stretch with seated back bends, side bends, wrist and forearm stretches, shoulder shrugs, and shoulder circles. You might also consider investing in a standing desk or height-adjustable workstation.

Turn to Yoga

Practicing yoga can help improve your posture and relieve neck and shoulder pain. Yoga postures can stretch your tight muscles and strengthen the weak ones. The practice also improves flexibility, boosts stability, and eases movement.

Here are some exercises to try…

• **Shoulder shrugs.** If you are seated, follow the guidelines above for proper posture. If you're standing, make sure your feet are shoulder-width apart and your weight is evenly distributed.

As you inhale, lift your shoulders toward your ears. As you exhale, drop them down. Repeat three to five times, synchronizing your movement with your breath. Keep your arms relaxed. For variety, try circling your shoulders in one direction for a few breaths and then switch directions.

• **Tree pose.** Stand with your feet hip-width apart and focus your gaze on a fixed point. Envision roots growing from your right foot into the ground. Bend your left knee and place your heel against your right ankle, keeping the ball of the foot on the ground. Bring your palms together and extend your arms upward, keeping your shoulders down and relaxed. Balance for a few breaths before switching sides. To increase the challenge, move the sole of your left foot up your leg and place it anywhere but on your knee.

• **Chair pose.** Sit toward the front of a chair with both feet firmly on the floor. Take an easy full breath and exhale as you hinge forward from the hips (not the waist). Keep your back lengthened, not rounded. Press your feet into the floor and use the strength of your legs to come to a standing position. Stand in front of the chair, inhale, and as you extend your arms forward to shoulder height, bend your knees and hinge forward from your hips. At the same time, stick your bottom out and lower yourself slowly into the chair. Repeat five to 10 times, coming to a standing position then lowering back down. For more challenge, hover a few inches from your seat before going all the way down.

• **Legs up the wall.** Sit on the floor about one hand-width from the wall. Swing your legs up onto the wall and ease your back onto the floor. Adjust the distance between your bottom and the wall so you feel comfortable and take several deep breaths.

Feeling Dizzy? Get the Correct Diagnosis

Study titled "Asking About Dizziness When Turning in Bed Predicts Examination Findings for Benign Paroxysmal Positional Vertigo," by researchers at University of Gothenburg, Sweden, published in *Journal of Vestibular Research*.

Benign paroxysmal positional vertigo (BPPV) is a medical mouthful but an important condition to know about—especially because it's often challenging to get a proper diagnosis for this common type of dizziness.

When you break down the medical terms of BPPV, each one describes a key element of the condition—benign means it's not life-threatening...paroxysmal means it starts and stops suddenly...positional means symptoms are triggered by position changes...and vertigo, which is the main symptom, refers to the unpleasant sensation of feeling like you or the room is spinning.

Because dizziness, a general term used to describe vertigo, light-headedness and/or impaired balance, is estimated to affect three of out every 10 people age 70 and older, it's crucial to correctly diagnose the problem so it can be treated appropriately. With BPPV, X-rays and other diagnostic tests don't identify the condition. Instead, a special type of physical exam that many health care providers may not be familiar with must be used for a proper diagnosis. The good news is that once BPPV is diagnosed, it's fairly easy to treat (see below), and you don't need to take medication.

To help physicians home in on BPPV and the dangers of its related fall risk in older adults, researchers at the University of Gothenburg asked 149 older adults being treated for dizziness to answer a 15-question survey about their symptoms in addition to receiving a physical exam.

The key question: "Do you get dizzy when you lie down or roll over in bed?" was most often associated with the correct diagnosis of BPPV. Patients who answered "yes" to this question were about 60 percent more likely to be diagnosed with BPPV than those who answered "no."

Patients who said they had "continuous dizziness" were less likely to be diagnosed with BPPV than those who had dizziness "lasting seconds," according to the research, which was published in *Journal of Vestibular Research*. Short periods of dizziness are linked to BPPV.

Effective treatment for BPPV: While the exact cause of BPPV has not yet been determined, doctors know that the condition occurs when calcium crystals, known as otoconia, break loose from sensory hair cells in-side the inner ear. BPPV usually goes away on its own within a few weeks, but you can eliminate it sooner by doing simple exercises called the Epley maneuver.

This treatment involves positioning your head and body in ways that help the otoconia settle inside the inner ear. The maneuvers can be done by a health-care provider (such as an ear, nose and throat doctor, or otolaryngologist, or an audiologist). They take only a few minutes to complete, and they usually relieve BPPV after a few sessions. Go to YouTube.com and search "Epley manoeuvre from BMJ learning" to see how the maneuver is performed.

Important: If you have sudden episodes of spinning vertigo triggered by movement, especially while lying down or turning over, you may have BPPV and should consult your health-care provider for a diagnosis. Other causes of vertigo include Ménière's disease (see next article) and labyrinthitis, which often results from an infection in the inner ear. Treatment depends on the cause.

To get a diagnosis and appropriate treatment for vertigo, start with your primary care provider. He/she may refer you to an otolaryngologist, who specializes in these conditions. To find an otolaryngologist near you, consult the American Academy of Otolaryngology-Head and Neck Surgery at ENTnet.org and click on "Find an ENT."

Vertigo: Not Just Dizziness

Oliver Adunka, MD, director of the division of otology/neurotology and cranial base surgery, and clinical professor of otolaryngology at the Ohio State University Wexner Medical Center in Columbus.

One of the hallmarks of Alfred Hitchcock's masterpiece *Vertigo* is the camera work that captured the overwhelming sensation of the world spinning out of control. That feeling is all too real for the one in three people who experience vertigo at some time in their lives.

What Is Vertigo?

Vertigo is the uncomfortable sensation of feeling like the room you're in is spinning around you, or that you are spinning within the room. It can be mild or severe and frequent enough to keep you from even the simplest activities of daily life. Vertigo is not as simple as feeling dizzy when standing too quickly or being off balance from poor muscle tone. Rather, it is a symptom of a problem within your vestibular system, a circuit linking parts of the brain and inner ear that works to control balance, eye movements and even posture.

The vestibular system may be impaired by a variety of factors, from a temporary injury to a progressive disease. Here are the most common vestibular disorders that can cause episodes of vertigo. Note that how long an episode lasts provides a great clue to the underlying cause.

Benign Paroxysmal Positional Vertigo (BPPV)

This is, by far, the most common cause of vertigo. With BPPV, vertigo episodes usually last for a matter of seconds up to one minute, often when you're lying in bed or when you lean over.

Typically, BPPV occurs when microscopic calcium deposits within the ear called *otoliths* come loose and float in one of the canals of the vestibular system. This can be caused by ear or head surgery (the vibration from surgical drills can cause otoliths to break free), trauma to the head or dental work. It may occur as an aftereffect of an ear infection or even the remnants of an upper respiratory infection. Often, no cause can be identified.

One way to manage BPPV is to use the Epley maneuver, a set sequence of head motions that is designed to change the balance in the canal and help put the otoliths back into place. You should learn how to do them and how often to do them from a trained

physical therapist or occupational therapist, but once you know them, you can do them on your own to manage symptoms (see previous article). The movements can feel somewhat awkward, but people do respond very well to them.

Ménière's Disease

This inner ear disorder stems from an imbalance of fluids in the inner ear and affects both balance and hearing. While it is a common cause of vertigo, it is relatively rare and is often overdiagnosed. Eight out of 10 people referred to me for Ménière's disease don't actually have it. Who develops it and why are still enigmas, and it seems to come out of the blue. Fluids in a tube in the inner ear that are not normally under pressure suddenly become pressurized.

There are four defining symptoms of Ménière's disease: episodes of vertigo that last between 20 minutes and two hours, ringing in the ear (tinnitus), hearing loss and the sensation of pressure or fullness in the ear—almost always on one side only. Vertigo episodes with Ménière's disease can happen infrequently or they can be daily, getting in the way of your normal life. The more frequent the attacks, the greater the chance of permanent hearing loss, so treatment is important.

Though Ménière's disease isn't caused by salt intake, salt can bring on an attack—people often get one right after eating a fast food meal, for instance, so a low-salt diet is part of the plan. Taking medications, such as a diuretic, can help reduce pressure, while a two- or three-day course of steroids can help prevent hearing loss during an attack. Pressure devices and surgical interventions can also reduce the frequency and severity of life-altering vertigo episodes.

Vestibular Migraines

Many people misdiagnosed with Ménière's disease instead have silent migraines. Vestibular migraines are characterized by daylong attacks of vertigo without actual migraine head pain. They can occur frequently or months apart. Some other signs are a lack of balance, problems with motion, like not being able to read a book in a moving car, and/ or a personal or family history of migraine. Hearing is not typically affected.

Vestibular migraines can be hard to diagnose because there's no single test to identify them. It may first be necessary to rule out other causes with imaging tests. Some people find relief by taking a migraine-prevention medication, an antihypertensive, a beta blocker or a low-dose anti-seizure drug. Finding the right medication can be trial and error, but it's reassuring just to know that this is a functional problem: It's not subtle, but it's also not dangerous.

Finding Help

Getting the right diagnosis can be a challenge, but there are many specialists who can help. Otolaryngologists, also called ENTs for ear, nose and throat, are skilled at treating problems with those structures. Some specialize in vestibular disorders. An otologist/neurotologist, for example, has additional training in how the ears and brain work together. Seek out a neurologist with a headache subspecialty if you have vertigo and other possible signs of vestibular migraine, such as double vision or seeing flashing lights. Depending on your diagnosis, you might be referred to a physical or occupational therapist as part of your treatment plan.

Medication May Be to Blame

It's important to distinguish between a drug that causes standard dizziness and one that causes vertigo because it's toxic to ear structures. A careful evaluation of all medications you're taking by your doctor or pharmacist can help pinpoint a possible culprit, and switching to a different drug could stop your symptoms. Exposure to environmental chemicals, like lead and mercury, can also damage the ear.

Stay Safe and Secure When You Live Alone

Kristina Butler, RN, founder of Comfort Keepers, an international care service for seniors and adults who need assistance with everything from errands to long-term planning and personal care so that they can remain at home for as long and as safely as possible. ComfortKeepers.com

Being able to stay in your own home as you age is the gold standard for many of us, but that ideal can be challenging to pull off when you live on your own and don't have family nearby to help.

The secret to doing it successfully: Preparing for a potential emergency, whether it's a natural disaster such as a hurricane…an injury such as a fall…or an acute illness.

Here are the steps to take now to help keep yourself safe and secure in any event in the future.

1. Get all your legal documents in order, and store them in one place in your home. This includes your health insurance cards and policy information, will, trusts, power of attorney and an advance health-care directive that states your wishes in the event that you become incapacitated. Also give a set of copies to someone you trust. I can't tell you how common it is for a scavenger hunt to ensue because no one knows where these documents are when an emergency occurs and first responders and medical staff don't know your wishes.

2. Wear a medical-alert pendant or bracelet. Even if you are active and healthy, wearing one of these devices gives peace of mind in case of emergency. You shouldn't just rely on a cell phone—you may not be able to reach it. And digital assistants, such as Alexa, currently can't call 911. Consider a plan that offers a mobile network with GPS technology that you also can use when you are away from home if you were to get lost or, say, suffer cardiac symptoms or an injury on a hike or bike ride. Buy a waterproof model that can be worn in the shower. The

Apple Watch is another option, although it can be difficult to set up for those who are not tech-savvy.

These devices aren't just for injuries and illness. You can use them to call 911 in the event of fire or flood or if someone is trying to break into your home.

3. Make a plan for responders to get into your home. What happens if you need emergency help and can't get to the door to unlock it? Besides a delay in your treatment, first responders are going to knock down your door or break a window to get inside, and the repair costs will be up to you. Giving a neighbor a key—and including him/her on the contact list for your medical-alert provider—is one way to avoid that. Add an extra level of security by getting a lockbox to hold your keys on your front or back doorknob. (This is the gadget that realtors use in order to enter a house that is for sale.) Or install a keypad lock that requires only a numerical code. Give the access code to a neighbor and to your local police and fire departments. This way, it's in the dispatcher's instructions to first responders if you call 911.

4. Make your kitchen emergency central. One of the first places responders look for info is the refrigerator door. Post a list there of what responders should do in an emergency. Include the people to contact and their phone numbers, the location of those important legal documents you've stored in one place, preferred doctor and hospital information, and the medications you take and where they are located.

Also helpful: Keep all those meds (prescription and over-the-counter) in a visible container on your kitchen counter.

5. Stock up on provisions. Make sure you have at least one week's worth of medications on hand at all times—set up auto refills and delivery service with your local pharmacy. Keep about two weeks of nonperishable foods (canned soups and vegetables, pasta, cereal, peanut butter, etc.) on hand, as well as personal-care items, a supply of batteries and a working fire extinguisher.

6. Get involved in your community. Social support and companionship have been shown to improve physical and mental health, and there's another plus for those who live alone—it extends your care network. Attending a regularly scheduled event might raise a red flag if you don't show up one week, for example. You also can develop a buddy system with other people in the same situation and check in on one another daily with a call or text—just as you should be doing with faraway family members. YWCAs/YMCAs typically offer many programs, as do many church and religious organizations and local community centers. Seek out local clubs for your personal interests.

7. Interview home care agencies well before you need them. Most people call for professional assistance only in an emergency—after an injury, returning home after rehab or when they suddenly realize that they need help. If you investigate care providers when you're well, you can decide which one you prefer and have your information in its system so that it is ready to go when you are.

Home care isn't just for the immobile or cognitively impaired. Services such as grocery shopping, transportation to the doctor, light housekeeping and companionship also come in handy.

8. Stay on your feet. One out of every four adults age 65+ suffers a fall annually. It is the leading cause of injury and death in this age group, according to the Centers for Disease Control and Prevention (CDC). Prevent falls by having your bathroom outfitted with grab bars, shower benches, nonslip mats and elevated toilet seats—these items can be useful for anyone, not just for seniors. As a precaution, always wear your medical-alert device while in the bathroom.

You'll also want to remove any area rugs with corners you can trip over...make sure that you have plenty of lighting (including nightlights)...eliminate clutter on floors and steps...and arrange furniture so that you have plenty of room to maneuver. Eldercare and home-safety companies often will have safety pros available who can come to your home, usually for an hourly rate, and do an assessment of what you need. You also can find checklists online, such as from the CDC at https://bit.ly/2AaGPQp.

And, of course, stay physically active. Exercise helps prevent injury by maintaining strength and balance.

9. Consider working with a geriatric-care manager if you become infirm. These professionals are typically licensed nurses or social workers who specialize in geriatrics—though they can help people of any age. They are sometimes referred to as "professional relatives" because they can take over a lot of what family members might help manage—assessing your assistance needs, helping develop a care plan, hiring help and acting as your advocate. They usually charge by the hour and typically aren't covered by insurance. The cost may be worth it, however, because they can ensure a more positive outcome and reduce medical costs down the road, lessen the need for distant family members (if you even have them) to engage in emergency travel and save the time spent trying to coordinate care. Ask about nearby care managers at your doctor's office, elder-care companies that probably have them on staff and local senior programs...or go to Eldercare Locator at Eldercare.acl.gov.

Sugar Shortens Lives—but Not Necessarily Through Obesity

Study by researchers at MRC London Institute of Medical Sciences, UK, published in *Cell Metabolism*.

Excessive sugar causes buildup of the natural waste product uric acid that can lead to gout, poor kidney function and kidney stones.

Recent finding: Fruit flies fed excess sugar developed metabolic diseases similar to ones in humans—but the uric acid buildup appeared to correlate with earlier death.

You're Never Too Old for Cavities

Louis Siegelman, DDS, board-certified dentist anesthesiologist in New York City. Dr. Siegelman is assistant director of the dental anesthesiology residency program at NYU Langone Medical Center and clinical assistant professor at NYU College of Dentistry. DentalPhobia.com

Most people think one's "cavity-prone years" end in your teens. But guess what...that's not true.

Growing risk: Compared with earlier generations, older adults today are at greater risk for cavities because more are keeping their teeth. In the early 1970s, about 55 percent of adults ages 65 to 74 had at least some of their teeth. Now, 87 percent do. What about those over age 75? About three-quarters still have some of their teeth. The scary part is that about one in every five adults over age 65 has at least one untreated cavity, which can lead to tooth loss and other harms.

5 Cavity Traps—and Solutions

There's a lot you can do to prevent cavities as you grow older.

Here's a no-brainer: If you're a smoker, your dental health gives you just one more reason to quit—tobacco increases risk for tooth decay. *Other cavity promoters...*

• **Dry mouth.** A steady supply of saliva helps fight cavities by washing away food particles and coating your teeth with minerals such as calcium and phosphate. Hundreds of medications, however, contribute to inadequate saliva, also known as dry mouth.

Common culprits: Drugs used for pain, high blood pressure, depression and bladder control. Dry mouth also is common in people with diabetes and those undergoing chemotherapy or radiation treatments for cancer.

Self-defense: If you are taking a medication that causes dry mouth, ask your doctor about alternatives, including nondrug approaches.

Also: Be sure to drink plenty of water. Sugar-free dry-mouth lozenges, such as Thera-Breath, Biotène and Act Dry, can help but aren't a cure. (Lozenges with sugar increase your risk for cavities.)

• **Acid reflux.** When stomach acid backs up into your mouth, it can erode tooth enamel, setting the stage for decay.

Self-defense: If you have heartburn or bad breath or notice a sour taste in your mouth after eating, ask your doctor whether you could have acid reflux and, if so, get it treated.

• **Receding gums.** Tooth decay at the gum line is common with age because so many older adults have gum disease. As gum tissue gradually pulls away from teeth, pockets can form, creating a breeding ground for the bacteria that damage teeth. Even people who took excellent care of their teeth in younger years may brush and floss less often or less thoroughly because of physical challenges, such as arthritis.

Self-defense: Be sure to brush twice daily and floss at least once daily. Consider using an electric toothbrush to assist with effective brushing.

Also: Consider using a toothpaste that contains "remineralizing" agents, such as stannous fluoride, sodium fluoride and calcium phosphate. These ingredients can bond to weakened enamel, strengthening teeth and creating an extra shield against decay. If your gums have receded, these products help prevent cavities on vulnerable surfaces.

• **Sugary and acidic drinks.** Sweet drinks, such as soda, bottled tea and juice, are among the greatest threats to your teeth. In addition to large doses of sugar, many such drinks also contain high levels of corrosive acid. Even many unsweetened drinks, such as flavored mineral waters and teas, are acidic.

Self-defense: Make water your go-to beverage. When you do indulge in a favorite sweet drink, have it with a meal, then swish with plain water.

• **Processed foods.** A diet heavy on processed foods is, by default, heavy on sugars and acid and low in nutrients that support a healthy mouth.

Self-defense: Avoid processed foods, and opt for whole, nutrient-packed foods. Emphasize crunchy fruits and vegetables, such as apples, carrots and celery, that help remove food particles and promote saliva production.

Important: Some adults may cut back on dental visits when they retire, lose employer-paid dental insurance and learn that routine dental care is not covered by Medicare. Don't do that. Get cleanings and exams at least twice yearly. If you have periodontal disease, you may need four visits.

Surprising Danger of Earwax

Jackie L. Clark, PhD, clinical professor of audiology at The University of Texas at Dallas and past-president of the American Academy of Audiology.

If you have had trouble with your memory lately, there may be a simple answer…and it's not in your brain.

More than 30 percent of elderly people have excessive or impacted cerumen, the technical term for earwax, that can block hearing and accelerate cognitive decline because of associated disconnection from community and loneliness. If you can't hear, you can't make memories or exercise your brain through communication. Unfortunately, few people—and even some doctors—think to check the ears when investigating a failing memory. Hearing loss also can worsen behaviors associated with dementia, such as distress and depression.

Normally, earwax moves up and out on its own. It's best not to interfere with this natural self-cleaning function. Even cotton swabs such as Q-tips can force the cerumen migrating out of the ear back into the canal. And the FDA has warned against ear candles due to risk for injury, such as burns, ear-canal blockages and perforations.

Instead: Simply let new earwax form and push out the old on its own. If your ears feel full and sounds are muffled, place a few drops of mineral oil or commercially made drops into the ear to loosen wax. Or see an ear, nose and throat (ENT) doctor or an audiologist to have the wax removed. It is an extremely common ENT procedure.

Note: People who wear hearing aids are especially likely to accumulate earwax because the devices push wax down into the ear canal. Every day, use the pick and brush provided by your hearing professional to gently remove wax from the hearing aids. Wipe aids with a dry or slightly moistened cloth (with water only), and air-dry them overnight.

Heart-Healthy Diet May Save Hearing

Hugo Olmedillas, PhD, is professor of functional biology at University of Oviedo, Oviedo, Spain, and leader of a study published in *Journal of the Formosan Medical Association*.

A heart-healthy diet may also save your hearing, based on a review of 22 studies on nutrition and hearing loss. Key vitamins and minerals reduce inflammation and support the health of the small blood vessels crucial for hearing. Aim to fill half your plate with nonstarchy vegetables (such as greens, broccoli, onions and peppers) and/or fruit and half with whole grains, plant proteins and/or fish.

Poor Vision Linked to Dementia Risk

Study of 1,061 women, average age 74, led by researchers at Stanford University, published in *JAMA Ophthalmology*.

Postmenopausal women who wore glasses or contact lenses that corrected their vi-

sion to 20/40 or worse were from two to six times as likely to develop dementia within seven years as women whose corrected vision was 20/20. The vision problems were in at least one eye and could not be fully corrected due to various eye diseases. The highest dementia incidence was in women who scored 20/100 or poorer. Impaired corrected vision also was linked to risk for mild cognitive impairment, which sometimes turns into dementia. The association does not mean poor corrected vision causes dementia—both conditions may result from the same underlying factors. (For more about dementia and Alzheimer's disease, see chapter 2, Brain Health.)

Coping With Eye Floaters

Margaret Liu, MD, medical director of the Pacific Vision Surgery Center, Pacific Vision Foundation, San Francisco Eye Institute.

Eye floaters, the spots and strings that drift across your visual field, can range from an annoyance to a downright problem if they interfere with the ability to drive or read. They are more common in people who are over age 50 and those who are nearsighted.

Let's take a look at what is happening in the eye when these appear. Most of the eye is filled with vitreous, a gel-like substance that is about 99 percent water and 1 percent solid materials that include collagen. As we age, bits of collagen can cluster into masses that cast shadows on the retina, causing most floaters.

A large, ring-like floater, called a Weiss ring, appears when the condensed vitreous gel separates from the retina at the optic nerve.

The Risks

While floaters are most often a harmless result of aging, they can sometimes be a sign of something more serious, such as a sight-threatening retinal tear or detachment, inflammation in the back of the eye or bleeding in the eye from diabetes, hypertension, blocked blood vessels or injury.

If you experience a sudden onset or increase in the number of floaters, flashes of light or darkness in your peripheral vision, make an appointment with an eye doctor as soon as possible. Even if you don't have signs of a serious complication, it's a good idea to have an eye checkup whenever floaters appear. Once serious conditions are ruled out, it's perfectly safe to leave floaters alone. Over time, many people no longer notice them.

Coping Strategies

Not everyone adapts, however, and floaters can be maddening for some people. *Here are some tips to help manage the annoyance...*

•**Distract yourself.** If you are sitting idle, you are more prone to focus on the floaters. Distract yourself with an enjoyable activity, like riding a bike or going out with friends.

•**Wear brown,** polarized sunglasses. They can make the floaters less obvious, particularly in bright light.

•**Go dark.** Use dark mode and reduce the brightness on your electronic devices to make the floaters less visible.

•**Consider interior design.** White walls and bright lights accentuate floaters. If you can't repaint light walls, use art to create visual distraction.

•**Meditation** can help reduce your stress levels and allow you to gain control over your emotional response to floaters.

•**Change your diet.** Some people report that cutting out sugar and fatty foods can reduce the appearance of smaller floaters.

•**Rest your eyes.** Get enough sleep and take regular breaks from computer screens.

Treatment

For people who can't tolerate floaters or are debilitated by them, there are treatment options, but they're not to be taken lightly. Vit-

rectomy, a surgery to remove the vitreous, has risks including infection, retinal detachment or bleeding.

Laser treatment (vitreolysis) is a less invasive option. An ophthalmologist focuses laser energy onto the clusters that are causing the shadows and administers a burst of energy for a tiny fraction of a second about 150 to 300 times. This energy pulverizes some of the floaters into a gas that completely vaporizes them and breaks apart others into smaller pieces that are less bothersome.

The effectiveness of laser therapy varies. Studies show that some patients have complete resolution, some only partial, and some report worse symptoms. Because the treatment options are risky, eye doctors consider them only for very severe cases.

Many people have the hardest time with floaters during the first year after they appear. Often with time, the floaters will naturally settle down and become less noticeable as the brain learns to adapt.

Don't Miss Your Eye Appointment

Brian L. VanderBeek, MD, MPH, MSCE, assistant professor of ophthalmology, Scheie Eye Institute, University of Pennsylvania, Philadelphia.

Treatment for age-related macular degeneration (AMD), a leading cause of blindness, typically includes a monthly visit to an ophthalmologist for an injection of the drug anti-VEGF, which helps maintain or even improve vision.

Recent finding: Missing just one injection of this drug over a two-year period can result in the loss of visual acuity, according to research involving nearly 1,200 people with AMD.

This Eye Surgery Improves Driving Safety

When researchers used a driving simulator to test the driving skills of 44 patients before and after cataract surgery, near misses and crashes dropped by 35 percent after surgery on one eye…and by 48 percent after surgery on the second eye.

Explanation: Cataract surgery not only improves visual acuity (how well one sees an eye chart) but also contrast sensitivity (the ability to distinguish increments of light versus dark) and night vision.

Jonathon Ng, MD, clinical senior lecturer, School of Population Health and Global Health, The University of Western Australia, Nedlands, Australia.

Will I Ever See My Feet Again? A Flat-Belly Quest

Adriane Berg, Esq., an attorney who helped found the National Academy of Elder Law Attorneys and founder of Adriane Berg & Associates, a firm that helps companies market to mature generations. She is author of 14 books including *How Not to Go Broke at 102: Finding Everlasting Wealth.*

I have researched ways to rid myself of my middle bulge, which has haunted me from baby fat to teen tummy to my adult wardrobe of over-blouses, and I discovered a shocking eye-opener. I may never see my feet again.

For postmenopausal women, belly fat might be hormonal and biological, in a Darwinian sense.

According to Babak Moeinolmolki, MD, of Healthy Life Bariatrics, it's all a matter of childbearing physiology. Damn that estrogen…

"During puberty, the hormone estrogen tells the body to begin storing fat on the hips and thighs to prepare for pregnancy. While this subcutaneous fat isn't harmful, the excess fat can be challenging to lose," said Dr. Moeinolmolki.

"Menopause officially occurs a year after a woman has her last menstrual period. Around this time, the woman's estrogen levels plummet, which causes fat to be stored around the abdomen rather than on the hips and thighs."

And for anyone at any age, you can't diet off fat in one specific region of the body.

"It's essentially impossible to tell one specific region of your body to accelerate fat metabolism," says Chris DiVecchio, an NASM-certified personal trainer and author of *The 5 x 2 Method: Revealing the Power of Your Senses.*

So should I just give up the ship (SHAPE)? No. Belly fat, even though natural as we age, can be dangerous.

It's "the most dangerous location to store fat," says Lawrence Cheskin, MD, chair of the department of nutrition and food studies at George Mason University and adjunct professor at Johns Hopkins School of Medicine. Belly fat tends to increase sugar levels and thereby to increase the risk for heart disease and type 2 diabetes.

So how should I go about finally seeing my feet?

For me, a lot of the basics are already in place. That's why I am at my ideal weight of 117.2 (I don't mean to brag!). *Still, let's just list some of these essentials, lest you forgot how to diet…*

● **Limit sugary foods and beverages, and watch calories.** Before you know it, that single serving can lead to an excess of fat in and around your stomach. Calorie control is hard—one good bit of online help is "25 Ways to Cut 500 Calories a Day" at Prevention.com/weight-loss/20-ways-to-cut-500-calories-a-day/

● **Limit alcohol.** Unfortunately, excess calories from alcohol are partly stored as belly fat. (Hence, the well-known term "beer belly.") Honestly, I drink a glass of wine almost every day…but I play around with calorie-free spritzers and two tiny glasses instead of one big one, as I typically like to pour.

● **Avoid trans fats.** Trans fats, derived from animal proteins and dairy, can cause

19

inflammation, which can, in turn, lead to insulin resistance and an excess amount of belly fat.

• **Move.** Sitting more than moving raises the rates of obesity, especially abdominal obesity. And studies have also shown that inactivity can contribute to regaining belly fat after losing weight.

• **Walk every day.** One small study published in the *Journal of Exercise Nutrition & Biochemistry* found that obese women who did a walking program for 50 to 70 minutes three days per week for 12 weeks slashed their visceral fat compared with women in a sedentary control group. Check out Freewalkers (Freewalkers.org), and walk with us or form your own local chapter.

It was these habits that got me to my lower weight…which is…well, you know. So, what more can I do?

Add fat-burning foods, such as…

• **Avocados**
• **Yogurt**
• **Berries**
• **Chocolate skim milk**
• **Green tea**
• **Citrus**
• **Chia seeds**
• **Fibrous foods,** such as whole-grain bread, oats, vegetables, beans, legumes and chia seeds

• **De-stress to lower cortisol.** Cortisol, the "stress hormone," leads to weight gain, particularly around the abdominal area. Significantly, cortisol-induced weight gain, instead of spreading out the storage across the entire body, gets stored right where you don't want—on your belly. Analyses have shown that women who have a larger waist-to-hip ratio secrete more cortisol when stressed.

• **Do core exercises more religiously.** According to Dr. DiVecchio, "There are literally dozens of muscles between your shoulders and your hips that are involved in every movement you do. The fastest way to create a lean midsection begins with choosing the right moves." There are tons of different ab workouts you can do right in your home. Choose the YouTube class that suits you best. Although exercise won't spot-reduce the fat, you will look toned when the weight comes off.

• **Get a good night's sleep.** Sleep is huge when it comes to your weight-loss success—and that's both if you sleep too much or too little.

And finally, the hardest new habit…

• **Roll with the punches.** I may have to accept the fact that with regard to my chance to be a supermodel, that ship has sailed. Or maybe…I can change the image of what is beautiful. For example, the standard for beauty could become, let's say, someone who is 72, in good shape, has a bit of a belly…and of course, weighs 117.2!

Intermittent Fasting and Older Adults

Roundup of physicians quoted in Harvard Health Letter.

In recent years, various eating strategies that involve regularly interspersed periods of fasting have become popular in weight-loss and healthy-lifestyle circles. While research does point to benefits of intermittent fasting, it has mostly been conducted on young, healthy people. If you're older and are considering it, talk to your doctor first. Many older people need to eat at regular intervals to take medications with food or to maintain stable blood-sugar levels. Fasting also may cause dangerous imbalances in potassium and sodium for those taking heart or blood pressure meds.

Chapter 2

BRAIN HEALTH

Train Your Brain for Better Memory and Greater Joy

News headlines make it sound like scientists are completely stumped by the mysteries of Alzheimer's disease and other forms of dementia. While there's still no cure for these devastating diseases, new discoveries are continually being made when it comes to improving the brain's "plasticity" —perhaps the strongest known defense in protecting our memory and ability to think clearly.

Plasticity refers to the brain's capacity to create new neural connections and networks in response to changes in one's environment, including those in your body and your experiences. Simply put, how you live your life defines the anatomy of your brain. With positive changes, you can improve your memory, mood, attention and zest for life—while negative habits result in a "sluggish" brain.

My personal journey: A few years ago, I realized that my intense focus on my work as a neuroscientist, surprisingly, had left vast parts of my brain unused. At the same time, I constantly worried about possible negative outcomes—a thought pattern that causes the body to chronically pump out excessive levels of the stress hormone cortisol, which over time kills neurons and impairs memory. On top of that, my lack of physical movement in my lab led to a 25-pound weight gain!

Adding more movement in my life not only turned everything around for me but also led to my current research focus on the effects of exercise on brain function. To help people make the same transition I did from couch potato to regular exerciser/gym rat, I came up with a series of four-minute brain hacks. These allow anyone who is time-challenged to add little chunks of brain boosters throughout the day.

***STEP #1:* Do brain-body exercise.** Exercise is the mother lode for fortifying your body and your brain. Just one workout boosts your brain power by improving focus, attention, mood and reaction time. If you regularly do aerobic exercise that causes you to work up a sweat, over a period of weeks, months and years, you'll gradually

Wendy Suzuki, PhD, professor of neural science and psychology in the Center for Neural Science at New York University in New York City. She is the founder of NYU's Suzuki Lab, which focuses on the effects of exercise on brain functions, and the author of *Healthy Brain, Happy Life*. WendySuzuki.com increase the brain-boosting effects, thanks to exercise-induced neurochemicals, such as growth factors that promote the survival and growth of neurons (neurogenesis).

These changes lead to new brain cells in the hippocampus, where new long-term memories are formed…and new synapses in the prefrontal cortex, critical for planning, problem-solving and decision-making. Strengthening these areas can help ward off dreaded cognitive decline.

For a greater brain boost: When exercise is physical and mental—for example, you're fully engaged and/or feel passionately about it—you'll improve your emotional health and self-confidence…and prime your brain for more plasticity. Inspired by high-energy movements from such disciplines as kickboxing and martial arts, I dubbed this "intentional exercise" because it requires deep focus combined with motivational affirmations spoken out loud.

Here are two powerful moves and affirmations that work for me—do each for one minute daily for a mental boost that fuels other positive habits…

Affirmation #1: **As you punch your arms forward like a boxer (right and left), say, "I am strong now!"**

Affirmation #2: **This time, throw an uppercut alternating between your right and left arms and say, "I am inspired now!"**

My own research shows that it takes three or four 30-minute workouts a week to achieve enhanced alertness and decision-making.

My personal approach: Three weekly aerobic exercise sessions (such as spin, kickboxing and dance classes) and two yoga classes per week for mindfulness practice.

Four-minute exercise brain hacks…

●**Walk up stairs to an upbeat song,** such as "Happy" by Pharrell Williams.

●**Set your timer for four minutes,** and clean as much of your office or home as you can.

●**Challenge someone to an arm-wrestling match.**

●**Dance around your living room or kitchen to one of your favorite songs.**

STEP #2: **Get creative.** The prefrontal cortex and the hippocampus are crucial to our creativity. Most people don't realize that everyone has this ability and that there are two main ways to express creativity. Invention creates new ideas and finds solutions… and divergent thinking challenges you to bring novelty to the way you've been doing something for years.

Four-minute creativity brain hacks for invention…

●**Think of two ideas to make your day more efficient**—for example, switch the order in which you do chores.

●**Cook a dish from a new spicy cuisine**—for extra benefit, take time to appreciate the aromas (the olfactory bulb is a key site for neurogenesis).

●**Make up lyrics for a favorite song.**

●**Create free-form cutouts with colored paper à la Matisse.**

Four-minute creativity brain hacks for divergent thinking…

●**Think up four ideas that use an object in a way it wasn't intended,** such as using a toothbrush to get crumbs out of your keyboard.

●**Come up with a new, efficient way to get to your workplace or the supermarket.**

●**Devise three new ways to play with your pet.**

●**Drink your coffee in a different way,** maybe with a straw or a new added spice.

STEP #3: **Try meditation.** Long term, meditation increases the size of various brain areas. The improvements are deeper for Buddhist monks who practice for hours a day than for the casual meditator. But you still can improve your brain by sitting quietly and focusing your mind on yourself or a mantra for just a few minutes. This practice will help enhance attention, working memory and recognition memory. For best results, it should be done daily.

Four-minute meditation brain hacks…

• **Start your day by reciting your intentions or goal for your life.**

• **Get lost in the details of a piece of art at a museum.**

• **Sip a cup of tea with absolutely no distractions.**

• **Focus quietly on your breath before you go to sleep.**

STEP #4: **Be generous.** Giving and receiving stimulates dopamine, resets the sympathetic and parasympathetic nervous systems to reduce anxiety...and makes the world a little better.

Pick something you do really well that's easy and enjoyable to do—and give it to someone else. One example for me is inviting my friends' kids to my lab and introducing them to science. For my friend Cheryl, an expert baker, it's making a pie for friends.

Four-minute generosity brain hacks...

• **Write a thank-you note or text to a loved one for being in your life.**

• **Find ways to "pay it forward"**—help a stranger or pay the toll for the driver behind you.

• **Be kind to someone you dislike.**

• **Smile and greet someone you don't know.**

Headaches? Memory Loss? Blame Menopause!

Dr. Suzanne Steinbaum is a cardiologist who has devoted her career to the treatment of heart disease through early detection, education and prevention. She is author of *Dr. Suzanne Steinbaum's Heart Book: Every Woman's Guide to a Heart Healthy Life.* DrSuzanneSteinbaum.com

Chances are, you value your brain more than just about any other part of you. It has gotten you this far, and you've come to rely on it a bit. Right? Maybe you have always assumed that it will be at your service, functioning as it always has, remembering things, staying alert, keeping track of your keys and your appointments, and nearly effortlessly recalling names, dates and words, whenever you need them. And maybe it has only rarely hurt beyond the occasional tension headache. It's there for you. You probably take it for granted. So, what the heck is going on now?

Menopause Headaches

Remember back in the day when "I have a headache" seemed like a perfect excuse to get out of intimacy when you were just too tired? Those occasional "headaches" may have been figments of your brain's imagination, but maybe now you are getting payback because...your head hurts!

Headaches, and often migraine headaches, are a common symptom of the period surrounding menopause. It's part of the hormone dance. Migraines in particular have been linked to hormonal fluctuations, so if you have them now in a way you never did before, don't panic. You probably don't have a brain tumor. It's probably just your changing hormones. That's not to say that a persistent new headache, blinding in nature, should not be investigated. It should be. Talk to your doctor. But the chances that it is menopause-related are pretty high, and there are treatments out there that can work. Signs that you are dealing with a migraine include intolerance to light, nausea or vomiting, and sometimes an "aura," which often involves visual changes that precede the pain—such as seeing lights, or wavy lines or other disturbances. There could also be issues with speech or numbness and tingling. When these symptoms are severe, definitely see your doctor, as these aura symptoms have been correlated with stroke later in life. But more often than not, menstrual migraines are just a pain in the brain, and something that may need treatment now, but which will come to an end when menopause does.

Tension headaches can also become more frequent with menopause. These are easier to deal with and are often a side effect of stress, both emotional and hormonal. You may find you can deal with them by taking a nap, a bath, doing some exercise or yoga, engaging in a good hearty crying session, or just popping a couple of naproxen, ibuprofen, aspirin or whatever you find wedged into the corners at the bottom of your pocketbook.

Menopause Brain

Maybe you're one of the lucky ones who doesn't get menopause headaches. But maybe you have other brain symptoms, and believe me, you would not be the only one. You know that thing that happens when your brain stops doing what it used to do? It's the other major brain issue. You know which one. What's it called? What's the word? Wait, wait, it will come to me! It's menopause brain!

So-called "menopause brain" is notorious—it is that sudden inability to concentrate...uncharacteristic forgetfulness... problems with word recall...and generalized brain fog that may feel like impending dementia but which is actually caused (like so many other unpleasant things) by your shifting hormones. If you are having trouble recalling all the details of life that you used to know instantly—those things you always knew that made you the quick-witted, go-to person everyone relied on for information like names, dates, times and places—these sudden "senior moments" can be disconcerting and even alarming. As described to me by a brilliant writer friend, it can feel like reaching for information in a file cabinet, but somebody put the file in the wrong spot. But again, all is not lost. *Menopause brain is a temporary condition, and you can help to alleviate its intensity by going back to the basics...*

• **Don't drink too much alcohol**—but do drink plenty of water to stay hydrated.

• **Get enough sleep.**

• **Stay moving and exercise as much as possible.**

• **Eat healthy food.**

• **Manage your stress.**

• **Don't get lazy with your brain activity.** Keep yourself engaged and stimulated, memorizing, creating, and speaking. Consider relearning that foreign language that was mandatory in high school. Travel. Talk to new people. Disrupt your routine.

All of these things can keep that brain machine of yours as well-oiled as possible. Your brain does not exist in a vacuum. Everything that is happening to you right now because of hormonal fluctuations—sleep disruption, hot flashes, fatigue, stress, depression, anxiety, weight gain, bloating, and just not feeling like yourself—has an impact on your brain function. It can feel like a cruel joke, but it happens to just about everyone. And it is temporary.

Breathe. You will get through it. When menopause is over, if you are still having cognitive issues, then you should get evaluated by a physician. But until then, just as with headaches, chances are that it is all just part of the old menopause dance. Once you come out the other side, you will usually get your brain back.

So, do what you need to do to keep yourself healthy. Breathe. Make healthy choices. Talk to friends, a therapist, the women next door in her 70s who can remember when it happened to her, or a psychiatrist, if you need one. Keep some ibuprofen in your bag. And, definitely do not count the minutes. It will give you a headache!

The 3 Steps to Worry Less...and Enjoy More

Mark Goulston, MD, host of the "My Wakeup Call" podcast. His books include *Why Cope When You Can Heal? How Healthcare Heroes of COVID-19 Can Recover from PTSD...Just Listen: Discover the Secret to Getting Through to Absolutely Anyone...*and *Get Out of Your Own Way: Overcoming Self-Defeating Behavior.* MarkGoulston.com

---

The word "neurotic" might conjure up images of lovable worry-warts such as *Seinfeld's* George Costanza or comic strip icon Charlie Brown, who famously lamented, "My anxieties have anxieties." But true neuroticism—a personality trait that describes people who are prone to anxiety, self-consciousness, irritability, emotional instability and depression—is no laughing matter. Neurotic individuals worry excessively, often about things that they have no control over, and they are more likely to develop a variety of psychological conditions, from mood disorders to substance abuse.

Now, a new study published in *Journal of the American Geriatrics Society* has linked neuroticism with an increased risk for a specific type of predementia called non-amnestic mild cognitive impairment (MCI), in which one's memory remains relatively unscathed but language, visual-spatial skills, decision-making, planning and/or other cognitive abilities become impaired.

Researchers followed 524 adults ages 65 years and older for three years, examining what effects, if any, their personality type had on their cognitive functioning. They focused on the "Big Five" dimensions of personality—agreeableness, extraversion, conscientiousness, openness and neuroticism. That last one proved to be the troublemaker, associated with a 6 percent increased risk for non-amnestic MCI.

Individuals with non-amnestic MCI, in turn, are thought to be at increased risk for Lewy body dementia, a disease in which abnormal protein deposits accumulate in the brain, impairing thinking, behavior, mood and movement.

What Is Neuroticism?

People tend to use the word "neurotic" loosely. In order to be clinically neurotic, one tends to ruminate constantly but that doesn't provide any relief from their anxiety. Instead, their worries simply beget more worries, and their thoughts often are tinged with negative emotions such as angst, sadness, anger or disgust. These people often have trouble leaving anything to chance and live life with a perpetually pessimistic point of view.

If a neurotic person was, say, waiting for his/her doctor to call with important test results, each passing moment without the phone ringing would be interpreted as, I must have cancer…that's why the doctor is taking so long. In contrast, someone who tends toward openness or agreeableness (two of the other Big Five personality traits) might think, *The doctor is calling other patients who do have cancer, and that's not me.* Interestingly, unlike neuroticism, openness is believed to be protective against dementia.

Chronic worry bathes the body and brain in the stress hormone cortisol. In short bursts, cortisol can help motivate people through challenging times and even keep them safe from danger—it's one of the key focus-sharpening hormones released when your brain senses a threat, such as a dog running toward you or a car cutting you off in traffic. But with chronic worrying, elevated cortisol levels damage brain cells and shrink the hippocampus, the brain's memory center.

Train Yourself to Be Less Neurotic

Just because you're a natural worrier doesn't mean that you're destined for cognitive trouble. There are ways to temper your neuroticism. The payoff may come not only in the form of healthier brain functioning but also as reduced anxiety, less pessimism, improved memory and/or focus. And this can lead to an overall improved quality of life.

STRATEGY #1: **Boost the bonding hormone.** During times of bonding, such as cuddling, breast-feeding or orgasm, the brain secretes the hormone oxytocin. Besides promoting attachment between two individuals, this so-called "love hormone" also helps reduce cortisol levels. That's one reason cuddling feels so relaxing and enjoyable. New research also suggests that oxytocin may have a preservative effect on brain functioning. It's a win-win!

When it comes to oxytocin, snuggling and sex get all the attention, but there's another way to get your love hormones flowing—by talking with someone you trust and who makes you feel heard. When you allow yourself to open up to a friend, family member or even a therapist and that person treats you with kindness and empathy, you experience a surge of oxytocin. As a result, you feel less alone and you help rewire your brain in a way that promotes openness, trust and optimism.

STRATEGY #2: **Try this spin on cognitive behavioral therapy (CBT).** CBT is a type of talk therapy that helps individuals change their distorted thought patterns and damaging behaviors. One popular CBT strategy involves catching yourself in harmful thinking in the moment and then reframing it in a more logical way. *Here's how you can do this without a therapist…*

• **Buy a journal, and paste a photo of a loved one**—someone who cares about you or someone you look up to—inside the front cover. This person can be living or deceased. When your neurotic worrying starts to ramp up, grab your journal, look at the photo, and imagine the person saying, *You can get through this.* Or, if it suits his/her personality, imagine him saying, with love, *Stop it! You're fine!!*

Now, picture that person asking you about your worrying and write down your answers. Questions can include, *What happened that got you worried?…How did you feel when it happened?…What does it make you want to do?…What would happen if you did that?… How likely is your worry going to come true?…* and *Look at me, take a deep breath, and tell me what would be a better thing to do?* Writing your responses acts as a neuroticism-release tool…and because you've invoked the image of a caring, empathetic person, you feel seen and heard, which sparks oxytocin.

STRATEGY #3: **Stop, look, listen, smell.** Long practiced by the military, this technique encourages you to pause and focus on your surroundings. The stop-look-listen aspect is widely known, and in the context of anxiety, these action items help force you to focus on something else.

The addition of smell makes it a game-changer when it comes to calming the nervous system. Smelling your environment requires inhaling deeply through the nose. Doing this also stimulates the vagus nerve, which connects the brain to almost every organ in the body. When stimulated, the vagus nerve initiates the body's natural relaxation response, eases anxiety and enhances mood. While you're smelling what you smell, make an internal association that is pleasurable—for instance, the smell of gasoline may remind you of pleasant road trips with your family or the smell of perfume or lotion may remind you of a scent you associated with a loving grandmother.

The next time you get caught up in a cycle of neurotic worrying, try the SLLS protocol…

Stop: Stop what you're doing…recognize your worrying is unproductive and spinning out of control.

Look: Look around you, and identify something you've never noticed or paid attention to. It could be the fabric on your couch, a tree, a button on an appliance. After observing the object for 30 seconds or so…

Listen: What do you hear? A neighbor's lawnmower? A bird chirping? Your freezer humming? Can you associate that noise with something positive, such as the backyard of your childhood home or tasty ice cream?

Smell: Smell something—coffee, perfume, a flower. Inhale slowly through your nose, expanding your belly to fill your lungs with air, then exhale through your mouth.

A note on medication: Sometimes neurotic worrying can grow so out of control that no amount of journaling or talking or professional counseling can tame it. In these cases, antianxiety medication may be an appropriate next step. For short-term help, your doctor may prescribe a fast-acting antianxiety drug called a benzodiazepine, such as Xanax (*alprazolam*) or Ativan (*lorazepam*). They work quickly to punch a hole in your anxiety but last only a few hours. In the longer term, selective serotonin reuptake inhibitors (SSRIs) such as Prozac (*fluoxetine*), Zoloft (*sertraline*) and Lexapro (*escitalopram*) can offer relief. I'm not advocating that you rush to medication—that can start you down the road of physical or psychological dependence and possible addiction. What I do suggest is, with your physician's agreement, perhaps using medicine that may calm your mind enough to begin to learn new and effective psychological coping mechanisms that you eventually are able to turn to without medication.

Strength Training Starts With the Brain

Study titled "Cortical, Corticospinal, and Reticulospinal Contributions to Strength Training," led by researchers at Institute for Neuroscience, Newcastle University, UK, and published in The Journal of Neuroscience, *July 2020.*

Resistance training is a type of exercise that causes your muscles to work against resistance. It is also called strength training because the goal is to make your muscles stronger. A classic example is weight-lifting. But a new study shows that before you can strengthen the muscles in your arm, you have to strengthen the nerve pathways from your brain to your arm.

Researchers at the Institute of Neuroscience at Newcastle University in the United Kingdom worked with two monkeys to get a better understanding of how resistance training works. They measured changes that occur in the motor cortex of the brain and in two pathways that carry motor signals from the brain, through the spinal cord, and out to the muscles of the upper arm. The motor cortex is the part of your brain that controls muscle movement. The two tracks are the corticospinal tract (CST) and the reticulospinal tract (RST).

The study is published in *The Journal of Neuroscience.* The investigators trained monkeys to pull a weighted handle with one arm. Over 12 weeks, the investigators gradually increased the weight on the handle to im-

prove muscle strength in the arm. To check the progress of the strengthening exercise, they stimulated the motor cortex of the monkeys and measured how well nerve signals passed down the CST and RST. They found that although the CST did not change, the RST nerve signals increased gradually over the training period. At the end of the study, although RST tracks go to both sides of the body, only the tracks to the exercised arm got stronger.

The researchers concluded that the RST is more important than the CST for strengthening arm muscles, and that before the muscles actually grow and become stronger, this nervous system pathway must change and adapt to exercise. The monkeys needed a stronger nerve pathway before they could get stronger arm muscles.

Although the research was done in monkeys, it probably applies to humans also. So, if you have started strength training and you are wondering when you will see bigger muscles, don't give up. You are probably getting results in your brain. Those big, strong muscles should follow eventually.

How to Remember Names...

Cynthia Green, PhD, one of America's foremost experts on brain health and founding director of the Memory Enhancement Program at Icahn School of Medicine at Mount Sinai in New York City. Her company, Total Brain Health, develops evidence-based brain wellness classes and programs. TotalBrainHealth.com

You met Beth minutes ago but already you can't remember her name. Forgetting names is one of the top memory complaints of adults. *Here's how to get your brain in gear for better name recall...*

•**Prime your brain to pay attention.** If you know in advance that you will be meeting a lot of new people, make sure you're well rested. Your memory doesn't work as well when you lack sleep.

Also: Limit your intake of alcohol. Alcohol has been shown to impair our ability to learn new information. Too much caffeine or sugar can be overstimulating and make it harder to concentrate on what you're learning.

• **Repetition.** When you are introduced to Tom, say, "Hi, Tom. It's nice to meet you." Continue to repeat his name in the course of the conversation. Say, "Tom, where do you live?" Repetition is a simple and straightforward way to help you remember something.

• **Use a simple association strategy.** Find a connection to something familiar. If you meet a Barbara, think of Barbara Bush, Barbra Streisand or your cousin Barbara. Making a connection between something that you know and something that you're learning is a powerful way to remember.

• **Create a visual association.** If you meet someone named Robin, you might picture a red "robin" bird. By creating a snapshot in your mind, you are less likely to forget.

• **Tell yourself a story.** Make up a silly little one-liner to go with the name. Think, "Kristen kissed Kris Kringle." When you see her again, this line will come back to you. "Oh right, Kristen kissed Kris Kringle." If it's easy for you to be creative, storytelling is a great way to amplify your memory.

• **Make a mental movie.** If you meet someone named Frank Hill, you might imagine frankfurters marching over a hill. The more absurd and bizarre the image, the more memorable it's going to be.

When You Forget

In spite of all your best efforts, sometimes you are going to forget someone's name.

• **Make a deal with your significant other or someone from work**—"If I am talking to someone you don't know and I don't introduce you within 15 seconds, stick out your hand and introduce yourself."

• **Admit that you don't know.** Say, "I'm sorry, I don't remember your name." The person might turn around and say, "Gee, I'm sorry, I don't remember your name either." Everyone forgets sometimes.

Alcohol and the Brain

Bankole A. Johnson, MD, DSc, the Dr. Irving J. Taylor professor and chair of the department of psychiatry and the pharmacology director of the Brain Science Research Consortium Unit at the University of Maryland School of Medicine. He is the author of *Six Rings: Preparedness and Restoration: Beyond Imagined Borders of Brain Wellness and Addiction Science.*

Just eight drinks for women (and 15 for men) over the course of a week is considered excessive alcohol use, and research shows that it's associated with a host of illnesses, from gastrointestinal disorders to liver disease, high blood pressure to increased cholesterol, and heart attack to many cancers.

Drinking heavily can affect the part of the brain that is responsible for motivation, appetite, emotions and memory. Over long periods, it can cause short- and long-term brain damage that manifests as dementia, confusion, visual disturbance, hallucinations and delusions. It can alter brain chemistry, creating psychological conditioning that limits a person's ability to control the desire to drink.

If excessive drinking becomes uncontrollable, it can tip into alcohol use disorder (AUD). People with AUD develop tolerance to the effects of alcohol, suffer from withdrawal symptoms when they are not drinking, and may experience cravings and a compulsion to keep drinking after starting.

In the Brain

People drink because it feels good. It can ease stress, lower shyness and make things more fun. All of those positive feelings come from an increase in the neurotransmitter dopamine. As the production of dopamine molecules rises, receptors in the brain rush to meet them. This helps stimulate a system in the brain that governs emotions—the cortico-mesolimbic system. Three structures in this system are crucial elements in producing pleasure and can move some people from casual drinking to AUD.

• **The hippocampus** can remember everything about the experience of drinking alcohol with extreme clarity. It will capture the "high" as well as the people, places, objects, smells, and tastes associated with drinking. When a person drinks, the hippocampus triggers the production of dopamine by firing off another neurotransmitter, glutamate. Glutamate helps the brain receive a signal that it is about to experience something good.

• **The amygdala** then goes into overdrive, producing a strong, emotional response.

• **The insular cortex** plays a role in the way people consciously seek pleasure from food, alcohol, or drugs.

Over time, alcohol can damage this system and other parts of the brain, creating an imbalance between neurotransmitters, like dopamine, and their receptors. The brain's ability to interpret and respond to dopamine becomes dulled, so the cortico-mesolimbic system responds by demanding more input. For someone with AUD, that can translate to a craving for more alcohol.

Rethinking Treatment

Excessive drinking, then, is a brain disorder. The most common approach to treating AUD, however, is based on talk therapy and self-help, which ignores the biological underpinning of the disease. About 60 percent of AUD is biological. The most successful treatments address both biology and psychology with the use of medication.

Naltrexone

Drinking activates opioid receptors, and *naltrexone* (Vivitrol) is an opioid antagonist. It blocks those receptors and prevents the pleasurable response to drinking. If a person drinks while taking the medication, they simply won't get the high feeling. As a result, naltrexone can help reduce the number of days a person drinks each month, as well as the number of drinks consumed.

A course of the treatment can last three months to one year or longer. With several months of abstinence strung together, naltrexone essentially gives the brain a chance to reconfigure itself, separating good signals from bad ones and making more logical connections. A person whose life used to revolve around alcohol has an ever-increasing chance of long-term abstinence.

The Combining Medications and Behavioral Interventions for Alcoholism (COMBINE) study showed that a combination of the medication naltrexone and brief counseling curtailed drinking and enhanced abstinence among people with AUD. Side effects can include sleep problems, tiredness, anxiety, headache, joint and muscle pains, abdominal pain and cramps, nausea and vomiting.

Topiramate

Topiramate (Topamax) was developed to treat epilepsy, and it is approved by the U.S. Food and Drug Administration to prevent migraines. Psychiatrists have used it to treat bipolar disorder and counteract the weight gain associated with some antidepressants. It has also been investigated for use in treating obesity, binge eating, post-traumatic stress disorder, bulimia, obsessive-compulsive disorder, smoking cessation, cocaine dependence and AUD.

Topiramate appears to be particularly effective for reducing cravings and increasing abstinence in people who are still drinking. First, it blocks the ability of glutamate to increase dopamine. Since glutamate is involved in the process of long-term memory, blocking it holds back the pleasurable feelings associated with memories of drinking. Second, topiramate enhances the production of gamma-aminobutyric acid, which suppresses dopamine output, reducing the pleasurable effects of drinking.

In two large-scale clinical trials, topiramate helped improve all drinking outcomes. One of the studies reported that heavy drinkers were six times more likely to remain abstinent for a month when taking topiramate even in small doses. Participants taking topiramate had fewer drinks during a drinking day, fewer heavy drinking days, more days abstinent, and were less likely to binge drink when compared with the placebo group. Half of everyone in the topiramate group reported less craving for alcohol.

Topiramate is most effective when it is paired with brief counseling on a weekly basis. Most patients need to be treated for six months to one year to decrease the possibility of full-blown alcohol relapse. Topiramate can have side effects that include weight loss, fatigue, a feeling of pins and needles, mental slowness, and kidney stones.

Ondansetron

Ultra-low-dose *ondansetron* (Zofran), is a serotonin-3 receptor antagonist. Serotonin helps to regulate appetite, sleep, memory, learning and mood. The serotonin system modulates the effects of other neurotransmitter systems, including the cortico-mesolimbic dopamine system. Many antidepressant drugs act by regulating serotonin levels in the brain.

Blocking serotonin receptors decreases dopamine release and, as a result, lessens the craving for alcohol. This treatment is targeted for people with a specific genetic composition. It was shown to work for the subpopulation of 35 percent of people of European or Hispanic descent who have a specific genotype of key genes in the serotonin system. In a pivotal phase 2b clinical trial, ultra-low-dose ondansetron reduced the number of drinks per drinking day, increased abstinent days, and decreased the percentage of heavy drinking days in that specific population.

Ondansetron is currently used for the treatment of vomiting, but the lowest dose currently available commercially is 12 times higher than the dose required to treat AUD. That ultra-low dose of ondansetron is not

---

What's in a Drink?

In the United States, one drink contains roughly 14 grams of pure alcohol, which is found in...

- 12 ounces of regular beer
- 8 to 9 ounces of malt liquor
- 5 ounces of wine
- 3 to 4 ounces of sherry or port wine
- 1.5 ounces of distilled spirits
- 2 to 3 ounces of cordial liqueur

For different types of beer, wine, or malt liquor, the alcohol content can vary greatly. Check labels or the bottler's website for specific information.

---

commercially available, but it is in a phase 3 trial that is scheduled to be completed in 2022. Side effects can include headache, constipation and fatigue.

Acamprosate

Acamprosate works as a relapse-prevention drug. The glutamate system remains highly active and seeks out additional stimulation even after alcohol intake stops, causing negative emotions and sometimes withdrawal symptoms. Acamprosate is thought to restore normal glutamate activity in the brain. Acamprosate has been found to be most effective when combined with behavioral interventions focused on preventing relapse.

Side effects can include diarrhea, constipation, nausea, stomach pain, loss of appetite, headache, drowsiness, dizziness, weight changes, muscle/joint pain, change in sexual desire or decreased sexual ability.

A Makeover for Your Mind

Norman E. Rosenthal, MD, is a clinical professor of psychiatry at Georgetown University School of Medicine in Washington, DC. He is author of *Transcendence: Healing and Transformation Through Transcendental Meditation*. NormanRosenthal.com

Women's magazines love to feature beauty makeovers that turn Plain Janes into glamour girls. But what about a brain makeover? How valuable would it be if we could transform our minds into calmer, cleverer, more creative and more focused versions of ourselves?

Well, guess what? That's easily within reach…and it involves only minimal effort and a modest investment of time. The key is a particular form of meditation called transcendental meditation (TM).

TM has been shown to help people recover from the emotional anguish of traumatic experiences such as rape and physical abuse. TM can benefit not just trauma victims, but anyone who wants to elevate her or his cognitive skills in order to deal more successfully with life's everyday challenges. It's a brain makeover! In fact, TM's enthusiastic practitioners include superstars such as Oprah Winfrey, Jerry Seinfeld and director David Lynch.

Brain tune-up: According to psychiatrist Norman Rosenthal, MD, author of *Transcendence: Healing and Transformation through Transcendental Meditation*, TM actually helps optimize brain function. *For instance, numerous high-quality studies demonstrate that TM can help ability in areas such as…*

- **Creative problem solving**
- **Memory, concentration, alertness and mental clarity**
- **Prioritizing**
- **Stress management**
- **Interpersonal negotiations**
- **Maintaining a positive frame of mind**

As an example, Dr. Rosenthal cited a study from Norwich University in Vermont, which found that people who practiced TM for two months scored better than a control group of nonmeditators on a variety of psychological tests, including those measuring resilience, positive disposition, and levels of anxiety and depression. Such benefits could be especially helpful to women, Dr. Rosenthal noted. "Much more than men, women generally find themselves juggling an enormous number of challenges, including careers, homes, families and friends," he said.

The TM technique: There's nothing mystical, religious or cultlike about TM. The simple technique involves the silent repetition of a mantra, a particular sound with no meaning that serves as a vehicle to settle the mind into a profound state of restful alertness. When your mind wanders, you simply refocus on the mantra. Traditionally TM is practiced with eyes closed for 20 minutes twice daily.

Dr. Rosenthal likened the mind to the ocean—a choppy surface with miles of calm, still water beneath. "TM is like diving down into the deep," he explained. The practice helps the brain achieve a deeply restful level of relaxation that leads to greater mental clarity and enhanced performance.

Neurologically speaking, when people practice TM, the coherence of alpha brain waves throughout the brain is accompanied by slightly faster beta waves in the prefrontal region of the brain, behind the forehead. The alpha waves produce relaxation…while the beta waves improve focus and decision-making. Some physiological changes occur immediately, but people who practice TM regularly tend to have optimal results, probably due to increased synaptic connections (connections between brain cells). In other words, with practice, the brain may literally rewire itself.

Is there anything different in how a person who is meditating to improve her mind would approach her meditation, as compared with a person who is meditating to heal from trauma? Dr. Rosenthal explained, "The technique is done exactly the same way, but what happens in your mind is different. The brain 'plays' with your mantra in such a way that it does what it needs. So if all is well, your meditation works to make your mind even better…and if there is trouble, then that is where the energy goes."

Would any other forms of meditation be equally effective for tuning up the brain? Dr. Rosenthal said that they might also be helpful, yet mentioned several points that favor TM, in his opinion. For one thing, approximately 340 peer-reviewed published studies have demonstrated TM's various positive effects on body and mind. And different forms of meditation (such as focusing on the breath or an image) affect other parts of the brain and affect people in different ways, which may or may not provide similar benefits.

Also, despite its powerful effects, TM is especially easy to do.

To learn TM: You can find a certified TM teacher through the Maharishi Foundation USA (TM.org). (Dr. Rosenthal receives no financial compensation from this or any other TM organization.) Why seek out a teacher? Just as you can't truly master playing a sport or musical instrument by reading about it, you can't really learn TM from a book or article. Personalized instruction works much better.

Case Study: What to Do About That Failing Memory

Andrew Rubman, ND, is medical director of Southbury Clinic for Traditional Medicines in Southbury, Connecticut. SouthburyClinic.com He is author of the "Nature Doc's Patient Diary" blog at Bottom LineInc.com.

The patient: "Samuel" a 65-year-old retired Marine Master Sergeant.

Why he came to see me: Although Samuel was in "perfect health" according to his VA doctors, his memory was declining. Samuel had heard about me from another veteran who had great success in treating his issues and was hopeful that I could help him too.

How I evaluated him: I had Samuel bring over his medical folder from his team at the Veterans Administration and spent quite a bit of time reviewing the history and their findings, searching for some clue as to why this man, who still "ran five miles every morning at dawn no matter the weather" could be having problems with memory. His physical exams had been exemplary, his blood work "spot on," and X-rays and scans unremarkable. We did, however, discuss his having been close to "exploding ordinance" during one deployment in Iraq about 15 years ago. The vehicle that he was riding in had been destroyed by an exploding shell and he was knocked unconscious for a few minutes. He was evaluated by medics and later in the hos-

pital and there was no evidence of concussion. I thought that we had found a cause.

How we addressed his problem: I explained to Samuel that even though there was no discernable physical damage to his brain, that the shock could have produced sufficient disorientation of the "circuits" and that memory loss could occur later in life as a result. We discussed using a material called *piracetam*, which chemically resembles GABA (gamma-amino buteric acid), a substance used by the brain. This compound has been used successfully in Europe for victims of traumatic brain injury, helping one side of the brain integrate signals with the other side—so that a challenged area could recruit the parallel area on the other side of the brain to pick up the slack. (Natural doctors sometimes recommend piracetam for patients with dementia too.) He thought that this supplement made a great deal of sense and wanted to give it a try.

The patient's progress: Within a month, Samuel reported that not only had much of his memory issues abated but that the quality and richness of the memories had become enhanced. He was able to recall not only the images of past events, but often the associated sounds and even the smells present at the time. He said that although some of his past was extremely unpleasant that "the good outweighed the bad" and that he welcomed all of his past experience because taking on whatever comes "is what Marines do."

Treating Hypertension Could Reduce Dementia Risk

A meta-analysis of 12 trials with more than 92,000 patients shows that taking medication to lower your high blood pressure can reduce your risk for cognitive impairment and dementia by 7 percent.

Michelle Canavan, PhD, research fellow, National University of Ireland, Galway, and leader of a study published in *Journal of the American Medical Association*.

4 Natural Ways to Prevent Dementia

Michael Edson, MS, LAc, a licensed acupuncturist, certified herbalist and qi gong teacher based in Yonkers, New York. He is author of *Natural Brain Support and Natural Parkinson's Support*. EdsonAcu puncture.com

Much of the research on Alzheimer's and other forms of dementia focuses on pharmaceuticals, which often fail to reduce risk for dementia or improve symptoms.

Problem: About one-third of people who live to age 80 or older suffer from dementia.

Good news: Licensed acupuncturist and certified herbalist Michael Edson says there are safe, gentle, nondrug therapies that help delay the onset of symptoms and slow their progression…approaches that are supported by a growing body of evidence. *His four favorites**…

Juicing

Every minute of the day, you are exposed to environmental toxins, such as smoke and pollution. Your body also produces toxins as it goes about the very important job of keeping you alive. These toxins, known as free radicals, essentially "rust" your brain's wiring. Antioxidants—which are abundant in fruits and vegetables—neutralize free radicals, preventing them from causing damage.

Finding: Studies of centenarians have linked a high-antioxidant diet with reduced free radical damage and lower incidence of dementia.

Juicing or smoothie making concentrates a high amount of neuroprotective antioxidants into a tasty beverage. Start with green leafy vegetables such as spinach or kale. Then add a handful or two of berries. Berries and

*Combine these with a healthy, whole-foods–based diet and plenty of aerobic exercise. Stop smoking if you currently smoke. Discuss any supplements and dietary changes with your doctor, particularly if you are on blood-thinning medications or have low blood pressure.

pomegranate are high in polyphenolic compounds, most prominently anthocyanins, which have powerful antioxidant and anti-inflammatory effects.

Other brain-healthy vegetables to include are broccoli, avocado and red beets. Other healthful fruits include apples, black currant, citrus (especially lemon), kiwi and grapes. For even more brain-healthy nutrients, add some garlic, ginger, chia seeds, parsley, ginseng, walnuts, yogurt, coconut oil and/ or honey. Experiment to find your favorite combinations.

Antioxidant Supplements

In addition to an antioxidant-rich diet, those with a family history of dementia also should consider taking these supplements…

• **Acetyl-L-carnitine.** Several Alzheimer's medications work by increasing this neurotransmitter. It is vital for processing memory, learning and focus but is decreased in people with Alzheimer's. Acetyl-L-carnitine fuels the production of acetylcholine. It also reduces the buildup of dementia-predisposing waste products in the brain. Acetyl-L-carnitine is found in meat, fish, poultry, milk, nuts, seeds, cheese, asparagus and broccoli. Taking a 500-milligram (mg) supplement daily on an empty stomach will ensure that you get enough.

• **Curcumin.** This spice increases the production of new brain cells. It also may slow age-related cognitive decline by inhibiting the buildup of beta-amyloid plaques, clumps of proteins that accumulate between neurons and, over time, can interrupt cell function and pave the way for Alzheimer's. Curcumin gives curry powder its golden hue. This may help explain why the rate of Alzheimer's is so low in India—just 1 percent of those age 65 and over have it. Try a daily 500-mg to 1,200-mg supplement.

• **Ashwagandha root extract, also known as Indian ginseng.** Chemical changes in the brain caused by chronic stress reduce brain plasticity. This, in turn, can kick-start an irreversible cascade of neuronal death, a characteristic of many brain diseases including dementia. Ashwagandha may reduce neuronal death and beta-amyloid buildup.

Ashwagandha leaves are thought to enhance cognitive performance.

Scientific evidence: In one study, subjects either took 300 mg of ashwagandha twice daily or a placebo for eight weeks. At the end of the study, those in the ashwagandha group showed greater improvements in both immediate and general memory as well as improved executive function, attention and information-processing speed. Try 300 mg twice per day, taken with meals.

• **Vitamin D, zinc and magnesium.** Low levels of the first two may result in cognitive difficulty and learning impairment and even may mimic symptoms of dementia. Most seniors have been found to be significantly deficient in vitamin D—a blood test can determine your level. Higher magnesium levels have been associated with a lower risk for dementia.

Recommended: 5,000 IU/day of vitamin D...40 mg/day of zinc...and 500 mg/day of magnesium.

Essential Oils

Certain essential oils have been shown to support memory and cognition...boost circulation...reduce inflammation...reduce anxiety...and support healthy sleep, all critical for avoiding dementia.

• **Lemon balm.** This bright, sunny scent has been shown to improve cognitive function in patients with mild-to-moderate Alzheimer's. Lemon balm also has been used for centuries as a calming agent. Used at night, it can help promote sleep.

Why sleep matters: In the short term, inadequate sleep (less than seven hours a night) can lead to forgetfulness and other cognitive impairment. During sleep, the events of the day are consolidated and turned into memories...and accumulated waste products in the brain are flushed away. It's believed that this cleaning process is linked with a lower dementia risk because clumps of these same waste products typically are found in the brains of people with Alzheimer's.

• **Frankincense.** This iconic Christmastime scent has been shown to increase communication between neurons in the hippocampus, one of the brain's memory hubs. It also may help enhance concentration and focus and even promote sleep.

• **Rosemary.** This essential oil contains several compounds shown to enhance long-term memory.

Scientific evidence: In a British study, 150 healthy individuals over age 65 were divided among three rooms—one scented with rosemary, one with lavender, one unscented—where they were presented with a series of memory challenges. Those smelling rosemary experienced significantly improved memory compared with the others.

How to use oils: Dilute one drop of a quality essential oil brand such as Rocky Mountain Oils, dōTERRA or Aura Cacia in one teaspoon of a carrier oil such as coconut oil or jojoba oil. Apply to the skin of your neck, above the eyebrows, temples, behind the earlobes, chest and abdomen, arms, legs and/or bottoms of feet. Alternatively, use a diffuser to disperse the scent in your room.

Important: Before full application, apply a small amount of diluted oil to the skin and check for an allergic reaction after at least 24 hours.

Socialize

Poor social engagement was linked with significantly increased dementia rates in a recent review of 33 studies encompassing nearly 2.4 million people.

Socializing—even via a video or phone call—provides mental stimulation. It also reduces feelings of loneliness, which are stressful and inflammatory. In fact, loneliness is associated with a two-fold increase in incidence of dementia.

Danger for Women: Dehydration and Dementia

Betsy Mills, PhD, senior program manager, aging and Alzheimer's prevention, Alzheimer's Drug Discovery Foundation, New York.

Is there a link between dehydration and dementia? It turns out there is. And women are at high risk.

The human body is made up of over 50 percent water, and it requires this water to carry out all of its essential day-to-day functions, including cognitive function. When the brain cells don't have enough water, they have to work harder, so they end up operating at a slower pace, which results in mental fog.

The cognitive symptoms of dehydration differ depending on the age, sex and overall health of the person. Young, healthy people tend to experience fatigue and irritability, while older individuals are more likely to experience a reduced ability to focus and a slowing of processing speed, which is the time it takes to complete a mental task.

Although both men and women can experience cognitive symptoms of dehydration, they tend to be more pronounced in women. Women and the elderly may be more vulnerable to the negative effects of dehydration due to decreased muscle mass. Muscle tissue is composed of nearly 80 percent water and can buffer against dehydration by releasing its stored water when fluid levels get low. Therefore, in addition to eating a well-balanced diet containing many water-rich fruits and vegetables, engaging in muscle strength-building exercises is a good way to protect against dehydration.

The effects of dehydration on cognitive function are usually temporary and should resolve once the body is adequately hydrated. However, dehydration is a state of stress for the brain, and if it persists, then the brain cells could sustain long-lasting damage, which can pave the way for permanent cognitive dysfunction. Temporary cognitive dysfunction in response to dehydration is generally not considered a sign of dementia, but dehydration may exacerbate cognitive symptoms in people with dementia.

Additionally, dehydration can accelerate cognitive decline in individuals with dementia. The sensitivity to thirst declines with age, so elderly individuals, especially those with dementia, may not recognize that they are dehydrated. Since individuals with dementia are more prone to becoming dehydrated, it may be necessary to keep track of their fluid intake. Importantly, the brain can also be harmed by excessive water consumption, because it can lead to a dangerous drop in sodium levels. For more information on brain health and avoiding risks, please visit CognitiveVitality.org.

Promising News About Dementia Risk from Parkinson's Treatment

The study "Dementia and Subthalamic Deep Brain Stimulation in Parkinson Disease," led by researchers at Grenoble Alpes University in Grenoble, France, and published in *Neurology*.

Even though Parkinson's disease is best known for causing physical symptoms, such as difficulty walking and tremors, up to 80 percent of those affected by the movement disorder eventually develop dementia.

This sobering fact creates a dilemma when a treatment known as deep brain stimulation (DBS), which some research has suggested increases dementia risk, is recommended for people with Parkinson's disease.

Why use DBS? In cases of more advanced Parkinson's, the treatment has been shown to work better than medication at controlling motor symptoms caused by the disease, such as disabling tremors. DBS requires a surgical procedure to implant electrodes into areas of the brain that control movement, and a pacemaker-type device is implanted into the chest area. The pacemaker sends electrical signals to the brain to reduce abnormal movements.

Analyzing the risk: To better understand the potential dementia risk posed by DBS, researchers followed 175 people (average age 56) with Parkinson's disease who received DBS implants after being diagnosed with the disorder for an average of 12 years. The study participants were checked for evidence of dementia at one, five and 10 years after the DBS implant. The key results of the study were published in *Neurology*, a journal of the American Academy of Neurology (AAN)...

•**After one year,** 2.3 percent of patients developed dementia.

•**After five years,** 8.5 percent of patients developed dementia.

•**At 10 years,** nearly 30 percent had developed dementia.

"These rates are not higher than those reported in the general population of people with Parkinson's," said study author Elena Moro, MD, PhD, professor of neurology at Grenoble Alpes University in Grenoble, France, and a fellow of the AAN. "The few studies that are available with similar disease duration have reported higher rates of dementia."

Caveats: The lower rate of dementia in those who received DBS may be due, in part, to the younger average age group of study participants. The lower incidence of dementia also could be explained by the relatively high percentage of participants who could not be located or failed to respond to the researchers' requests for follow-up. For example, at the study's 10-year mark, only 104 of the 175 study participants were available for testing.

The researchers also evaluated risk factors for dementia. As with all people with Parkinson's disease, study participants who were male, older, had experienced hallucinations or scored low on thinking tests prior to the DBS surgery were more likely to develop dementia. The only risk factor that could be linked specifically to DBS was bleeding into the brain (cerebral hemorrhage) at the time of implant surgery.

"These results are very encouraging for people with Parkinson's and their families that they can take advantage of the benefits of deep brain stimulation without worrying about it increasing the likelihood of developing dementia," explained Dr. Moro.

Takeaway: Even though DBS does not cure or slow down the progression of Parkinson's disease, it does improve quality of life for many people. This study shows that the treatment may be safer than some previous research has suggested.

Dementia Alerts
Atypical Dementia Is Hitting Younger People

Doctors are increasingly seeing evidence of dementia in people in their 40s, 50s and 60s. Early-onset dementia now is about 5 percent of total cases. The symptoms of cognitive impairment are similar, but it can be harder for families of people with early-onset dementia to convince doctors of the problem, because dementia is considered a disease of old age.

Research led by scientists at Indiana University School of Medicine's Indiana Alzheimer's Disease Research Center, Indianapolis, published in *Alzheimer's Research & Therapy*.

New Form of Dementia Discovered

A mutation in the valosin-containing protein (VCP) gene causes vacuolar tauopathy, a newly discovered neurodegenerative disease characterized by a buildup of tau proteins and the accumulation of neurons with holes in them. The genetic link suggests that boosting VCP activity could help break up the protein aggregates in this and other diseases, such as Alzheimer's.

University of Pennsylvania School of Medicine

Parkinson's Patients Are Given Drugs That Work Against Each Other

Allison W. Willis, MD, MS, department of neurology, Perelman School of Medicine, University of Pennsylvania, Philadelphia, lead author of study titled "Patterns of Dementia Treatment and Frank Prescribing Errors in Older Adults With Parkinson Disease," published in *JAMA Neurology*.

If you get Parkinson's disease, there's a greater than 80 percent chance you'll have cognitive impairment within 20 years. So Parkinson's patients are commonly prescribed drugs to treat cognitive impairment. Alarmingly, a new study finds that these patients also are being prescribed drugs that work against their dementia drugs. Nor is it an occasional mix-up—it's happening to huge numbers of Parkinson's patients! Read on to learn how to protect yourself or your loved one.

Treating Parkinson's cognitive impairment, one of the major reasons for someone with the disease to end up in a nursing home, is critical. The cognitive drug most commonly prescribed is *donepezil hydrochloride* (Aricept), which belongs to a class of drugs called acetylcholinesterase inhibitors. Other drugs in that class include *rivastigmine tartrate* (Exelon) and *galantamine hydrobromide* (Razadyne). These drugs work by increasing levels of acetylcholine, a brain chemical that supports cognition.

However, Parkinson's primarily affects older adults, an age group that is prone to other medical problems such as depression, bladder incontinence, heart problems and allergies. So it's very common for Parkinson's patients to also be prescribed drugs to treat these conditions—and some of the drugs most often prescribed are anticholinergics such as *paroxetine* (Paxil) and *oxybutynin* (Ditropan). These drugs can decrease cognition, especially in people who are cognitively vulnerable—for instance, people with Parkinson's.

Researchers from Perelman School of Medicine at University of Pennsylvania reviewed one year of Medicare prescription records for Parkinson's patients and identified 65,000 who had been prescribed at least one acetylcholinesterase inhibitor. They found that about 45 percent of these patients had also been prescribed an anticholinergic drug for some other health condition.

The researchers further found that the risk for being prescribed these pharmacologically opposing drugs varied by region of the country and by race or ethnicity of the patient. Highest risks were in southern and midwestern states and among Hispanic patients.

Taking an anticholinergic along with an acetylcholinesterase inhibitor is like drinking an energy drink with a sleeping pill. It's a "prescription" that the researchers say should never happen. They also point out that many anticholinergic medications are available over the counter, and the study did not include these—for example, allergy, cold, flu, motion sickness and sleep-aid drugs can contain *diphenhydramine* (Benadryl), which is an anticholinergic. So the likelihood that Parkinson's patients are taking pharmacologically opposing drugs may be even greater.

Pharmacologically opposing drugs are bad enough for the Parkinson's patients themselves.

Even worse: Such widespread co-prescribing of drugs that work against each other may also be interfering with Parkinson's research. Most studies assume that cognitive decline is due to death of brain cells or build-up of certain proteins in the brain—when at least some symptoms of cognitive decline among these patients may be side effects from anticholinergic drugs.

If you or a loved one is being treated for Parkinson's, discuss with your doctor and/or pharmacist all medications—prescription and OTC—that are being taken. If it turns out that you're taking both an acetylcholinesterase inhibitor and an anticholinergic, discuss with your doctor whether another medication combination might be better for you.

Dementia Patients Often Get Ineffective Drugs

Donovan Maust, MD, is geriatric psychiatrist at University of Michigan, Ann Arbor, and leader of a study published in *JAMA*.

Among more than 700,000 people with dementia, nearly three-quarters had been prescribed an antidepressant, opioid painkiller, epilepsy drug, anxiety medication or antipsychotic drug—which have limited evidence that they ease dementia-related behavior problems and which all carry significant risks.

If your loved one has dementia: Ask the doctor what symptoms the proposed drug is supposed to alleviate and about its proven effectiveness.

A Novel Way to Identify Alzheimer's and Predict Its Progression

Study titled "CSF Tau Microtubule Binding Region Identifies Tau Tangle and Clinical Stages of Alzheimer's Disease," by researchers at Washington University School of Medicine in Saint Louis, published in *Brain*.

A protein in cerebrospinal fluid that could possibly indicate Alzheimer's disease in its earliest stage and predict its progression has been discovered by researchers at Washington University School of Medicine in Saint Louis.

Background: Two proteins that build up in the brain have been linked to Alzheimer's disease, the most common form of dementia. Amyloid protein plaques form between neurons, and tau tangles form inside neurons. Both of these proteins often begin to develop several years before cognitive impairment. Amyloid plaques or tangles can be found on a PET scan. However, PET scans are expensive and often difficult to obtain.

The researchers looked at a form of tau protein called microtubule binding region (MTBR) tau 243, in the fluid that surrounds the brain and spinal cord, known as cerebrospinal fluid (CSF). CSF can be obtained by doing a spinal tap. Since tau tangles often form before symptoms of cognitive impairment, finding MTBR tau 243 in CSF may diagnose Alzheimer's at its earliest stage. The research findings are published in the journal *Brain*.

Study details: The researchers collected CSF from 100 people age 70 or older. MTBR tau 243 was abundant only in people with cognitive impairment or dementia. They followed 28 people from the original group for two to nine years and found that MTBR tau 243 also increased in those who had been diagnosed with Alzheimer's disease. To test the ability of the MTBR tau 243 to predict the stage of Alzheimer's, they compared MTBR tau 243 levels with PET-scan imaging in 20 people with Alzheimer's. The CSF levels of MTBR tau 243 matched the amount of tau tangles found on the scans.

Benefits of early detection: The significance of their discovery, say the researchers, is that diagnosing Alzheimer's at an early stage could make treatment more effective. Levels of MTBR tau 243 could also be used to study how well an existing or future treatment is working. Finally, an interesting finding was that some MTBR tau 243 were found outside neurons. This raises the possibility that MTBR tau 243 may spread tau tangles from one neuron to another. If that's the case, it may be a target for new drugs to attack and stop the spread of the tangles that make Alzheimer's so insidious.

Multiple Sclerosis Symptoms Improve With Mindfulness Meditation

Studies titled "Mindfulness Training for Emotion Dysregulation in Multiple Sclerosis: A Pilot Randomized Controlled Trial," published in *Rehabilitation Psychology*...and "Effects of 4-week Mindfulness Training Versus Adaptive Cognitive Training on Processing Speed and Working Memory in Multiple Sclerosis," published in *Neuropsychology,* both by researchers at The Ohio State University, Columbus.

People who have multiple sclerosis (MS) deal with more than just physical problems—the disease also causes emotional and cognitive problems. Now, thanks to a new study, there may be an easy way for MS patients to improve both their mental and emotional health.

Bonus: It costs nothing and is drug-free.

MS is a neurodegenerative disease that damages the central nervous system. It affects nearly one million Americans, causing among other symptoms, unsteady gait, slurred speech, numbness, tingling, cognitive changes that make it take longer to understand and complete mental tasks and emotion dysregulation—difficulty managing negative emotions such as depression and anxiety. In fact, up to half of people with MS experience some type of psychiatric disorder.

In a small pilot study, researchers at The Ohio State University looked at whether people with MS would benefit from mindfulness meditation. This kind of meditation, which is known to help with depression and anxiety, focuses perception on awareness and acceptance of the present moment.

Study: Three groups of people with MS (61 total) received four weeks of either mindfulness meditation training...or adaptive cognitive training...or they were placed on a wait list and received no training (the control group). All participants had their cognitive impairment and self-reported emotional control evaluated before and after the four-week intervention.

Mindfulness training consisted of two hours of in-person training each week, plus 40 minutes of daily exercises to perform at home—such as breathing awareness, body scanning, sitting meditation and focusing on thoughts, emotions and sensations.

Adaptive cognitive training also included two hours weekly of in-person training plus 40 minutes of different daily exercises to perform at home—reading and video games focused on processing speed (time it takes to understand and react to information), attention, working memory (capacity for retaining information short term in order to perform mental operations using the information) and executive function.

Results: At the end of four weeks, participants in the mindfulness meditation group were significantly better able to manage negative emotions than the participants of other two groups.

An additional analysis looked at processing speed and working memory. While working memory was unchanged for all three groups, the researchers were surprised to find that the meditation group showed significant improvement in processing speed—surpassing adaptive cognitive training, currently a common and considered effective therapy for MS-caused cognitive impairment.

Since this research involved only a small number of participants, the researchers are hoping to do a larger study to test their findings. Meanwhile, results of the current study are encouraging. Mindfulness meditation is easy to learn and practice—and shows potential to be an important tool to improve the quality of life for people with MS.

Strenuous Physical Workouts Tire the Brain Too

Study by researchers at Pitié-Salpêtrière University Hospital, Paris, published in *Current Biology*.

In addition to making the body feel tired, a heavy training load leads to mental fatigue—reducing activity in the lateral prefrontal region of the brain, which is responsible for making decisions.

More TV Viewing, Greater Cognitive Decline

Analysis of data on 3,662 adults, ages 50 and older, by researchers at University College London, UK, published in *Scientific Reports*.

People who regularly watched television for more than 3.5 hours a day had poorer verbal memory six years later than those who watched three hours daily or less. And the greater the amount of TV watched above the 3.5-hour level, the larger the decline in this form of cognition.

Chapter 3

CANCER CARE FOR WOMEN

3-D Mammography Is Best for Breast Cancer Screening

Women have a few choices when it comes to screening for breast cancer. They can test with mammograms printed on X-ray film, digital mammography or with a newer imaging technology called digital breast tomosynthesis (DBT). In many screening centers, digital mammography, or two-dimensional (2-D) mammography, has actually replaced X-ray film mammograms.

Recent development: A growing body of research suggests that DBT, also known as three-dimensional (3-D) mammography, may provide better results than standard digital mammography. Now, a new study comparing digital mammography against DBT supports DBT as the better screening method for breast cancer.

Digital mammography allows the radiologist to make X-ray images darker or lighter—this helps find breast cancer, especially in dense breasts. These images can be viewed on a computer and the images can be made larger to focus on specific areas. DBT also uses computer imaging, but the images are taken as a camera arcs over the breasts taking pictures from different angles. This allows for a 3-D image and eliminates overlapping breast tissue that can hide a cancerous tumor.

Studies show that DBT misses fewer cancers than digital mammography. If a screening exam does not find a cancer (a negative exam), but a cancer is found within the following year, the exam is called a false negative. It's been shown that DBT provides a lower rate of false-negative exams, which may mean screening with DBT can find cancers earlier and increase survival because these cancers are less advanced and easier to cure.

Research details: To compare false-negative results from digital mammography versus DBT, researchers from 10 academic and community screening centers reviewed more than 380,000 screening exams. The exams were divided almost equally between digital mammography and DBT. *These were the key findings…*

• DBT had a false-negative rate of 0.6 per 1,000 exams compared with a rate of 0.7 for digital mammography.

Study titled "False-Negative Rates of Breast Cancer Screening With and Without Digital Breast Tomosynthesis," led by researchers at Yale School of Medicine, New Haven, Connecticut, published in *Radiology*.

• **DBT had a higher sensitivity rate (89.8 percent) than digital mammography (85.6 percent).** Sensitivity indicates how likely a test is to detect a condition when it is actually present in a patient.

• **DBT had a higher specificity rate (90.7 percent) than digital mammography (89.1 percent).** Specificity is the ability of a test to rule out the presence of a disease in someone who does not have it.

• **DBT had lower odds of missing an advanced cancer than digital mammography.**

Takeaway: Based on its improved sensitivity, specificity and ability to detect invasive cancers before they spread, screening with DBT is superior to digital mammography, according to this study. The researchers anticipate that DBT will eventually become the standard of care for breast cancer screening.

Earlier Breast Cancer Screening Saves Lives

Study titled "Effect of Mammographic Screening from Age 40 Years on Breast Cancer Mortality (UK Age Trial): Final Results of a Randomized, Controlled Trial," led by researchers at Queen Mary University of London, published in *The Lancet Oncology*.

It's well-established that women who receive mammograms to screen for breast cancer reduce their risk of dying from the disease, but when to start that screening has long been controversial with guidelines varying by country.

In the US, for example, the American Cancer Society (ACS) recommends that women receive mammograms to screen for breast cancer starting at age 45, while guidelines from the US Preventive Services Task Force, an independent panel of national experts in disease prevention and evidence-based medicine, advises women to begin screening at age 50. Both groups say that women should have the option to start breast cancer screening at age 40 with yearly or biennial mam-

mograms, depending on their personal risk factors.

In the UK, as well as many other countries, breast cancer screening is offered to women ages 50 to 70 every three years. The thinking behind this and other such recommendations is that screening with mammograms before age 50 will find more tumors that turn out to be benign, and the risk for overtreatment, with biopsies and other testing, will outweigh the benefits of screening.

Recent development: To further investigate the validity of the UK's breast cancer screening recommendation, researchers at Queen Mary University of London conducted a 23-year study to see how women fared when they began receiving mammograms at age 40 versus age 50.

To begin the study, which was recently published in *The Lancet Oncology,* researchers randomly assigned nearly 60,000 women to a study group that started receiving yearly mammograms at age 40. More than 100,000 women were assigned to a control group that would wait until age 50 to begin standard breast cancer screening with mammograms every three years.

Study findings: After the first 10 years of the study, 83 women in the study group had died from breast cancer compared with 219 deaths from the disease in the control group. This translates into a 25 percent reduced risk of dying from breast cancer when screening started at age 40 instead of age 50.

After the first 10 years of the study, the women who had started their breast cancer screening earlier adopted the same standard mammography screening schedule that the control group followed. During this part of the study, however, both groups had roughly the same risk of dying from breast cancer.

Takeaway: Based on these findings, the researchers conclude that the benefits of starting mammograms at age 40 outweigh the risks of overtreatment. They also note that the benefits may now be even greater than those shown in the research due to improvements in mammogram technology since the study began.

Some well-respected medical institutions in the US, such as the Mayo Clinic in Rochester, Minnesota, do recommend starting mammogram screening at age 40. This study suggests that lowering all official guidelines to age 40 could save lives.

Important: Women should discuss their breast cancer screening schedule with their doctors to ensure that they are doing all they can to help protect themselves against the disease.

A Fasting Diet May Boost Breast Cancer Treatment

Study titled "Fasting-Mimicking Diet and Hormone Therapy Induce Breast Cancer Regression," by researchers at University of Southern California, IFOM Cancer Institute and University of Genoa, published in *Nature*.

A diet with periods of calorie restriction, called a fasting-mimicking diet, may make hormone-sensitive breast cancers more responsive to hormone treatments, according to research from the University of Southern California (USC) and Italy's IFOM Cancer Institute and University of Genoa.

Background: About eight out of 10 breast cancers have female hormone (estrogen or progesterone) receptors on their cells that can drive breast cancer growth. Drugs such as *tamoxifen* and *fulvestrant* block female hormones from binding to cancer cells and are an integral part of breast cancer treatment. But these therapies can become less effective as the body develops a resistance to them over time.

Recent finding: Researchers initially worked with mice and found that a fasting-mimicking diet reduces blood levels of binding hormones that increase cancer growth. These binding hormones include insulin, insulin-like growth factor 1 (ILGF1) and leptin. The diet also enhances the ef-

fectiveness of tamoxifen and fulvestrant and delays resistance to these drugs. The researchers further described a long-lasting tumor regression in two mouse studies.

In these mouse studies, another benefit was that the diet reduced a known and limiting side effect of tamoxifen called endometrial hyperplasia, which is a thickening of the inside lining of the uterus. Endometrial hyperplasia is hard to treat, may increase the risk of endometrial cancer and limits the use of tamoxifen. This benefit from the diet could extend the use of tamoxifen if it holds up in human trials.

As a follow-up to the mouse studies, a small trial—known as a feasibility study—was conducted in women with hormone-receptor-positive breast cancers receiving hormone therapy. A feasibility study indicates whether further research on humans is warranted. When the women started a fasting-mimicking diet, they experienced reductions in insulin, leptin and IGF1 that paralleled the mouse studies. The results of both the mouse and human studies are published in the journal *Nature*.

Conclusion: The researchers would like to power up future studies to include about 300 to 400 women. Researchers at USC are currently conducting breast cancer trials that include fasting-mimicking diets. If the results hold up, adding this diet to other therapies would be a safe and non-toxic boost to breast cancer treatment.

Menopause Help for Breast Cancer Survivors

Andrew M. Kaunitz, MD, University of Florida Research Foundation Professor, associate chair of the department of obstetrics and gynecology, University of Florida College of Medicine, Jacksonville.

Breast cancer treatment often comes with a host of unwelcome side effects. One you may not expect from the treatment that has saved your life is the sometimes sudden and often intense onset of menopausal symptoms, such as hot flashes, night sweats, brain fogginess and vaginal dryness. Some women experience such debilitating symptoms that they skip preventive "adjuvant" cancer therapies just to avoid them. More than half of women in one recent study did just that—a decision with potentially dire consequences down the road.

A better approach: After doing everything possible to prevent a recurrence of breast cancer, explore the many safe ways you can minimize menopausal symptoms.

How Breast Cancer Leads to Menopausal Symptoms

Breast cancer and its treatment doesn't always bring on menopause or make symptoms worse. But it often does. The great majority of women in their 40s receiving chemotherapy for breast cancer, for example, will experience cessation of menstruation, which often is permanent. *Here are the main reasons…*

• **Chemotherapy may have harmful effects on your ovaries.** Chemo drugs attack cancer cells, but they can also damage your ovaries (and your eggs). The result can be a sudden drop in estrogen…and the immediate onset of menopausal symptoms. If you're premenopausal, your periods may stop or become irregular and may not return after treatment.

• **Surgery to remove the ovaries triggers immediate menopause.** Some women with breast cancer are also at a high risk of developing ovarian cancer, particularly those who have the BRCA gene. If your treatment included surgical removal of your ovaries, you'll experience "surgical menopause," which often causes more intense symptoms than natural menopause.

• **Hormonal therapy for some kinds of cancer can make menopause symptoms worse.** Some types of breast cancer are hormone-receptor positive. Receptors—tiny gatelike proteins in the cancer cell—respond to hormones. One treatment for this kind of breast cancer are drugs called selective es-

trogen receptor modulators (SERMS). These drugs, such as *tamoxifen* and *raloxifene*, can lead to hot flashes, vaginal dryness or other menopausal symptoms. Other hormonal treatments called aromatase inhibitors are used to treat breast cancer in postmenopausal women. They can halt all estrogen production, which worsens menopause symptoms.

Why Hormone Therapy Isn't Recommended for Breast Cancer Survivors

Many women ease menopausal symptoms using systemic hormone therapy—a combination of estrogen and progestin (a synthetic progesterone) for women with a uterus…estrogen alone for women without a uterus—that enters the bloodstream. These include pills and skin patches. But that type of relief may be off the table for breast cancer survivors, especially those who are taking drugs to prevent their cancer from returning.

Another type of hormone therapy, vaginal rings, deliver hormones through the vagina. One type of ring, Femring, is not considered suitable for women with a history of breast cancer because it releases hormones into the bloodstream. But another low-dose ring (Estring) may be OK for some breast cancer survivors because it releases lower levels of hormones and isn't considered systemic. More on these below.

In the 1990s, a major study looking at combined estrogen and progestin therapy for menopause symptoms was halted when breast cancer survivors suffered recurrences. Another study going on at the same time didn't show that same increased risk, but researchers called it off anyway to be on the safe side. The US Food and Drug Administration required a "black box" warning on hormone therapy that included an increased risk for breast cancer, prompting women with a history of breast cancer to avoid it. Is it estrogen alone that may affect the safety of hormone therapy for breast cancer survivors, or is it estrogen combined with progestin? The jury remains out.

Treating Menopause Symptoms Safely

So what should women who have a history of breast cancer do about their bothersome menopause symptoms? Start by talking to your oncologist. Together you can create a treatment plan that works with, not against, your breast cancer treatment or prevention therapy.

For vaginal dryness and painful intercourse...

• **Vaginal moisturizers are available over the counter.** They help to restore moisture to the lining of the vagina. Many are formulated to maintain the vagina's normal pH balance, which can help you avoid infection and irritation.

• **Lubricants ease discomfort during sexual intercourse.** Several types are available—oil-based (which should not be used with latex condoms), silicone-based and water-based. You may need to try a variety of lubricants to find one that you and your partner are happy with. Some women use coconut oil as a lubricant. Keep in mind that while moisturizers are used on a regular basis (regardless of sexual activity), lubricants are used specifically with sexual activity.

• **If these nonhormonal approaches aren't enough, you may want to consider low-dose estrogen therapy**—in the form of vaginal creams, tablets, and, as mentioned above, one brand of vaginal ring (Estring). Because the estrogen is absorbed into vaginal tissues and little makes it into the bloodstream, it's considered a safer option for women who have had breast cancer. Although some oncologists are comfortable with their breast cancer patients using low-dose vaginal estrogen therapy, be aware that the FDA states that even low-dose local vaginal estrogen therapy should not be used in women with a personal history of breast cancer. Talk to your doctor, especially if you take an aromatase inhibitor—because even a small increase in estrogen can be a concern. Women taking tamoxifen to prevent a breast cancer recurrence, on the other hand, may be better candidates for low-dose estrogen therapy. (*Editor's note*: You may also want to ask your doctor about Intrarosa, FDA-approved DHEA suppositories, which create estrogen in vaginal tissues but not in circulation.)

For hot flashes...

• **Avoid spicy foods such as hot peppers.** They have a thermogenic effect, which means they can actually raise your body temperature. Caffeine and alcohol may also trigger hot flashes.

• **Alternative therapies such as deep, paced breathing can lessen the frequency of hot flashes or help you get through them.** Practical solutions such as dressing in layers you can peel off and keeping a fan nearby are also smart. (*Editor's note*: See also the article at BottomLineInc.com, "Neroli Oil Soothes Menopausal Symptoms"—a nonhormonal botanical. Discuss its possible use with your doctor.)

• **A low dose of an antidepressant**—either a selective serotonin reuptake inhibitor (SSRI) or a selective norepinephrine reuptake inhibitor (SNRI)—may work to treat hot flashes without affecting hormones. *Paroxetine* (Brisdelle) is one low-dose SSRI that is FDA-approved to treat menopause symptoms, including in breast cancer survivors.

• **Some medications have been shown to be effective nonhormonal treatments for hot flashes,** but they are not FDA approved for this purpose. These include *venlafaxine* (an SNRI), the antiseizure medication *gabapentin* (Neurontin), and *clonidine* (Catapres), a blood pressure medication. These may be options to discuss with your doctor.

Keep in mind that these nonhormonal medications are not as effective as hormone therapy for treating hot flashes, and their side effects may be different from hormone therapy.

Bottom line: If you're a breast cancer survivor and have menopause symptoms, you don't have to suffer in silence—or forgo potentially life-saving posttreatment therapies. With the right information and support from your health-care team, you can find the right treatments for you to feel better both physically and emotionally without increasing your risk for a recurrence.

Honeybee Venom Kills Hard-to-Treat Breast Cancer Cells

Study titled "Honeybee Venom and Melittin Suppress Growth Factor Receptor Activation in HER2-Enriched and Triple-Negative Breast Cancer," led by researchers at Harry Perkins Institute of Medical Research and The University of Western Australia, both in Perth, published in *Nature Precision Oncology.*

When it comes to medical treatments, apitherapy may not be on everyone's radar. But this alternative treatment, which involves the medicinal use of products made by bees, is being increasingly studied and used to treat a variety of health problems.

Bee venom is one of the most popular products used as apitherapy and is sometimes given as an injection to treat such conditions as rheumatoid arthritis, nerve pain (neuralgia) and multiple sclerosis. Bee products such as honey, pollen and propolis can be used to treat everything from sore throats and cough to allergies and wounds.

Now: While laboratory studies have shown that a specific type of bee venom (honeybee) is effective at killing several types of cancer cells, including those from lung, brain, ovarian and pancreatic malignancies, researchers have recently found that this venom appears to have another important benefit—it rapidly and effectively destroys certain types of breast cancer cells.

Study details: The laboratory study, which was published in *Nature Precision Oncology,* investigated the effects of honeybee venom on normal breast cells and the cells of specific types of breast malignancies (triple-negative and HER2-enriched breast cancers), which are usually resistant to normal treatments.

The researchers also extracted from the honeybee venom a substance called *melittin,* which makes up about half of the venom. After studying the structure of melittin, which is a type of amino acid, the researchers were able to reproduce it synthetically. Both the honeybee venom and melittin were found to have significant effects on both triple negative and HER-2 enriched breast cancer cells.

"The venom was extremely potent," said Ciara Duffy, PhD, study author and a researcher at Harry Perkins Institute of Medical Research and The University of Western Australia. The honeybee venom, when used at a specific concentration, killed 100 percent of the breast cancer cells tested with little effect on the normal breast cells.

The melittin was found to destroy the membranes of breast cancer cells within 60 minutes. It had the added ability to create small holes in breast cancer cells that allowed an existing breast cancer chemotherapy drug, called *docetaxel* (Taxotere), to enter the cells and kill them. When tested in mice, the combination of melittin and docetaxel was "extremely efficient" at reducing tumor growth in mice, according to the study.

Interestingly, when venom from bumblebees was tested, it had no effect on the breast cancer cells. Both the honeybee and bumblebee venoms used in the study were harvested from bees in Perth Western Australia, Ireland and England.

Takeaway: Before honeybee venom or melittin can enter clinical trials as a treatment for breast cancer, future research will need to investigate how to deliver the venom and melittin to humans at a dose that does not cause toxicity. Because the study found that both potential treatments caused minimal damage to normal breast cells in a laboratory setting, the researchers are hopeful that these findings may someday lead to a real breakthrough in breast cancer treatment.

New Treatments Are Increasing Lung Cancer Survival

Study titled "The Effect of Advances in Lung-Cancer Treatment on Population Mortality," by researchers at National Cancer Institute, published in *The New England Journal of Medicine.*

A new study from researchers at the National Cancer Institute (NCI) is good news for people diagnosed with the most common type of lung cancer, non-small cell lung cancer (NSCLC). The study finds that new, genetic-based treatments are improving survival rates.

Since 1990-2000, reduction in the use of tobacco has caused a steady decline in the number of people diagnosed with NSCLC as well as the other common type of lung cancer, small-cell lung cancer (SCLC). The number of people diagnosed with a disease is called the disease incidence. Now, for the first time, deaths from NSCLC are declining even faster than NSCLC incidence.

The NCI researchers believe that the decline in deaths is due to better treatments available only for NSCLC, treatments that target specific genetic changes in the cancer's tumors. The researchers used statistics from NCI's Surveillance, Epidemiology and End Results cancer registry. Their key findings are reported in *The New England Journal of Medicine*...

•**From 2013 through 2016,** the yearly death rate for NSCLC decreased by 6.3 percent.

•**Two-year survival rates for NSCLC increased from 26 percent** for people diagnosed in 2001 to 35 percent for people diagnosed in 2014.

•**The increased survival rate corresponds to the time period when genetic testing and genetic-based treatments became available for NSCLC.**

•**Although a decrease in smoking reduced the incidence of both NSCLC and SCLC,** there has not been an increase in the two-year survival for SCLC.

People with NSCLC are now routinely checked for genetic tumor mutations that enable tumors to grow, called *epidermal growth factor receptor* (EGFR) and *anaplastic lymphoma kinase* (ALK). People with EGFR or ALK-positive tumors can be treated with drugs that inhibit these genes.

The researchers expect to see an even better reduction in death rates for NSCLC with a type of cancer drug called an immune checkpoint inhibitor. This drug takes the brakes off a person's immune system, giving it more power to attack and destroy tumor cells. Since NSCLC accounts for 76 percent of all lung cancers, these trends are good news for a disease that has been the number one cause of cancer deaths for both women and men.

How to Protect Your Colon: The 5 Essentials

Robert Bresalier, MD, vice chair for research in the department of gastroenterology, hepatology and nutrition at University of Texas MD Anderson Cancer Center, Houston. He has been a member of several national and international advisory committees aimed at reducing mortality from colorectal cancer.

With the recent death of actor Chadwick Boseman at age 43 from colorectal cancer and the early retirement of Japanese Prime Minister Shinzo Abe at age 65 due to ulcerative colitis, colon health is on many people's minds. How can you best take care of your colon?

That's not a simple question. The colon is not just a simple tube. It is a living, constantly changing organ whose microbiome (the mix of bacteria that call it home) is associated with many forms of serious disease besides cancer and colitis, including neurodegenerative disorders such as Alzheimer's and psychiatric conditions such as depression and anxiety. I'm happy to report that colon health is a very active area of medical research, but mostly what we have now are associations between lifestyle choices and outcomes rather than hard, scientifically proven causations.

Still, with each new finding, recommendations continue to focus in the following very basic areas to give your colon the best fighting chance…

•**Pay attention—even if it's gross or embarrassing.** In recent years, young-onset colorectal cancer (affecting people under age 50) has been on the rise. It is both a preventable disease and one that is highly treatable when it's caught early—but too many young people ignore symptoms that would allow for early intervention.

Understand that when it comes to bowel habits, there is a wide spectrum of "normal" in terms of how often you move your bowels, what the consistency is and so on. Feeling like you're outside of the norm is not cause for alarm, but seeing a dramatic change in what is normal for you should get your attention. Don't ignore significant and persistent changes in bowel habits such as blood in the stool, constipation or abdominal pain, any of which could indicate a problem. If a close family member—parent, grandparent, sibling—has had colorectal cancer, be especially vigilant.

•**Get screened.** Even if you have no symptoms, you still should be screened for colon cancer. If you're age 50 or older, most private insurance will cover a colonoscopy every 10 years or less. If you're between ages 40 and 50, check with your provider—colonoscopy typically is covered earlier when there is a family history and then again every five years. Medicare will pay for screening (including colonoscopy) in people age 65 and older or otherwise Medicare-eligible.

You may have heard of alternative screening methods such as fecal immunochemical testing (FIT), which looks for hidden blood in the stool…"virtual colonoscopy" (actually called CT colonography)…or at-home stool tests such as Cologuard, which analyze stool DNA in addition to FIT. These types of tests avoid the small risk associated with the invasive colonoscopy, and the stool tests avoid the unpleasant prep process. Those are fine if you're not in a high-risk group and are symptom-free. Note that insurance usually won't pay for virtual colonoscopy as a first test and coverage varies for Cologuard, but the cost may be substantially less than for colonoscopy. If you don't have insurance or if you have a high deductible that you never meet, you may come out ahead financially with one of these tests, assuming that you are a good candidate for them. Depending on the results, you may need to follow up with an actual colonoscopy. Whatever you do, don't put this off. Early detection is the best tool we have for fighting these cancers.

•**Don't stir up the microbiome unnecessarily.** Doctors are learning more and more about treating bacterial infections such as C. difficile and conditions like irritable bowel syndrome with "good" bacteria (probiotics or, in the case of C. difficile, fecal transplantation from a healthy donor). That has led some people to consume probiotics religiously, thinking that they'll proactively promote bacterial diversity and correct imbalances between "good" and "bad" bacteria in their gut. But they do so without any baseline knowledge about their existing levels and composition of bacteria before they start messing with it. While most probiotics are safe, they vary in their mix of bacteria, and it is unclear what the effects will be on your system and how long they will persist.

Other people undertake "colon cleanses" thinking that they'll flush out bad bacteria and make room for more good bacteria to grow. In fact, what tends to happen after a colon cleanse is that the exact same mix of bacteria grows back. So you may be wasting your money and putting yourself through discomfort for nothing.

Now, if you've been on an antibiotic and experience bowel issues such as diarrhea, it may be worth trying a live-culture yogurt or probiotic supplement to help get things back in balance. But even that is something the medical community needs to learn more about. Although there is a large body of research, the evidence is far from definitive. Persistent symptoms, however, require evaluation by your physician to rule out more serious disease.

• **Engage in physical activity and get plenty of sleep.** We know there's a strong association between regular exercise and colon health, and researchers currently are studying the link between sleep and a healthy colon. As a rule of thumb, things that are good for your heart also are good for your colon, and aerobic exercise is the best example of that. Research shows that physical activity in the form of regular exercise may prevent up to 15 percent of colon cancers and is effective in reducing symptoms of irritable bowel syndrome and other digestive issues.

• **Watch your diet.** It should come as no surprise that what you put into your body matters. Nutrition affects every cell of your body, of course, but it has a direct impact on the gut. Eat a diet with plenty of fruits, vegetables, whole grains and the omega-3 fatty acids found in fish oil and olive oil. Limit intake of red and processed meats and alcohol. Fiber intake in the form of fruits, vegetables and whole grains is associated with a lower risk for colorectal cancer across populations, but the reason for this is multifaceted. Other dietary components such as calcium, folate and vitamin D have been found beneficial. A general "eating well" approach is preferable to targeting specific nutrients. In one study, adherence to a Mediterranean-style diet, as described above, lowered risk for colorectal cancer by up to 11 percent.

• **Limit—or eliminate—unhealthy fats such as from fried foods, red meat, refined sugars and processed foods.**

If you are a young person, don't cheat yourself by waiting until you're older to clean up your diet. Nutritional interventions are not only most effective when you're young, they also lay the groundwork for a healthier future.

A Chinese Herb May Reduce the Risk of Colon Polyps

Study titled "Berberine Versus Placebo for the Prevention of Colorectal Adenoma: A Multicenter, Double-Blind, Randomized Controlled Study," by researchers at Shanghai Jiao Tong University School of Medicine, Shanghai, China, published in *The Lancet*.

If you had an adenoma polyp removed during a colonoscopy for colon cancer screening, you may already know that these polyps can come back and that they can become colon cancer. You were probably told to return for another colonoscopy in a few years, because up to 30 percent of adenomatous polyps come back. About 5 percent turn out to be cancer.

A recent study from China has found that a traditional Chinese herbal medicine called berberine may significantly reduce the risk of regrowing these polyps, and reduce the risk of colon cancer.

The study was done in seven hospital centers across China. It included about 1,000 patients. All these patients had adenomatous polyps removed during a screening colonoscopy. About half the patients were randomly assigned to take berberine twice per day and the other half were given a placebo. After two years, there was a significant difference in polyp regrowth found during colonoscopies: 155 patients had new growths in the treatment group, compared with 216 in the placebo group. The study was reported in *The Lancet*.

In China, berberine is extracted from the herb *coptis chinensis* and has been used in Chinese medicine for centuries to treat diarrhea and stomach bugs. In animal research, mice treated with berberine had reduced colon tumor formation. The researchers say that the results of their study are promising because berberine is inexpensive and safe, but more studies will be needed to confirm their findings. In fact, a new study has already started.

Berberine is also found in many herbal products outside of China, including barberry, goldenseal, goldthread, Oregon grape and tree turmeric. It is most commonly used to treat diabetes, high cholesterol and high blood pressure. Berberine is considered safe in normal doses. In the *Lancet* study, the only side effect was constipation, which occurred very rarely. The study used a dose of 0.3 grams twice per day.

Berberine is not recommended during pregnancy or breastfeeding and it may interfere with some medications. As with any herbal supplement, you should check with your doctor first before trying it on your own.

Colorectal-Cancer Screening Should Start Sooner Than You Think

Recommendation by US Preventive Services Task Force to the American Cancer Society. Cancer.org

Colorectal-cancer screening should start at 45, not 50, which has been the standard recommendation for many years. Most colorectal cancers are found in people age 50 and older, but there has been a significant rise in disease incidence among younger people—12 percent of colorectal cancers diagnosed in 2020 are expected to be in adults under age 50. Black men and women especially should be encouraged to be screened at 45, since African-American communities have high rates of the disease and higher death rates than other groups.

Gum Disease Raises Cancer Risk

After reviewing the records of nearly 150,000 adults, researchers found that periodontal (gum) disease and tooth loss were associated with a 43 percent increased risk for cancer of the esophagus and a 52 percent higher risk for stomach cancer.

Mingyang Song, MD, assistant professor of clinical epidemiology and nutrition at Harvard T.H. Chan School of Public Health and Harvard Medical School, Boston, and leader of a study published in *BMJ Gut*.

Severe Sunburn Can Make You Sick

Roundup of experts on sunburn, reported at Shape.com.

Severe sunburn can cause skin swelling, headache, fever, chills, nausea and vomiting. Seek medical attention if blisters cover at least 20 percent of your skin's surface...you have a fever of 102°F or higher...there is yellow drainage or red discharge from a blister... or sunburn does not heal within a week.

Caution: A single severe sunburn can double your risk for melanoma, so be sure to see a dermatologist regularly.

Routine CT Scan Predicts Heart Disease in Breast Cancer Survivors

Division of Imaging and Oncology at University Medical Center Utrecht, The Netherlands, research presented at the 12th European Breast Cancer Conference.

Three million women in the US are breast cancer survivors. Some of these women may experience a potentially serious side effect from treatment—an increased risk of developing cardiovascular disease (CVD).

Earlier research has shown that breast cancer patients treated with radiation therapy may be at increased risk for CVD. In rare cases, women treated with the breast cancer chemotherapy drug *anthracycline* may suffer heart damage.

Now: In a first-of-its-kind study, researchers from the Division of Imaging and Oncology at University Medical Center Utrecht, The Netherlands, have found a simple way to predict which breast cancer survivors may be at greatest risk of developing CVD. In some women, the risk of dying from CVD may be higher than the risk of succumbing to breast cancer.

The researchers discovered that a routine chest CT scan used to plan breast cancer treatment can also measure the amount of calcium in the walls of coronary arteries. This scan can help calculate a coronary artery calcium (CAC) score, which determines the risk of cardiovascular disease (CVD). These findings were presented at the 12th European Breast Cancer Conference.

Study details: In the study, which was done at three hospitals in The Netherlands between 2005 and 2016, about 14,000 breast cancer patients were followed for 52 months after their routine pre-treatment CT scans. All these women were treated with radiation therapy. *After calculating CAC scores, these were the key findings…*

•**In women with no calcifications (CAC score of 0),** 5 percent went on to be hospitalized with or die from cardiovascular disease.

•**In women with CAC scores of 1 to 10,** 8.9 percent were hospitalized with CVD or died from it.

•**In women with scores of 11 to 100,** the percentage was 13.5 percent.

•**In women with scores of 101 to 400,** the figure was 17.5 percent.

•**In women with scores over 400,** 28.3 percent were hospitalized with CVD or died from it.

•**After adjusting for age and year of diagnosis,** women with the highest CAC scores were 3.7 times more likely to be diagnosed with CVD than women with a CAC of 0.

In women treated with the chemotherapy drug anthracycline along with radiation, the link between a high CAC score and CVD was even stronger.

Conclusion: The researchers hope that their findings will provide a simple method to determine early risk factors for heart disease in breast cancer patients. Prevention strategies include close monitoring with a cardiologist and lifestyle changes, such as adopting a heart-healthy diet, losing weight and exercising.

Cutting-Edge Cancer Care

Katy Rezvani, MD, PhD, the Sally Cooper Murray Chair in Cancer Research, professor of medicine, chief of the section for cellular therapy, and director of translational research at MD Anderson Cancer Center in Houston. Dr. Rezvani's lab studies the role of natural killer (NK) cells in influencing immunity against blood cancers as well as solid tumors.

Long-used cancer treatments that "carpet-bomb" tumor cells systemically have increasingly given way to precision therapies that empower the body's immune cells to attack cancer.

But there's room for improvement even among these pioneering immunotherapy approaches. The newest advance takes a giant step forward by rapidly and precisely killing cancer cells with an off-the-shelf innovation.

A Brief History of CAR

In the late 1980s, researchers discovered that they could genetically alter T-cells to carry a molecule known as a chimeric antigen receptor (CAR) to help them recognize tumor cells. This immunotherapy treatment, called CAR T therapy, was translated to the clinic in the early 2000s. It provided new hope to people with hard-to-treat blood cancers, such as leukemia and lymphoma. Blood cancers are diagnosed in one person every three minutes in the United States.

Now, researchers are turning their attention to natural killer (NK) cells. These cells are extracted from donated umbilical cord blood and genetically engineered to express a CAR, which empowers them to recognize the CD19 protein found on the surface of specific malignant cells and, as a result, recognize formerly camouflaged cancer cells. Since NK cells are one of the most effective killers of cancer cells in our bodies—already primed to identify and eradicate invaders—this approach represents a potentially radical addition to the ever-changing landscape of cancer therapies.

Donated umbilical cord blood from a single birth can potentially generate hundreds of doses of CAR NK cells for therapy. CAR NK cells have the potential to be produced, frozen, and ready for any appropriate patient as an off-the-shelf treatment.

How It's Safer

While natural killer cells and T-cells are both powerhouses of our immune system, only NK cells can easily be shared between donor and recipient without worrying about tissue matching. This point is crucial because mismatched T-cells can provoke a potentially deadly complication known as graft-versus-host disease (GVHD) by attacking the recipient's body cells. On top of that, genetically altered T-cells can trigger a condition called *cytokine release syndrome*, which can cause a drop in blood pressure, shortness of breath, mental confusion, and, in rare cases, potentially fatal brain swelling. NK cells are apparently free of these potential perils, and the CAR modification means they target only cells expressing the CD19 protein—avoiding the toxic effects common to conventional chemotherapy, which attacks both cancerous and normal cells.

None of the 11 patients who participated in the first-in-human clinical CAR NK trial experienced GVHD or cytokine release syndrome despite a partial or total mismatch of their cell types with donors. Seven also

showed no evidence of disease at follow-up an average of 14 months later, although some of those patients also received additional therapy, such as a transplant, to maintain their response. While promising, it's too soon to know if CAR NK therapy might represent a cure for these or other patients.

Combination Approaches Offer Hope

Immunotherapy is hardly new, with the first attempts to unleash the power of the immune system to fight cancer dating back to the 1890s. But various types of immunotherapy have become standard treatment only in the past decade or so for a wide variety of malignancies, including melanoma and lymphoma along with lung, kidney, bladder, and head and neck tumors. Perhaps chief among these are so-called checkpoint inhibitors, drugs that essentially remove the "brakes" on the immune system that would otherwise stop it from attacking cancer cells.

Revolutionary as they are, engineered-cell therapies like CAR T and CAR NK treatment won't replace the cancer immunotherapies that predated them, but CAR NK therapy, if approved by the U.S. Food and Drug Administration, will beef up the arsenal of treatments available to patients. It may well be that combining two or more approaches proves to be the most effective one-two punch that knocks out some malignant tumors so they never return.

Future Direction

Right now, a first-in-human clinical trial is testing CAR NK therapy's power against certain types of leukemia and lymphoma. Patients with blood cancers participating in the CAR NK clinical trial first undergo three days of chemotherapy to prepare their bodies for the transformed NK cells. After a two-day break following chemotherapy, patients receive the cells in a single dose delivered like a blood transfusion. Then it's just a matter of time to see if those new cells do their intended job and beat back malignant cells by acting as "heat-seeking missiles."

Going forward, the plan is to test CAR NK therapy in other treatment-resistant and lethal cancers that have historically stymied scientists, such as the brain tumor glioblastoma. While solid tumors such as glioblastoma appear to be vulnerable to natural killer cells, many obstacles must still be overcome to prove the treatment's effectiveness in this realm.

One truism about cancer is there's no one-size-fits-all treatment. Different treatments are effective for different types of cancer. The hoped-for addition of CAR NK therapy to the ever-broadening landscape of options could help eradicate rogue cells for good.

A Psychedelic Drug Offers Years of Benefits to Cancer Patients

Antianxiety and antidepressant effects were still evident nearly five years after cancer patients were given a single dose of psilocybin, a substance found in certain mushrooms, combined with psychotherapy

Study by researchers at Palo Alto University, California, published in *Journal of Psychopharmacology*.

Cognitive Issues Linger in Breast Cancer Survivors on PPIs

Annelise A. Madison is a PhD candidate at The Ohio State University, Columbus, and leader of a study published in *Journal of Cancer Survivorship*.

Memory and concentration issues linger in breast cancer survivors taking proton-pump inhibitors (PPIs) for GI side effects. An analysis of three studies that included self-reported use of medications including PPIs (such as Prilosec) found that cognitive

issues were 20 percent to 29 percent worse for patients using the acid-suppressing drugs regularly. PPIs are designed for limited use, but many study participants were using them for between six months and two years.

If You Had One HPV Cancer, You're More Likely to Get Others

Andrew Sikora, MD, PhD, associate professor of otolaryngology, and codirector of the Head and Neck Cancer Program at Baylor College of Medicine in Houston, Texas, and coauthor of the study titled "Trends in Risks for Second Primary Cancers Associated With Index Human Papillomavirus-Associated Cancers," published in *JAMA Network Open*.

It's scary enough that HPV—the very common human papillomavirus—can cause cervical, vaginal, vulvar, throat, anal and penile cancers. Now a study done at leading cancer centers across the US has found that having one of these HPV-related cancers puts patients at a higher risk for a second one. These are not instances of metastatic cancer (when the original cancer spreads to another area). They are new cancers in a different part of the body.

Why does this happen? The most likely answer is that the virus infects multiple places in the body at once…but it takes different lengths of time for each cancer to develop. Research has also found that some people have variations in their immune genes that make them more susceptible to HPV-associated cancers.

The study, which looked at the records of about 73,000 female and 40,000 male patients with an HPV-related cancer, showed that the risk for getting a second cancer has grown over the past four decades…and that the risk varies depending on where the first cancer was located. The risk of a second HPV-related cancer was greatest in people who initially had HPV-related throat (oropharyngeal) cancer. And if the original cancer was not throat cancer, the most likely second cancer was throat cancer. But risk for any of the HPV-related cancers was elevated.

Here's how you can protect yourself if you've already had one HPV-related cancer...

• **Be vigilant about getting all recommended cancer screenings.** A colonoscopy can find signs of HPV-related rectal or anal cancer. Cervical cancer screenings for women uncover suspicious lesions, often before they have the chance to turn into cancer. Because the area susceptible to this type of throat cancer includes the base of the tongue, tonsils and soft palate, your dentist can visually check for signs of cancer in these areas— ask for this if it's not already part of every visit. And see an otolaryngologist if you experience any of the possible symptoms of throat cancer such as a persistent sore throat, trouble swallowing or a lump in your throat, neck or the back of your mouth.

• **Talk to your doctor about the HPV vaccine.** In October 2018, the FDA extended its approval of Gardasil 9 for people up to age 45. Scientists are also investigating whether it makes sense for people with a history of an HPV-related cancer to be vaccinated against HPV. The prevailing theory has long been that people are exposed to HPV when they are young and then develop cancer later in life. But it could be that later infection as well as infection with a different strain of the virus is occurring more frequently than previously thought and that vaccination could prevent cancer in these situations.

On the horizon: Clinical trials are currently looking at whether HPV vaccination can prevent existing precancerous lesions from developing into cancer and whether certain versions of the vaccine can decrease both the recurrence of an HPV-related cancer and the development of a second one when given as part of cancer treatment.

Seaweed May Treat Skin Cancer and MRSA

Studies titled "Bioactive Molecular Networking for Mapping the Antimicrobial Constituents of the Baltic Brown Alga Fucus Vesiculosus" and "Pyrenosetin D, a New Pentacyclic Decalinoyltetramic Acid Derivative from the Algicolous Fungus Pyrenochaetopsis sp. FVE-087," both by researchers at GEOMAR Helmholtz Centre for Ocean Research Kiel, Germany, published in *Marine Drugs*.

Among the many resources the sea offers humans are drugs—including life-saving cancer drugs—derived from marine organisms. Unfortunately, the process for developing such drugs is complicated, expensive and time-consuming, making it impractical to take better advantage of this rich resource.

Breakthrough: Thanks to cutting-edge new technology, scientists were able to dramatically shorten the research process...and discovered compounds that can treat skin cancer and a deadly skin infection in a common type of seaweed.

Normally, it takes up to four years to discover and identify bioactive compounds extracted from algae that might be effective against human diseases. But research scientists at Helmholtz Centre for Ocean Research in Kiel, Germany, used automated computer algorithms to map and analyze the massive chemical and molecular complexity of a type of seaweed called bladder wrack in just months. The algorithms also allowed the team to quickly and accurately identify known and new compounds...and to predict the bioactivity of molecules.

Bladder wrack (*Fucus vesiculosus*) is a brown alga that grows along coastlines of many oceans, including Kiel Fjord, an inlet of the Baltic Sea in Germany and the source for the bladder wrack used in the study. Bladder wrack and other algae living in intertidal zones of oceans develop protective molecules to defend against constant attack from millions of microorganisms found in seawater. Some of these molecules also happen to be active against human bacteria.

Study results: Some of the molecules in bladder wrack were found to inhibit the growth of methicillin-resistant Staphylococcus aureus (MRSA), skin bacteria that cause a potentially deadly infection. In another study, the researchers also examined the symbiotic fungi called Pyrenochaetopsis that naturally grow on bladder wrack and found important bioactive microorganisms that were able to efficiently kill melanoma skin cancer cells.

The researchers pointed out that bladder wrack's therapeutic potential is not limited to drugs. The seaweed is edible and also could be used to make food supplements.

They further predicted that computer-aided learning tools such as used in their study will accelerate the discovery of other active marine compounds that can be used for drug development—and may lead to an unprecedented number of new medications.

An Aspirin a Day May Make Cancer More Dangerous for Older Adults

Study titled "Effect of Aspirin on Cancer Incidence and Mortality in Older Adults," by researchers at National Cancer Institute, Bethesda, Maryland, published in *Journal of the National Cancer Institute.*

Low-dose aspirin is no longer the go-to preventive measure to ward off heart disease in healthy older adults. Now, a recent study shows that daily aspirin therapy may cause more harm than good for these individuals, especially when it comes to cancer.

Background: From 2010 through 2014, a clinical trial compared 100 mg of daily aspirin with a placebo pill in about 20,000 adults over age 65 who did not have cardiovascular disease, dementia or a physical disability when the study started. It was called the ASPREE (ASPrin in Reducing Events in the Elderly) trial. Previous trials in middle-aged adults had suggested that taking one low-dose aspirin each day could reduce heart disease risk and the risk for colorectal cancer.

This trial wanted to see if the same benefits were found in older adults. Three years into the trial, the researchers were surprised to find there was an increased risk of death from cancer in the aspirin group. Results of the ASPREE were reported in 2018.

Recent development: A new study from researchers at Massachusetts General Hospital, Berman Cancer Center in Minnesota and Monash University in Australia analyzed the data from ASPREE to learn more about older adults' risk of taking daily aspirin. Their study was recently published in the *Journal of the National Cancer Institute.*

The new analysis found that in the ASPREE trial, 981 cancers occurred in the aspirin group compared with 952 cancers in the placebo group. The researchers did not find this to be statistically significant, and they concluded that aspirin does not increase the risk of cancer. However, in patients with cancer, the aspirin group was 19 percent to 22 percent more likely to have spreading or stage IV cancer, resulting in a higher risk of death.

Takeaway: The researchers conclude that older adults with cancer may be at higher risk for death from more advanced cancer if they're taking daily low-dose aspirin—especially if they begin taking it later in life. Why this occurs is not known, but researchers suspect that aspirin may act differently on cancer cells in older people.

Important: The researchers do not advise people who are taking daily low-dose aspirin to stop this therapy without consulting their doctor, nor does the study suggest that low-dose aspirin recommendations should not include older adults, who generally get more benefits than risks from it if they have a history of heart attack, stroke or heart surgery. But the researchers do advise elderly individuals to proceed with caution and review aspirin intake carefully with their doctor, especially if they have cancer.

Combining Cancer Drugs Improves Leukemia Survival

Study titled "Azacitidine and Venetoclax in Previously Untreated Acute Myeloid Leukemia," by researchers at The University of Texas MD Anderson Cancer Center in Houston, published in *The New England Journal of Medicine.*

Acute myeloid leukemia (AML) is a rare cancer that begins in the white blood cells and bone marrow. It makes up about 1 percent of cancers. Because AML is hard to treat, the five-year survival rate is only 25 percent. A trial that combines two cancer drugs may change treatment for some individuals with AML. This combination was shown to be safe, and it improved overall survival.

The trial results were virtually presented by researchers at The University of Texas MD Anderson Cancer Center to the European Hematology Association Annual Congress and also published in *The New England Journal of Medicine.*

In the trial, 431 AML patients were randomly assigned to receive the cancer drug *azacitidine* and a placebo (single-drug therapy) or azacitidine and the cancer drug *venetoclax* (combination therapy).

Azacitidine is an injection drug used to treat AML and other bone marrow diseases. It works by killing abnormal bone marrow cells. Venetoclax is an oral drug that treats several types of white blood cell cancers. It works by blocking a type of protein that cancer cells need to survive.

Study results: During the trial, patients in the combination therapy group had a better response than patients in the single-drug group. Specifically, the combination therapy group had a rapid response, with 43 percent of patients responding to the first treatment cycle. Patients in the combination therapy

Beware of Cancer Treatment Side Effects

One in three cancer patients say they wish they'd known more about the potential side effects of their treatment, according to a survey of more than 400 women and men. Nearly 40 percent who reported severe side effects, such as fatigue, skin irritation, weakness and gastrointestinal disturbances, said they felt uninformed, compared with 4 percent of those whose side effects were minimal.

Good news: Nine out of 10 patients were happy with their treatment decision, even if they needed more information about side effects.

Takeaway: Ask about all potential side effects before undergoing cancer treatment.

Reshma Jagsi, MD, DPhil, professor of radiation oncology, University of Michigan, Ann Arbor.

group had an average survival of about 15 months compared with about 10 months for patients in the single-drug group. Although many patients did eventually relapse, 66 percent of patients in the combination therapy group had a complete remission of their cancer compared with only 28 percent in the single-drug group.

The combination therapy was found to be as safe as the single-drug therapy. The researchers see the combination therapy as an improvement for AML patients who are older and would not tolerate more aggressive treatments such as stem-cell transplantation.

Takeaway: AML affects about 20,000 people every year. The average age at diagnosis is 68. For many older patients, a tolerable, effective treatment has been elusive. The researchers plan to use this new therapy as a "backbone" treatment to which other new drugs may be added. This may improve survival for patients at highest risk with AML.

Chapter 4

DIABETES AND BLOOD SUGAR CONTROL

The Hot Flash/Diabetes Connection

Like a fingerprint, menopause is unique for every woman. Take hot flashes and night sweats. For some women, the "lucky few," they are momentary and mild—or don't happen at all—but for many women they are bothersome and last for years...even decades. For some women, they are truly severe and debilitating.

Your pattern for these symptoms, it turns out, may be a road map for your risk of type 2 diabetes.

Background: The risk of developing type 2 diabetes increases after a woman hits menopause (average age 51). Simply getting older is one reason—after all, risk for men also rises with age. But there is growing evidence that the pattern of hormonal disturbances related to the menopause transition—as revealed by "vasomotor" symptoms such as hot flashes and/or night sweats— also plays a role. Certain patterns signal increased risk for diabetes that develops later on, often years after symptoms subside.

Study: Researchers used data from the large Women's Health Initiative that includ- ed about 150,000 middle-aged women who did not have diabetes at the beginning of the study. The women were followed for an average of 13 years and reported if, when and how long they endured hot flashes and night sweats...and whether they were diagnosed with diabetes. In analyzing the data, the researchers controlled for obesity and other known risk factors for diabetes.

Results: Over those 13 years, more than 18,000 of the women developed diabetes. The risk of being diagnosed with diabetes was associated with the presence and duration of vasomotor symptoms, but especially their severity...

• **Women who reported mild vasomotor symptoms were 13 percent more likely to develop diabetes than women with no vasomotor symptoms.** But women with moderate symptoms were at 29 percent increased risk—and those with severe symptoms were at 48 percent increased risk—compared with women who had no such symptoms.

• **Women whose vasomotor symptoms started only after menopause were at 12**

JoAnn V. Pinkerton, MD, medical director of Mid- life Health Center, professor of obstetrics and gynecol- ogy and vice chair of academic affairs at the University of Virginia, Charlottesville. She is a former executive director of The North American Menopause Society.

percent increased risk, compared with women who did not have vasomotor symptoms.

• Women who had night sweats but no hot flashes were at 20 percent increased risk. Those with both symptoms were at 22 percent increased risk, on average.

• Each five-year increase in vasomotor symptom duration increased diabetes risk by 4 percent.

Surprising finding: Among white women, for each incremental increase in severity, risk for diabetes increased by 15 percent. But among black women, risk increased by only 7 percent. The reasons aren't clear.

Bottom line: This research reinforces the potential to use menopausal symptoms to understand risks for chronic disease—and to leverage the menopause transition to take steps to protect yourself.

While even a large observational study such as this one can't establish cause and effect, the researchers argue that a major way these symptoms contribute to diabetes is by interrupting sleep. Insomnia and other chronic sleep problems are well-established risk factors for diabetes. Night sweats in particular can wreck sleep, which may explain why night sweats were a risk factor for diabetes even when there were no hot flashes.

Although genetics plays a role in the risk of developing adult-onset diabetes, diabetes is a largely preventable illness, with poor diet and lack of activity playing key roles in its development. Women with persistent and, especially, severe hot flashes and/or night sweats may want to ask their health-care providers to check them for diabetes. Preventive steps include minimizing menopausal weight gain with reduced intake of calories and refined carbohydrates…making time for both aerobic and strength-building exercise…and getting adequate sleep of at least seven hours a night.

Probiotics Help People With Type 2 Diabetes

Study by researchers at Sri Adichunchanagiri College of Pharmacy, Karnataka, India, published in *Natural Science, Biology and Medicine.*

Probiotic supplementation improved study subjects' fasting blood sugar, after-meal blood sugar and insulin sensitivity, leading to better health-related quality of life after three months. The improvements were most pronounced in patients ages 30 to 40. Older patients had fewer benefits but still showed some improvement.

New Option for Preventing Diabetes

Michael Hochman, MD, MPH, associate professor of clinical medicine at Keck School of Medicine and director of Gehr Family Center for Health Systems Science and Innovation at University of Southern California, Los Angeles.

Are pharmaceuticals the answer to America's diabetes problem? One group of diabetes researchers recently reported on a novel approach—give people with prediabetes, those who are close to developing full-blown diabetes, three different drugs, including one that needs to be self-injected as often as twice a day.

It sounds extreme, but it worked. In the study, published in *The Lancet*, 81 overweight participants took the diabetes drugs metformin, *pioglitazone* (Actos) and a GLP-1 receptor agonist (Byetta, Victoza and others). On average, they were treated for 32 months. None of them got diabetes. In contrast, 11 percent of those in the study's "lifestyle only" group, who were given diabetes-prevention advice on diet, weight loss and exercise and followed for 32 months, on average, developed diabetes.

So is lifestyle a failure? Don't jump to conclusions from this study. Some of the people in the lifestyle group lost weight, but others gained weight. And losing weight if you are too heavy is a linchpin of preventing diabetes.

Maybe changing your diet, exercising and therefore losing weight—and keeping it off—is hard. But taking three medications for the rest of your life has plenty of downsides. Metformin often causes gastrointestinal problems...pioglitazone is associated with fluid retention and heart failure...and the GLP-1 medications may trigger nausea and headaches.

And the lifestyle changes above give you benefits well beyond keeping your blood sugar "number" down. They help prevent heart disease, stroke and other "complications" of prediabetes. It's good that we have the prediabetes drugs for people who need them. But it's better to improve our health ourselves and not have to take them.

The Gut Bug That Protects Against Diabetes

Study titled "Indolepropionic Acid and Novel Lipid Metabolites are Associated With a Lower Risk of Type 2 Diabetes in the Finnish Diabetes Prevention Study" by researchers at University of Eastern Finland et al., published in *Scientific Reports*.

Andrew Rubman, ND, naturopathic physician, Southbury Clinic for Traditional Medicines. Southbury Clinic.com

Here's a diabetes paradox. While most people who get type 2 diabetes are overweight or obese, some overweight/obese people never get diabetes—even those with elevated blood sugar levels and prediabetes!

What's protecting them? One possibility is the beneficial bacteria living in their guts. Ironically, the best way to foster these good-for-you bugs may be to eat foods that you may be trying to avoid in the search for diabetes prevention!

Background: There is growing evidence that the "gut microbiome"—the collection of helpful organisms living in the gut that play a key role in digestion—influences type 2 diabetes risk.

Study: Researchers from Finland and Sweden compared two groups of people who had participated in the Finnish Diabetes Prevention Study, which began in the 1990s with more than 500 adults who were at high risk of developing diabetes because they were overweight and had high blood sugar. Like the American Diabetes Prevention Program, the Finnish program focused on lifestyle change to stop progression to diabetes. Fifteen years later, 52 percent of the participants remained free of the disease.

The researchers compared 104 individuals who remained diabetes free for 15 years with 96 individuals who developed diabetes within the first five years of the study. They looked closely at levels of various metabolites—by-products of digestion—to see whether there were big differences between the two groups. They compared diets, too.

Results: In participants who had not developed diabetes, there were much higher blood levels of *indolepropionic acid*. This compound, produced by beneficial bacteria in the gut, is known to protect the ability of beta cells in the pancreas to secrete insulin. The compound also improves insulin sensitivity—making insulin more effective. Both reduced insulin sensitivity and flagging insulin production are linked to developing type 2 diabetes.

Surprising finding: Higher levels of indolepropionic acid were also associated with lower levels of C-reactive protein, a marker of inflammation throughout the body. High levels of C-reactive protein can signal an increased risk for heart disease.

Diet connection: When the researchers looked at the participants' diets, they found that higher levels of indolepropionic acid were associated with high fiber intake... particularly from whole grains, especially rye. And, as it turns out, whole grains' fiber stimulates gut bacteria that convert the amino acid tryptophan from protein-rich foods into…indolepropionic acid.

These results not only back up the observation that people who have high-fiber diets are less likely to develop diabetes, but they also help explain why high-fiber diets are protective against diabetes.

Bottom Line: Weight loss and exercise remain the cornerstones of diabetes prevention. But a healthy diet that supports "good bugs" is important, too.

Many people, when they find out they're at risk for diabetes, cut way back on carbohydrates—often as a way to lose weight. That can backfire by cutting out sources of gut-friendly high-fiber foods. A diet rich in fiber and whole grains, such as whole-grain rye and steel-cut oatmeal, is good for everyone, but it may be especially protective if you're at high risk for diabetes.

For a healthy microbiome, according to Bottom Line medical editor Andrew Rubman, ND, you'll also want to include plenty of fresh fiber-rich fruits and vegetables—both raw and cooked—as well as beans.

Acid Reflux Drugs May Increase Diabetes Risk

Study titled "Regular Use of Proton Pump Inhibitors and Risk of Type 2 Diabetes: Results from Three Prospective Cohort Studies," by researchers at Sun Yatsen University, Shenzhen, China, published in *Gut*.

Proton pump inhibitors (PPIs) are popular drugs used to treat acid reflux, ulcers and indigestion. Many are available over the counter with brand names that include Prilosec, Nexium and Prevacid. PPIs are among the top 10 most commonly used drugs worldwide, despite evidence of their potential dangers. They have been linked to an increased risk for bone fractures, kidney disease, gut infections and cancer.

Now, recent research has found a possible connection between PPIs and type 2 diabetes. Although some past studies have linked the use of these drugs to an increased risk for type 2 diabetes, the association remained unclear.

To get more clarity, researchers from Sun Yat-sen University in China reviewed information provided by three long-term health studies in the US. Their findings, published in the medical journal *Gut*, found a significant increased risk.

The research: The long-term studies used by the researchers are two US Nurses' Health Studies and the Health Professionals Follow-up Study. Every two years, participants have been reporting on their health conditions and medications. Since 2000-2004, depending on the study, this has included the use of PPIs. The researchers looked at nine to 12 years of the studies, during which just over 10,000 nurses reported a diagnosis of type 2 diabetes.

After factoring in other risks for type 2 diabetes, such as hypertension, high cholesterol, smoking, family history and physical inactivity, the researchers calculated that PPI use increased the risk of type 2 diabetes by 5 percent if used for less than two years…and by 26 percent if used regularly for more than two years.

This type of observational study does not prove that PPIs cause diabetes in the same way that a randomized controlled study could, but the results are important because of the large number of participants. The findings add to growing evidence linking PPIs to type 2 diabetes.

Takeaway: The researchers conclude that doctors should be cautions about prescribing or recommending PPIs for an extended period of time, and patients who have been taking PPIs for a long time should be screened for type 2 diabetes with blood glucose testing.

The Hidden Risks of Normal-Weight Obesity

John A. Batsis, MD, a staff geriatrician at Dartmouth-Hitchcock Medical Center in Lebanon, New Hampshire, and an associate professor of medicine at Geisel School of Medicine at Dartmouth. He is also director of clinical research at Dartmouth-Hitchcock Weight & Wellness Center. Dr. Batsis has authored or coauthored more than 120 scientific papers that have appeared in leading medical journals, such as *Obesity, American Journal of Cardiology* and *Mayo Clinic Proceedings*.

Your weight is "normal." So why are you at higher risk for heart attack, stroke and diabetes? *Here's why—and what to do…*

Normal-weight obesity (NWO) may sound like an oxymoron, but that doesn't make it any less harmful.

Obesity (or, in many cases, simply being overweight) is a well-established risk factor for a slew of health problems, including hypertension, elevated cholesterol and high blood sugar—which, in turn, increase your odds of having a heart attack, stroke, type 2 diabetes and other serious medical conditions.

The grim link between excessive body weight and poor health is why scientists have carefully defined who is overweight and who isn't, creating three main categories—normal weight, overweight and obesity—based on a formula called the body mass index, or BMI.

Here's the rub: Your BMI can be normal, but you can still have the same weight-related health risks as a person with obesity—something known as normal-weight obesity, or NWO.

For important insights on this commonly overlooked phenomenon, we spoke with John A. Batsis, MD, a noted authority on NWO…

Understanding Body Weight Labels

NWO occurs when a person has excess body fat that the BMI fails to take fully into account. The type of fat found in NWO is almost always excess abdominal fat, commonly called "central obesity" or "visceral fat" because it surrounds the viscera, or the internal organs of the abdominal cavity.

There are varying estimates on the extent of this problem in the US, but a scientific paper published in *Nutrition Reviews* stated that 30 million Americans have NWO.

A Risky Type of Fat

The scientific evidence linking NWO to poor health is very strong…

•**Metabolic syndrome, cardiovascular disease and diabetes.** Metabolic syndrome is a cluster of conditions—including hypertension, high blood sugar, elevated cholesterol or triglycerides and central obesity—that increases your risk for heart disease, stroke and type 2 diabetes. In a study published in *European Heart Journal*, people with NWO were four times more likely to have metabolic syndrome than those without NWO.

•**Functional decline.** As one ages, function—the ability to get out of bed, walk, do everyday activities and take care of yourself—is paramount. As function declines, risk increases for frailty, falls, fractures… and placement in a nursing home. When researchers at Dartmouth-Hitchcock Medical Center analyzed six years of health data for nearly 4,500 adults age 60 and older, they found that women with NWO had a much greater decline in function than women with a normal BMI and waist circumference.

•**Premature death.** Among more than 7,000 patients age 65 and older with heart disease, those with NWO were 29 percent more likely to die during a 7.1-year period than those without NWO, according to a study published in *Mayo Clinic Proceedings*. In research published in *Annals of Internal Medicine*, men with NWO were twice as likely to die over a 14-year period as men who were overweight or obese.

Why would NWO be even more harmful than obesity alone? The main reason is that the component of central obesity that characterizes NWO is particularly inflammatory—and inflammation drives chronic disease, such as heart disease, diabetes, cancer, kidney disease, fatty liver disease, autoimmune disease and neurodegenerative disorders such as Parkinson's disease.

Do You Have NWO?

NWO is common, but most people don't know they have it because primary care physicians rarely diagnose it. NWO can be identified by determining your BMI and measuring your waist circumference.* If your BMI is "normal"—between 18.5 and 24.9—but your waist circumference is greater than 40 inches (for men) or more than 34.6 inches (for women), you have NWO.

That may sound like an easy determination, but measuring waist circumference accurately is not that simple. Ideally, a nurse or other trained health professional should do it. But you also can measure your waist circumference by using a cloth tape measure and following these steps (*Note*: this method may not be 100 percent accurate)…

Put the tape measure at the top of your hip bone. Loop the tape measure around your waist, level with your belly button and level all the way around your body, front and back.

Important: Make sure the tape measure is snug but not too tight…breathe easily while measuring—and don't hold your breath… take the measurement right after you exhale.

How to Prevent or Reverse NWO

If you have NWO or are concerned about belly fat, you can reverse the condition—or prevent it. *My advice…*

• **Diet.** Follow a nutritionally balanced, evidence-based weight-loss and weight-maintenance diet, such as a Mediterranean-style diet or the DASH (Dietary Approaches to Stop Hypertension) diet. Both plans emphasize fruits and vegetables, whole grains, beans, poultry, fish and low-fat dairy products, with a minimum of lean, red meat and avoidance of fried foods, refined carbohydrates and processed foods.

*To determine your BMI, go to NIH.gov and search "BMI Calculator."

Important: When losing weight, it's important to lose fat, not muscle. To do that, you need to consume enough muscle-building protein—typically a daily protein intake of 15 percent to 25 percent of total calories. Good protein sources include chicken, meat and nuts.

Caution: Avoid very low-calorie diets for weight loss, which in older adults can cause imbalances in fluids and electrolytes (calcium, magnesium, potassium and sodium). Never consume less than 1,200 calories daily unless your doctor recommends this and you are under medical supervision.

• **Exercise.** Aim for at least 150 minutes of moderate-to-vigorous exercise every week.

Examples: Walking for moderate exercise…and jogging for vigorous exercise. Ideally, your routine should also include resistance-training two to three times weekly, along with stretching and balance training.

• **Take vitamin D.** This nutrient is crucial for maintaining muscle mass and strength. Ask your doctor to test your blood level, which should be no lower than 30 ng/mL. If your level is low, your doctor can recommend a supplement dosage tailored to your needs and recheck your vitamin D levels in about eight weeks.

• **Set and monitor goals.** Making and sustaining behavioral changes is difficult, but it can be done. You must decide what you're going to do…track your progress with a daily diary…and adjust your routine to stay on track.

Flax and Pumpkin Seeds May Fight Diabetes

Recent study: When rats with induced diabetes were fed a mixture of flax and powdered pumpkin seed, their blood chemistry normalized, becoming more like that of rats without diabetes.

Study by researchers at Institut Supérieur de Biotechnologie de Sfax, Tunisia, published in *Journal of Diabetes and Its Complications.*

COVID-19 Causes Dangerous Spikes in Blood Sugar

George L. King, MD, is chief scientific officer at Joslin Diabetes Center, Boston, commenting on a Chinese study published in *Diabetologia*.

Nearly half of hospitalized COVID-19 patients studied had blood sugar readings similar to those with type 2 diabetes/prediabetes even if they'd never had diabetes. This spike nearly doubles risk for death from COVID. Hospitalized COVID patients should have blood sugar tested daily...and those with diabetes should be put on constant glucose monitoring. If you're home with COVID, ask your doctor to test your glucose level and, if it is high, follow instructions to control it.

Diabetes Makes COVID-19 Worse and Possibly Vice Versa

"Kings College London, Study of New-Onset Diabetes in Covid-19," letter written by 17 leading experts involved in CovidDiab Registry project, published in *The New England Journal of Medicine*.

It is known that having diabetes tends to make COVID-19 worse. In fact, between 20 percent and 30 percent of people who die from COVID are diabetics. There are also reports of people who never had diabetes developing that condition during a COVID infection, and reports of diabetes becoming more severe and harder to manage during an infection.

Both COVID and diabetes are epidemics that are occurring around the world. An international group of 17 diabetes experts are warning about the clash of these two epidemics. The warning appears in a recent let-

ter published in *The New England Journal of Medicine*. The letter announces the establishment of a new global registry for COVID-related diabetes.

It is not surprising that having COVID makes diabetes worse, because any stressful illness makes diabetes worse. The big questions are does COVID cause diabetes in a person without diabetes and does COVID change the natural long-term course of the disease. In other words, does diabetes continue to get worse after COVID goes away? The diabetes experts are warning that emerging evidence suggests diabetes and COVID may be bidirectional. That means diabetes makes COVID worse and COVID makes diabetes worse.

The experts have a theory of how this may happen. COVID enters the body's cells by binding to proteins on cells called ACE-2 receptors. These receptors are found in the lungs, which is why people with COVID often get pneumonia. ACE 2 receptors are also found in tissues such as the pancreas, small intestine, fats cells and liver that are important for glucose metabolism. Disruption of glucose metabolism can cause diabetes.

Goals of the Global Registry

The international experts hope that pooling information on patients with diabetes and COVID around the world will allow researchers to answer these questions...

• **Does COVID cause new-onset diabetes?**

• **Does COVID cause type 1, type 2 or a new type of diabetes?**

• **How common is new-onset diabetes with COVID?**

• **Does new onset-diabetes continue or resolve after COVID?**

• **In people who already have diabetes, does diabetes continue to get worse after COVID?**

• **Does COVID increase future risk of diabetes?**

• **What is the best way to treat a combination of diabetes and COVID?**

The diabetes experts hope that answering these questions will add to our knowledge of both of these important epidemics. Leaning how COVID causes or worsens diabetes may also lead to new ways of understanding and treating diabetes in all people.

Statins Raise Diabetes Risk

Data on 4,683 subjects showed that prolonged use (two years or more) of the cholesterol-lowering drugs more than tripled the risk for type 2 diabetes.

But: Statins are very effective at preventing cardiac events among patients with indications for their use (both primary and secondary prevention). So discuss risks and benefits with your doctor.

Victoria Zigmont, MPH, PhD, is an assistant professor of public health at Southern Connecticut State University in New Haven. Her peer-reviewed research was published in *Diabetes/Metabolism Research and Reviews.*

Stem-Cell Treatment May Cure Diabetes

Study by researchers at Washington University School of Medicine, St. Louis, published in *Nature Biotechnology.*

Mice with severe diabetes that were given insulin-secreting beta cells had normal blood glucose levels within two weeks, and levels stayed that way for months. The beta cells were converted from stem cells using a new process that researchers hope will eventually work in humans.

Weak Grip Strength Can Predict Type 2 Diabetes Risk

Elise Brown, PhD, is assistant professor of wellness and health promotion at Oakland University, Rochester, Michigan, and leader of an analysis of data on more than 5,000 patients, published in *American Journal of Preventive Medicine.*

Exact grip thresholds depend on body weight, sex and age. Grip strength, measured by an electronic handgrip device, can be performed during annual checkups in order to identify patients who may need further diabetes diagnostic testing and lifestyle intervention.

Diabetes Vaccine Under Investigation

Virginia Stone, PhD, assistant professor, Karolinska Institutet Center for Infectious Medicine

Researchers suspect that a subgroup of viruses called Coxsackie B (CVB) contribute to the development of type 1 diabetes, and they've developed a vaccine to fight it. Animal studies have been successful, and human studies will soon begin. If proven safe, the vaccine will be given to children with a genetic risk profile for type 1 diabetes in the hopes that it can prevent the disease from developing. The vaccine would also protect against myocarditis and many viruses that cause the common cold.

Chapter 5

EMOTIONAL RESCUE

Surprising Cause of Anxiety...and How to Heal It

You may think that feelings of anxiety—excessive worrying... irritability...jitteriness...clammy hands...upset stomach...panic attacks—start in your brain. But you'd be wrong. The truth is that 80 percent of emotion-related signals begin in the gut and are then sent to the brain. Your ability to know "in your gut" whether something is good or bad is actually the same gut/brain connection that is at the root of many of our anxious moments. *Here's how it works...*

The Gut Controls the Brain and Our Bodies

You may think that the brain is the master of the body, but the gut is actually in the driver's seat when it comes to feelings of anxiety. The gut even makes some of the chemicals (neurotransmitters) like serotonin, dopamine and gamma-aminobutyric acid (GABA) that the brain uses to process its emotions and thoughts. It's a great point-to-point communication system—when the lines are clear. Unfortunately, complicating this delicate relationship are the many stressors of life that cause the fragile gut biome of bacteria to become out of balance.

You've heard a lot about it in recent years—the importance of a healthy gut and healthy "good" bacteria...the need to take probiotics...and the dangers of poor diet, stress, certain medications and more on these delicate microorganisms. Just as there is an entire sub-universe of life living in coral reefs, so too there is an entire sub-universe of life living in our guts. Allow algae to grow out of control and the reef dies. Similarly, if we allow bad bacteria to overgrow in our intestinal tract, the sub-universe gets stressed... and so do we.

Anxiety and other health problems can arise when the balance between the good and bad bacteria in the gut microbiome tips toward the bad. Chronic inflammation and infection in the gut itself and an imbalance of neurotransmitters can also lead to anxiety. Other causes include your genetics, excessive stress, medical conditions and a poor diet. Most medications, including anti-anxiety

Hyla Cass, MD, integrative physician in private practice in Los Angeles. She is author of several books, including *8 Weeks to Vibrant Health and Supplement Your Prescription: What Your Doctor Doesn't Know About Nutrition.* CassMD.com drugs, can also throw the gut microbiome out of balance by killing off good bacteria.

Relieve Your Anxiety

Recent data suggests that anxiety is on the rise. Nearly 40 percent of Americans reported feeling more anxious in 2018 than they did the year prior, according to the American Psychiatric Association. Luckily, there is a remedy—if you ingest the right nutrients, you can influence the chemical messengers in your brain that in turn work to prevent and relieve your anxiety. The seven-step formula below is the safest and most effective way to balance your body and relieve the very unpleasant symptoms of anxiety. *Here's what to do to help restore your gut—and your head—to health…*

• **Eliminate toxic foods from your diet.** The most toxic foods are non-organic, non-grass-fed red meat, which can contain antibiotics, and non-organic grains, which have most likely been exposed to the herbicide *glyphosate* (an ingredient in Roundup weed killer that has been linked to cancer).

Best: Eat organic, non-GMO (genetically modified organism), fresh foods.

• **Remove potentially allergenic foods from your diet.** These foods promote inflammation and lead to imbalances in the gut microbiome. Wheat, barley, rye and other grains, dairy products, eggs and soy are common allergenic foods. Sugar is highly inflammatory and causes yeast overgrowth.

Strategy: To identify what's bothering you, try an elimination diet. Stop eating the foods listed above for two weeks and then introduce them back one by one for a week. If you start to experience anxiety or other symptoms—you feel overly stimulated or alternately very tired or foggy-headed, for instance—when you reintroduce a food, you know your body doesn't tolerate that food well and you should avoid it. Be aware that the reaction may be delayed anywhere from a few hours to a day.

• **Avoid highly processed foods.** Most Americans consume too much sugar from products like sodas, baked goods, candy and ice cream. Sugar has been associated with a host of diseases, and it can directly affect your mood. The American Heart Association recommends limiting added sugars to 25 grams a day for women and 36 grams for men. This recommendation is for healthy people. If you have anxiety, cut out as much sugar as possible

• **Look at the ingredients list…**You have probably already heard the wise advice that if you can't pronounce the name of a chemical on a label, it's better not to eat it! Buy most of your food in the outer aisles of the supermarket where you'll find fresh fruits and vegetables. If you do buy prepared foods such as canned soup or a frozen entree, try to find ones that have just a few ingredients and that don't contain artificial flavorings/sweeteners or preservatives.

• **Consume fermented foods which contain good bacteria (probiotics),** including sauerkraut, pickles, yogurt, kefir, kombucha, kimchi, miso and tempeh. Ingest a couple of tablespoons of fermented foods daily to keep your gut microbiome in balance.

• **Take probiotic supplements.** In spite of encouraging reports about probiotics, research is still in the early stages. Many animal and human studies suggest a wide variety of benefits—especially emotional health benefits.

Example: A 2019 study of "stressed-out" adults who took a daily probiotic supplement containing *Lactobacillus plantarum DR7* found they had reduced stress and anxiety symptoms after eight weeks compared to subjects who received a placebo. Their cortisol levels (a measure of stress) were also lower.

Best: Look for a probiotic supplement that contains multiple strains of *Lactobacillus* and *Bifidobacterium*, both of which have been shown in research studies to reduce anxiety symptoms. Start with a dose of 15 billion live bacteria in the morning before breakfast and adjust upwards to 50 billion as long as you can tolerate the higher dose without experiencing gas and/or bloating.

The independent supplement testing group Consumer Lab ranks these brands well: Align, Culturelle, Florastor, Jarrow Formulas, Nature's Way Primadophilus Optima and Sigma-Tau VSL#3 The Living Shield.

• **Eat high-fiber foods like beans, oats, avocado and fruits with skins like pears and apples.** They provide nourishment for the probiotics in your gut. There's also emerging evidence in animal studies that high-fiber foods themselves may have antianxiety and antidepressant effects. A study published in *Biological Psychiatry* suggests a beneficial role of prebiotic treatment for stress-related behaviors. The government recommends that women over the age of 50 consume at least 22 grams of fiber daily and men over the age of 50 eat 28 grams.

Examples: A cup of black beans has 15 grams…a slice of whole grain bread may have about two to four grams. Since most people fall short of fiber consumption recommendations, also consider taking a fiber supplement to ensure the good bacteria in your gut are well fed.

Other Natural Anxiety Remedies

• **Aloe vera juice.** This plant is known for its healing properties for burns but a study found that aloe vera juice also promotes the growth of healthy Lactobacillus in the gut microbiome. Try consuming two to four ounces once or twice a day. You can notice a change within days.

• **Hemp oil.** Cannabidiol (CBD) is often labeled as hemp oil. The compounds found in hemp plants have been shown to have many healing properties and are now being sold widely throughout the US in a variety of forms from liquids and oils to creams. Hemp oils help to heal the gut lining and enhance the immune system, 70 percent of which is found in the gut. They also have been shown to manage anxiety and depression symptoms by enhancing the activity of neurotransmitters like serotonin that are essential to mood.

How to take it: Experiment with doses and formulations. I sell a hemp oil formulation on my website, and I suggest starting with the 500 milligram (mg) or 750 mg bottle and taking one dropper full (8.3 mg of 500

mg or 12.5 mg of the 750 mg bottle). Wait 30 minutes to see if your anxiety eases. If it doesn't, take another dropper full and then another (maximum four droppers per day).

To ensure quality when buying hemp oil, look for a label that says "GMP," which stands for good manufacturing practices. This means that an independent lab has verified the product's ingredients.

Stick to hemp products, which don't contain any of the psychoactive ingredient tetrahydrocannabinol (THC) that makes you high and is still illegal in most states without a prescription.

Note: CBD will have either 0 or under 0.3 percent THC. This will not make you high. But CBD can accumulate in your body and there is a chance that it could yield a positive drug test. This is a concern if your job has random drug testing.

Ways to Keep Anxiety from Spiraling

Deep diaphragmatic breathing: Hold one hand on your belly and the other on your chest. Expand your belly but not your chest when you inhale.

Dip your face in cold water: A 15-second dip can calm the body.

Touch something cold: It distracts you and interrupts your body's stress response.

Get moving: Outside is best, but any physical activity works—mow your lawn, clean your shower or do some sit-ups.

"5-4-3-2-1" method: Focus on five things you can see, four things you can touch, three things you can hear, two things you can smell and one thing you can taste. This can help you create some distance from the feeling of anxiety.

Progressive muscle relaxation: Clench then relax your toes, then calves, then thighs, etc., working your way up your whole body.

Roundup of experts quoted on Self.com.

Important: Hemp oils can interact with certain medications but generally only in higher doses, close to 100 mg a day. If you are on blood thinners, there are interactions so talk to your doctor before use.

The Narcissistic Partner

Candace V. Love, PhD, founder and president of North Shore Behavioral Medicine, Chicago, Illinois, and author of *No More Narcissists! How to Stop Choosing Self-Absorbed Men and Find the Love You Deserve.* DrCandacevLove.com

Are you in a relationship with someone who has an inflated sense of self-importance? Who requires excessive admiration? Who can't tolerate criticism? Someone who shows a complete disregard for your feelings and belittles or criticizes you for seemingly insignificant things? If so, you might be dealing with a narcissist.

A person with narcissistic personality disorder (NPD) is entirely motivated by an insatiable need to feel worthy and loved, and to avoid any feelings that threaten that need. They are unable to emotionally connect with others: They lack both empathy (the ability to understand the emotions of others) and compassion (the ability to feel the distress of another and to want to help). As a result, they can hurt others with impunity.

At the root of NPD is a childhood experience that made the person feel deeply shamed, worthless, or unloved. In some cases, it is because they were treated like a prince or princess and they don't want to lose that feeling of being special, so they become driven to seek excessive admiration.

To avoid feelings of vulnerability and pain, that child built a wall of defenses that became a pervasive and consistent way of interacting with the world. In the *Diagnostic and Statistical Manual of Mental Disorders, Fifth Edition*, the American Psychiatric Association outlines nine traits that come from that process (see box).

Make a Choice

Being in a relationship with a narcissist can erode your self-esteem and lead to anxiety and depression. It can make you feel like a shadow of your former self.

The first step, then, is to think about whether you want to stay in the relationship or leave. People stay in relationships with narcissists for various reasons, such as finances, children, societal position, and love, so it is a choice that only you can make. Although I respect an individual's decision, if there is physical abuse, I strongly recommend leaving the relationship.

Don't Expect Change

To guide your choice, you must accept that a narcissist will likely never change. It's not that they absolutely can't—some psychologists have treated NPD—but it is very rare. A person with NPD is rarely motivated to change because they don't think they have a problem. The majority of narcissists do not seek therapy. Those who do only do so to serve a personal need, such as to try to avoid a divorce or to blame marital problems on a spouse.

Narcissistic Traits

To be diagnosed with NPD, a person must have at least five of these. (Only a qualified, licensed mental-health professional can diagnose a mental health disorder.)

1. **Grandiose sense of self-importance**
2. **Fantasies of unlimited success, power, brilliance, beauty, or ideal love**
3. **Belief they are special and unique and can only be understood by,** or should associate with, other special or high-status people or institutions
4. **Need for excessive admiration**
5. **Sense of entitlement**
6. **Interpersonally exploitative behavior**
7. **Lack of empathy**
8. **Envy of others or a belief that others are envious of them**
9. **Arrogant or haughty behaviors.**

If you choose to stay in a relationship with a narcissist, then, you must have realistic expectations of what your relationship will look like: It will not be a partnership. It will be two people coexisting in a home. You will have to carve out a life that runs parallel to your partner and find ways to focus on yourself and seek out what brings you happiness.

Avoid Confrontation

You will rarely win an argument with a narcissist. Part of their disorder is the need to avoid anything that makes them feel pain or shame, so they will fight in any way they can to prevent that. They may redirect the conversation to get the focus off of themselves, shift the blame onto you, respond with exaggerated rage, or even retaliate. I advise my patients to just avoid confrontation, if possible.

That doesn't mean that you have to agree with whatever a narcissist asks of you. *If you must discuss something, try these suggestions…*

• **Make the other person feel heard and understood.**

• **Pick and choose your battles.**

• **Expect pushback, but think of it as an exercise in assertiveness.**

• **Try to address issues in a way that doesn't feel confrontational to the other person.**

• **Stay calm and avoid accusing.**

• **Pick a good time to talk.** A sunny morning is better than right before bed. Make sure no one is feeling rushed.

• **Stress how what you're asking for will benefit the narcissist.** Remember that NPD causes people to care only about their own needs and feelings.

Why You Choose Narcissists

Some people unintentionally but repeatedly choose romantic partners who share narcissistic traits. To break that pattern, you must first understand where it came from.

Our childhood experiences cause us to have certain beliefs about ourselves that affect how, as adults, we relate to our environment and intimate relationships. These beliefs are called core beliefs.

A person's core beliefs can lead to what psychologist Jeffrey Young, PhD, calls life traps: They trap you into self-destructive patterns of behaviors.

Life traps feel familiar, so if you had a parent who was unable to address your emotional needs, you may then grow up to seek the same trait in a partner. There are seven life trap and core belief combinations that make people particularly vulnerable to falling in love with a narcissist (see table on page 70).

Here's an example of how a core belief and life trap could play out. As a small child, Ann perceived that her parents valued boys more than girls, so she believed, "I'm not as valuable as boys." Over time, that belief festered and developed into the core belief, "I am not valuable." Ann's belief led her into a life trap of not feeling adequate or worthy of love, which made her highly susceptible to the initial charms of a partner with NPD. (Narcissists are often very charming and attentive at first.) But when the NPD started to show through, Ann's feelings of inadequacy led her to think it was her fault that the relationship was souring. After the relationship ended, Ann was still in the same life trap that led her to be attracted to another man with NPD, perpetuating the cycle.

Break the Cycle

The only way to stop the cycle is to address core beliefs and life traps head on. It's not easy. Our core beliefs are at the root of our automatic thoughts. Those thoughts are like a Jeep going down a dirt road. They create deep ruts, so we keep going back to them over and over. But it's possible to turn the wheel and work toward getting out of the rut and develop new paths. When we do, we make new neural pathways in the brain.

By working with a trusted psychologist, we can break free of destructive thought patterns and, ultimately, of narcissists, too. It takes time, patience, and commitment to learn strategies to survive and/or leave an

NPD relationship. For a more thorough discussion, read *No More Narcissists! How to Stop Choosing Self-Absorbed Men and Find the Love You Deserve.*

Table: Life Traps		
LIFE TRAP	**FEELING**	**CORE BELIEF**
Abandonment	You feel rejection.	People always leave you.
Mistrust/Abuse	You feel hurt.	People hurt or manipulate you.
Emotional deprivation	You feel misunderstood.	No one is there for you.
Defectiveness/shame	You feel inadequate or unworthy.	You're not good enough to love.
Subjugation	You supress your wants and needs to please someone else.	If you don't meet someone's needs, they won't care about you.
Self-sacrifice	You feel like you must take care of others, but also resent having to do so.	You need to help or fix others.
Unrelenting standards	You feel that you must try to be the best at everything.	What you do will never be good enough.

Are Your Clothes Ruining Your Mood? How to Dress to Feel Your Best

Dawnn Karen, pioneer in the field of fashion psychology and founder of the Fashion Psychology Institute in New York City. She is author of *Dress Your Best Life: How to Use Fashion Psychology to Take Your Look—and Your Life—to the Next Level.* Dubbed "The Dress Doctor" by *The New York Times*, she is assistant professor in the social sciences department at the Fashion Institute of Technology in New York City and has a private therapy practice. FashionPsychology Success.com

W hen you get dressed each day, external forces typically dictate what you wear. We dress for the weather…specific occasions…for work or a party. We rarely dress just for ourselves, and even

if we do, we may not feel like our best selves in the clothing we're wearing.

Example: Wearing baggy sweatpants all day can put you into an all-day emotional slump.

Many of us are continuing to spend more time at home since the COVID-19 pandemic made it more feasible and rarely, if ever, donning that fitted dress or suit and tie to feel empowered. Even if you don't need to dress for the office, why not take this time as an opportunity to re-examine your clothing choices? To align your internal and external selves to find clothing that truly reflects who you are and what makes you feel good about yourself? This is a great opportunity to move beyond old dressing habits and dress for what makes you feel confident and proud.

As a pioneer in the social science of fashion psychology, an emerging field that looks at the ways in which clothing impacts mood and behavior, Dawnn Karen has seen how wardrobe choices impact people's lives. She has helped hundreds of clients achieve better self-esteem and a happier outlook by changing what they wear. *Here are her tips for dressing to feel your best, wherever you are…*

●**Figure out your signature style.** Is Halle Berry (elegant, glamorous) your style icon, or are you more of a Jennifer Aniston (classic, relaxed, minimalist) or Jennifer Lopez (colorful, fashion forward, trendy) type of dresser? For the man in your life, does he identify with Brad Pitt (ultra-cool, artsy and bohemian) or Will Smith (sporty, colorful, streamlined), or is he a Clint Eastwood type (rugged, casual)? By identifying the style you (or your mate, if you want to give him a boost) gravitate toward and that you feel is most authentically you, you can home in on your best clothing options while also leaving room for creativity and experimentation.

●**Clean out your closet.** You may not realize it, but you have a relationship with everything in your wardrobe, some of which may have been hanging there for many years and through assorted phases of your personal growth. Take some time to go through each item you own to assess if it is serving you well now. You even may want to do a fashion show for yourself and try it all on to gauge how you feel.

If you don't plan to wear something again, choose to get rid of it or understand why you might want to hold onto it. If it's a piece you're keeping for only sentimental reasons, how would you feel if you were to get rid of it? Is holding onto it an emotional drain? Maybe giving it away—or even throwing it away—will be a needed emotional release.

If you love a piece that is in good shape but not currently in style, I suggest that you keep it if you have the room! Styles come back around, and you may never be able to replace a beloved piece.

For the balance of your wardrobe, ask yourself if you want to see yourself wearing each item again. Is it in sync with your signature style and the image that you want to project? Is it demotivating or motivating to wear? Does it make you feel confident and powerful...or nervous and meek? And remember—just because you like something aesthetically doesn't mean that it looks good on you. A kind and trusted friend may be able to give you some helpful feedback when you're not sure. Feel good about giving away the pieces you no longer want—there's someone out there with that style who will enjoy owning those clothes.

●**Change your outfit.** During the pandemic, we didn't have the option of going out to a lot of places, but even if you're home most of the time, changing your outfit at least once a day creates an emotional boundary between work and leisure time.

Example: Beyoncé told Oprah about how her attitude and mind-set change when she puts on the clothes and wig of her stage character Sasha Fierce. "My posture and the way I speak and everything is different," she said. Likewise, donning a favorite outfit will energize you for dinner with your partner or a video call with friends...luxurious, soft loungewear will signal your mind and body that you are in the off mode, and it's OK to calm down and release the stressors of the day.

●**Boost your mood.** Actors and performers will tell you that when they put on a character's clothes, they start to embody that character more fully. I recommend dressing to enhance your mood—to chase away the blues or feel more energized, for example—and faking it until you make it. Whatever the season, wear your favorite colors, patterns, prints and styles, even if that means wearing white in winter and black in summer.

Example: Jim, a lawyer in his mid-40s, was getting divorced. He looked rumpled and undone, with untied shoelaces and untucked shirts. He avoided looking in mirrors because they reminded him of the person he had become—a divorced man disconnected from the people he loved most. But ignoring his appearance only added to his anxiety and damaged his self-esteem. During our sessions, he began to be more conscientious about wearing ironed, unstained clothing and tucking in his shirt, which led him to stand taller—a small tweak that improved his feelings about himself.

Think about how you feel when you wear different shades and hues. Yellow typically makes people feel happy...red, sexy and empowered...orange, fresh and alert...blue, calm and peaceful...green, upbeat. Figure out the colors that make you feel the best. No matter your skin tone, there is a hue of any color that will look good on you.

Example: One of my clients was a doctor who was feeling depressed. She was treating COVID-19 patients at work and just throwing on whatever was clean to wear under her white coat. I worked with her to wear happy colors like yellow and professional clothing like a dress and nice shoes under her hospital coat to boost her confidence and energy. I also suggested that she buy pretty loungewear to switch into at home to help her relax without feeling frumpy.

●**Eliminate ruts.** Extroverts typically enjoy switching up their outfits and introverts, like Mark Zuckerberg (t-shirt and jeans), feel anxious if they have to select a new outfit each morning. Having a uniform actually boosts introverts' productivity.

But: If you're reaching for the same clothes because it's convenient—not because you like them—you're in a rut. And you can get yourself out.

Example: Patricia was laid off from her job at a nonprofit after-school program. Her work uniform had been leggings and sweaters paired with sneakers or flats—and she was wearing the same outfits while at home. But now, these clothing items reminded her of her lost job and exacerbated her feelings of sadness and failure. I advised her to get out of her rut by putting aside her former work clothes and dressing in an outfit that would put her in a confident frame of mind—a button-down shirt, gray slacks and heels that would encourage her to sit at the computer and look for a new job.

When You Shop

Before buying a new item, ask yourself these questions…

Does this make me feel great?

Does this project my personal style?

Do I like the way I look in it?

Will I still love it in a year or two…or five?

Is this an impulse buy that I will later regret?

Do I need it?

Can it update my look and replace something else in my closet?

What do I already have that will work with it?

After you buy: To keep your closet from being overrun, get rid of one old item for every new item that you buy.

Fashion psychology is not retail therapy and buying brand names. Rather, it's about selecting clothing that reflects who you are, raises your spirits and makes you feel stronger, safer or more empowered.

Art Relieves the Stress of Caregiving

Spending 45 minutes filling in a coloring book or creating original art brought feelings of greater pleasure and enjoyment—and less anxiety and tension—to professional caregivers and to family members who are taking care of loved ones.

Girija Kaimal, EdD, associate professor, College of Nursing and Health Professions, Drexel University, Philadelphia, and leader of a study of caregivers, published in *European Journal of Oncology Nursing*.

Adults With ADHD Are More Likely to Get into Car Crashes

Study by researchers at University of Ottawa, Canada, published in *Journal of the American Academy of Child and Adolescent Psychiatry*.

Adults with attention deficit/hyperactivity disorder (ADHD) had 1.45 times the risk of getting into a car wreck compared with the rest of the population. Research also shows that adults with ADHD have more traffic and speeding violations, license suspensions and risky driving behaviors.

A Faux Commute Could Be Good for You

Roundup of experts on home-life balance reported at CTVNews.ca.

If you now are working from home and find yourself missing your daily commute, you're not crazy. That downtime that we used to complain about actually was psychologically healthy, because it allowed us to plan our workday, decompress and establish a clear boundary between work life and home life. Even though there's no travel involved, you still can set up a routine that serves the same purposes. Walking for an hour before or after work…exercising before logging in… meditating for 15 minutes at the beginning and end of each workday…or just listening to music can help you with recovery and make working from home more sustainable over the long haul.

Social Anxiety May Affect Your Memory

Study by researchers at University of Waterloo, Ontario, Canada, published in *Cognition and Emotion*.

People who experience social anxiety have a harder time than less socially anxious people remembering the details of social scenarios that end well. This may be because positive social experiences do not conform to their expectations. Socially anxious people also did not have better memory for social situations that ended poorly. No matter what level of anxiety participants report, they all had similar memories for nonsocial scenarios. The study was based on self-reported levels of social anxiety and on hypothetical social and nonsocial situations, not ones that the participants actually experienced.

Remember in a New Way

Peggy St. Jacques, PhD, is assistant professor of psychology at University of Alberta, Canada, and leader of a study published in *Cortex*.

Remembering in the third person helps us to see memories in a new way. Recalling troublesome events as an observer instead of from our own point of view helps us keep psychological distance. Also, it changes the interaction between different parts of the brain, helping us to view the past from a new perspective.

Time and Money Traps That Can Rob You of Happiness

Ashley Whillans, PhD, assistant professor at Harvard Business School, Boston, and a leading scholar in the time and happiness research field. She is author of *Time Smart: How to Reclaim Your Time and Live a Happier Life*. AWhillans.com

When thinking about the future, it's very easy to think about our decisions—both major ones, such as a job change or a new home, and small, everyday ones such as where to fill up your gas tank—in terms of dollars and cents, yet it is very hard to think about what it costs to give up our time to have that money. This money-focused mind-set can have seriously negative consequences for our happiness. Research shows that being willing to give up money to have more leisure time is a predictor of greater happiness, better relationships, less stress, even being more physically fit.

Researchers define "time poverty" as the feeling of having too many things to do—both professional and personal—and not enough time to do them. An astonishing 80 percent of working Americans report feeling time-poor. My research shows that the emotional impact of being time-poor can be greater than the emotional impact of being unemployed. We all should strive toward greater time-affluence, which is the opposite of time-poverty. Another way of thinking about time-affluence is that if you could write out the time spent in your ideal day in terms of social, work and leisure, your ideal day and your actual day would be congruent with one another.

Here are a few of my favorite tips for bringing more time-affluence into your life…

Account for Your Time

It's critical to account for your time because it easily goes missing.

Try this: At the end of next Tuesday (I suggest a Tuesday because Tuesdays tend to be average workdays), fill out a time diary to observe how you spend your time. What activities did you do? How positive did you feel those activities were? How meaningful? If you find that you're stuck in frustrating meetings or other activities that zap your energy 80 percent of every day, is that really how you want to spend your life?

Then think consciously about choosing time over money. We know very well, from decades of research, that a $10,000 raise will give you a half-point bump on a 10-point happiness scale. But there are many other things we can do that will give us a similar happiness boost. So think about each tiny decision you make in a day as having an income equivalent in terms of happiness. For example, just shifting your mind-set from valuing money to valuing time—in the absence of changing your behavior at all—is worth the income equivalent (in terms of happiness) of making $2,200 more personal income a year. Spending 30 minutes exercising every day will give you a mood bump that our research shows is equivalent to earning an additional $1,800 a year. For people who tend toward valuing money over time, being mindful of these dollar equivalents on activities helps improve life balance.

Avoid These "Time Traps"

A time trap is something that makes you time-poor but that you might not even be aware you're doing. *Learning to recognize and correct for these traps can ratchet up your time-affluence…*

•**Technology trap.** The reason we're all so time-poor isn't necessarily because we're working more hours. We actually have more leisure time than we used to. The problem is that our leisure time gets broken into small, unsavory moments of free time that are easily lost because our technology is constantly pinging us. Our brains are sucked out of the present moment and thrown into the online environment, which undermines our enjoyment of the present. (I call these shredded-up bits of freedom "time confetti.") The solution is simple—when it's time for leisure, turn off your phone and choose to focus on something you really want to do rather than piddling it away on social media.

•**"Yes…Damn!" effect.** As part of human nature, we believe that we'll have more time in the future than we do in the present, so we overcommit our tomorrow even though we're very busy today ("Yes, I'll help you move next Saturday…Damn! I didn't know I'd be this busy."). To avoid this trap, ask yourself, If I couldn't do it in the next two hours, should I really be saying yes to doing it next week?

•**Undervalued time.** People who value money over time often will spend hours researching a purchase for days in order to save 50 bucks or will choose a flight with lots of connections in order to save $75 in airfare. It's easy to understand why we make such choices—we readily comprehend the value of $50 or $75 but have a harder time valuing the time lost. Yet such decisions do have a cost.

For example, I've calculated that habitually driving six minutes farther to save five cents per gallon of gas will, in a year, have saved $108 and cost nearly five hours of time. That puts a price on your time of $22 per hour and does not account for the opportunity cost of the happiness-inducing activities you might have spent your five hours on.

Solution: Train yourself to recognize the moments when you're making "cheaper" decisions, and weigh that savings against the time it will cost you and what else you might do with the extra time.

•**Idleness aversion.** Humans are hardwired to not enjoy the feeling of doing nothing, sitting alone with only our thoughts. When we have an important, thinking-heavy task before us, we'll often focus instead on smaller tasks, such as reading e-mail. Responding to a message makes us feel like we're doing something proactive. It gives us a sense of self-efficacy and of being in control of our lives—even though it's not moving the needle on truly important activities.

Solution: Put "focus blocks" into your calendar, and don't let anything else in there. Thinking time is thinking time. No mail, no distractions, only heads-down stuff.

The secret to doing this successfully: Create three such blocks for your week. Set aside the first of them (say, 15 to 30 minutes on Monday morning) exclusively for planning what you'll do in the other two. Treat that time like it's the most important doctor's appointment in the world.

• **Merely urgent.** Any possible use of your time can be assessed along two axes—urgency, requiring immediate attention…and importance, contributing to your long-term goals. Ask yourself, If I had to classify this activity, in which quadrant is it located? Is it urgent but not important? Urgent and important? Not important? Not urgent? Being mindful of those two measures helps us avoid a lifetime of chasing after things that are urgent but ultimately unimportant, while the things that we care about but don't require immediate attention are put off forever. To make sure you get to those important-but-not-urgent tasks (writing that novel, revamping your budget, setting up your kid's college savings plan), you have to schedule them in to what I call "proactive time." Maybe they go into the focus blocks described above or maybe they're their own category, but they must be sacrosanct and inviolable.

If you find that a task is not important and not urgent, why are you doing it? Such tasks—home repairs, for example—are great candidates for delegating or outsourcing. If you're hesitant about spending money on such a "luxury," it might help you to know that outsourcing your most unpleasant tasks is worth the happiness equivalent of an $18,000 salary increase.

A "Gratitude Jar" Can Help Lift Your Spirits

Ruth Williams, business psychologist and former director of Department Store for the Mind, where people can explore ideas and emotions, and author of *The Mind Remedy: Discover, Make and Use Simple Objects to Nourish Your Soul.*

Making a "gratitude jar" to acknowledge the things and people we're grateful for can foster contentment and healing.

For individuals: Each day, jot down something that you're thankful for on a slip of paper and drop it into the jar. This practice will increase your happiness and make you more satisfied with life.

For families: Make a gratitude jar accessible for everyone in the family. At intervals—perhaps during a holiday—pull out the slips of paper, and celebrate the things you're thankful for together.

For couples: Telling your beloved what you appreciate about him/her can strengthen your bond. If you feel like you have been growing apart, this can remind you of what you see in the other person. Reviewing the notes can put you in a good mind-set before you face difficult discussions.

"Doomscrolling" Makes a Bad Time Span Worse

Amelia Aldo, PhD, clinical psychologist, New York City, quoted at NPR.org.

Many people are constantly scrolling through news stories, Twitter comments, Facebook posts and opinion pieces about COVID-19, serious economic turmoil, protests, national and international tensions and more. This harms mental health by keeping doomscrollers in a constant state of anxiety and fear.

Self-defense: Set a timer for yourself—create an artificial boundary for the amount of time you will spend getting information on the many negative events of the current year. Use your phone and computer for specific information—instead of clicking constantly from one article or post to the next, decide what you want to know about, get that information and then stop. Find ways to balance the negatives with positives.

Depression After Surgery

Amy Vigliotti, PhD, founder of SelfWorks: Therapy Professionals, quoted on Health.com.

Although it's seldom talked about, depression after surgery is quite common even when the operation is small and successful. Postsurgery depression—feelings of hopelessness extending two weeks or more after the operation—can interfere with recovery and continue for months if left untreated. Experts say it may be caused by feelings of vulnerability and trauma.

What to do: After surgery, be sure you have a good support system. Spend as much time as possible outdoors, and eat and sleep well. If depression does find you, talk to a therapist promptly.

Use Instagram to Lift Your Spirits

Better Homes & Gardens. BHG.com

Use Instagram to lift your spirits by following feel-good accounts from celebrities and influencers and about animals. *Jennifer Garner's* feed often features celebrities reading children's books and acting them out.

Golden Retrievers is nothing but cute photos and videos of those specific dogs. *My Therapist Says* is sarcastic and filled with puns, memes and jokes. *Chunk the Groundhog* shows footage of a real groundhog that walks up to a backyard camera, stares at it and keeps eating from the homeowner's vegetable garden. *Kristin Bell* offers a mixture of humor and thoughtfulness. *Upworthy* shows ways in which people are helping each other, fighting climate change and contributing to the common good. *Tank's Good News* offers similar content.

Make a Big Change in Small Increments

Small shifts in behavior can lead to big changes over time. Instead of worrying about your ultimate goal, ask yourself, Can I do 5 percent more? Do 5 percent more exercise? Relax 5 percent more? Be 5 percent more open-minded?

Shauna Shapiro, PhD, clinical psychologist and professor of counseling psychology at Santa Clara University, California, and author of *Good Morning, I Love You.* DrShaunaShapiro.com

Finding Meaning After the Death of a Loved One

David Kessler, grief specialist based in Los Angeles and founder of the website Grief.com. He was a protégé of the famed grief and death researcher Elisabeth Kübler-Ross and coauthor with her of *On Grief and Grieving.* His most recent book is *Finding Meaning: The Sixth Stage of Grief.*

Candy Lightner, whose daughter was killed by a drunk driver, launched Mothers Against Drunk Driving to save other lives. John Walsh, whose son was murdered, created and hosted the TV series *America's Most Wanted* to help catch killers.

Not everyone who suffers the loss of a loved one finds meaning through such dramatic actions. But finding meaning in some form is an essential step in the grieving process and dealing with the pain of the loss, according to grief specialist and author David Kessler. *He recently told us why finding meaning can be considered a crucial stage in that process...*

The Sixth Stage

When I coauthored *On Grief and Grieving*—published in 2005—with my mentor, Elisabeth Kübler-Ross, we discussed the five stages that she had originally identified in her 1969 classic *On Death and Dying*. They are denial, anger, bargaining, depression and acceptance. However, those stages of the healing process do not represent the entire journey for most people.

To find a path forward from their grief, even after they have experienced the five stages, survivors often need to identify some kind of greater meaning in the lives and/or deaths of their loved ones. Their pain doesn't disappear when this happens, but it is cushioned. They find that thinking about the deceased no longer brings only pain—it now brings a mixture of pain and love.

The meaning that survivors find does not fit a single form or framework. While Lightner and Walsh launched crusades, other people find meaning by reflecting on the positive influence that the deceased had during life... by using the death as inspiration for positive changes in their own lives...through belief in an afterlife...and in various other ways. The pursuit of meaning doesn't have a predictable time frame, either—some survivors find meaning almost as soon as the death occurs, while for others it takes months or years.

Six ways to find meaning...

Changed Behaviors

•**Create stronger bonds with fellow survivors.** The death of a loved one can draw survivors together, presenting an opportunity to tighten weak relationships and overcome long-standing differences. These improved relationships can serve as a legacy for the deceased. *Examples...*

A pair of siblings who have been estranged for years reconnect at their mother's funeral "because that's what mom would have wanted."

An office worker mentions that she will be out for her mother's funeral. A colleague expresses her condolences and says that her father died only a few months earlier. These coworkers provide support and understanding to one another in a time of need, and their shared experience of grief creates a lasting bond where previously none existed.

•**Treat the death as a wake-up call in your life.** Are you living the life you want to be living? If not, the death of a loved one could serve as a reminder that our time on Earth is short and that, whatever we want to achieve, we'd better get started achieving it. If you follow through and make useful life changes, those changes will always be linked in your mind to the deceased loved one, imbuing his life and death with a deep, positive meaning.

Example: A woman quits smoking after her mother dies of lung cancer.

Tributes

•**Become the legacy.** Grieving people often lament that "a part of me died when he did." Maybe so, but consider the flip side as well—part of him lives on in you. Think about what made this person wonderful—what were his very best qualities? One way to find meaning is to make a conscious effort to expand this part of yourself in his honor. *Examples...*

A man always respected his brother for pulling over to offer assistance whenever he saw a motorist stranded by the side of the road. After his brother died, this man began doing the same thing.

A woman's father was a big tipper—he had worked as a waiter to pay his way through college and knew how much waiters and waitresses depend on this money. After his death, she decided to henceforth tip 30 percent in his memory.

• **Find a physical touchstone that shifts your focus to a positive legacy.** Our brains have a negativity bias—they're much better at recalling bad things than good ones. That's one reason why it can be difficult to escape negative emotional triggers when a loved one dies—our brains recall the negative of the death much more readily than the positives of the life. A lasting physical memorial can serve as an enduring reminder of the good of the life. If your mother enjoyed watching the sun set in a local park, finance a park bench with a plaque bearing her name in her favorite spot. If you have a photo of your husband that always makes you smile and recall a happy time, have this photo enlarged, framed and hung in your home.

The memorial even can be something that no one but you will notice or understand.

Example: A woman purchased many sheets of postage stamps featuring a picture of comedian Danny Thomas and put these on all of her mail. Each time she used one, she smiled at the pleasant memory of her deceased father's sense of humor and his story about the day he met Thomas.

Donations

• **Contribute to good works in the deceased's name.** Wealthy families sometimes create nonprofit foundations in the name of the deceased. It's an effective way to create a meaningful legacy—and it's possible on a more modest scale, too. Make donations in honor of your loved one to a cause that he/she cared about…or to a nonprofit working to solve the problem that led to his death. The recipient doesn't even have to be a nonprofit—you might help out local families in need or young people struggling to pay college tuition, if you believe your loved one would have wanted to help these people. The amounts you give don't have to be large if your budget is tight—you could periodically contribute $5 or $10 to charity drives and

think, That's for you, mom. Helping is healing even in small denominations.

Another option is to do good works rather than donate money. Volunteer your time to a cause that the deceased gave his time to during his life…or participate in a project connected to the loved one or his death.

Examples: A man in India whose son died in an auto accident caused by a pothole started filling potholes in his spare time.

• **Reflect on the lives that might have been saved by the loved one's donated organs.** A woman who was devastated by the death of her 17-year-old son hired a house painter a few years later—and made the remarkable discovery that her son's kidney had saved this man's life. (This unlikely fact was confirmed through the transplant center.) Without her son's death, the painter's sons might have grown up without their father—and that was only one of the organs that her son donated.

Most people never get to meet the people saved by a loved one's organ donations, but knowing that these people are out there can bring meaning to the loss. More than half of Americans have signed up to be organ donors. It sometimes is possible to exchange messages with organ recipients through organ-donation programs if both the recipient and the donors' family are interested in doing so.

"Mind Over Matter" Can Reduce Inflammation

George Slavich, PhD, is associate professor of psychiatry and biobehavioral sciences at University of California, Los Angeles, and leader of a study published in *JAMA Psychiatry*.

Cognitive behavior therapy (CBT), which is commonly used to treat anxiety and depression by changing how we think about ourselves and the world, also shows promise for reducing inflammation, which has been linked to heart disease, cancer and other deadly diseases. Benefits lasted six months after treatment.

Are You a Precrastinator?

David A. Rosenbaum, PhD, professor of psychology, University of California, Riverside, quoted at BHG.com.

It is the opposite of procrastination, putting things off—it means doing things more quickly than necessary, such as answering non-urgent e-mails as soon as they arrive. It usually is the result of wanting to get rid of the mental overload of having so much to do. Getting anything finished, even something unimportant, feels like an accomplishment. Precrastinators do get things done—but often at the expense of crafting thoughtful or more useful replies and often in a way that prioritizes less important tasks over ones that take longer to accomplish.

Helpful: Tell yourself to wait a bit before tackling a non-urgent task...spend time gathering information before taking action.

How to Prevent Problems Before They Erupt

Dan Heath, senior fellow at Duke University's CASE Center in Durham, North Carolina, which supports entrepreneurs who are working for social good, and author of *Upstream: The Quest to Solve Problems Before They Happen.* HeathBrothers.com

---

Two men standing by a river notice a child struggling to stay afloat, so they dive in to save him. Then they see a second child in the river and a third. One of the men continues saving children, but the other rushes to shore and runs up the bank. When asked where he's going, he responds that he's headed upstream to stop the guy who is throwing kids into the river.

This parable is used in public health circles to raise an important point—we often become so focused on coping with the problems in front of us that we fail to consider whether we need to look "upstream" and prevent those problems before they occur. That's why some people seek medical care only when they feel horrible rather than focusing on preventive measures that could have kept them healthy. It's also why many homeowners don't install a security system until after they've been robbed.

Here are four strategies to shift from reacting to problems after they occur to avoiding them before they occur...

•**Stop allowing a minor irritation to repeatedly fly under the radar.** People often just endure seemingly trivial annoyances—it doesn't seem worth devoting the time, attention and/or money that would be required to solve them. But that little thing you chronically bicker about with a friend or family member could expand into a major relationship rift. That odd sound your car is making could lead to a breakdown that leaves you stranded and with a costly repair bill. That mild recurring ache could develop into a major medical problem.

Even if a minor problem never escalates, the drip-drip-drip of mild irritation the problem causes over time often means that it would have been wise for you to solve it rather than let it continue.

What to do: The third time you notice a problem, take it as a sign that it isn't going to go away on its own. Consider what's at the root of the problem, and brainstorm potential permanent solutions—even if this approach takes significantly more time than the temporary fix you have been using.

Example: A husband's habit of leaving the hall light on was a recurring source of mild friction with his wife. When he finally took a moment to think about this problem, he realized that he could install a timer switch on the light, permanently removing this irritation.

● **Focus on the problems that almost emerged, not just those that did.** When a major mishap occurs, most people try to figure out what went wrong and how they can prevent it from happening again. But when people have a near miss with a major mishap, they often think, Well, that was a close one, count themselves fortunate and get on with their day. But today's miss could foreshadow tomorrow's disaster—luck might not be on your side next time.

What to do: Take the time to carefully review your near misses, not just your mishaps. Some savvy hospitals have made this a standard practice, holding daily "safety huddles" during which staffers discuss errors almost made in addition to errors actually made. If you don't have a group with which you can discuss your near misses, take a quiet walk and think through whatever nearly went wrong while it's still fresh in your mind. Try to develop a plan to reduce the odds that a near miss actually could come to pass.

Example: If you nearly have an auto accident at a dangerous intersection that you regularly cross, you might want to take a different route to avoid this intersection in the future...or always wait an extra moment at this intersection to confirm that drivers coming the other way see that they have a stop sign.

● **Recognize the power of social norms to spur yourself to take preventive measures.** Most people are terrible at finding time for preventive measures. They know there are things they should be doing to reduce the odds of future problems, but they're so busy dealing with more pressing tasks that these future-focused actions never reach the top of their to-do lists.

Example: Many homeowners chronically fail to apply a pre-emergent crabgrass preventer and fertilizer to their lawns as growing season begins each year, even though doing so could significantly reduce the problems the lawn faces later in the season.

There is a glaring exception to this tendency to neglect the prevention of future problems—dental care. Most Americans brush once or twice almost every day to prevent future dental problems, even on days when they're busy or tired.

Why are people so much more responsible with problem prevention in this area than in most other facets of life? Of course, one of the reasons is that it is drilled into our consciousness that not doing this can be very harmful.

But another key factor is that it has become the social norm to take this preventive step. You wouldn't want to admit to anyone that you don't brush every day—it would make you feel weird and would seem inappropriate to others.

What to do: You can increase the odds that you will take preventive measures in other areas as well—if you can convince yourself that just about everyone else is already doing these things and that it would be embarrassing and inappropriate not to.

For your grass, if you focus on the difference between your lawn and your more diligent neighbor's lawn, you will be more likely to find the time to take preventive measures that produce a more attractive lawn.

● **Assign responsibility for preventing a potential future problem.** It's often obvious whose job it is to fix a problem that has already materialized but much less clear whose job it is to prevent that same problem from happening down the road.

Example: It's the responsibility of the police to catch criminals...but who has the primary responsibility for taking steps that could reduce future crime rates? Is it the police? Politicians? Social workers? Schools? Parents?

What to do: If you have the power to fix a problem, assign yourself responsibility for it. If you are unable to prevent a future problem on your own, try to determine who has the influence and/or skills to do so, then assign yourself responsibility for convincing that person or those people to take on this role.

Example: In 1975, a pair of researchers calculated just how massive of a problem car safety had become for kids—in America, car accidents were the leading cause of death for

Happiness Lies in Change

When 20,000 people were allowed a coin toss to determine whether to make a change in their lives (leaving a job, ending a relationship, etc.), those who were instructed by the coin to quit the status quo were happier six months later. If you're on the fence about a choice, opting for change may be wiser than maintaining the status quo.

Steven Levitt, PhD, is professor of economics at The University of Chicago and leader of a study published in *The Review of Economic Studies.*

young children. These researchers lacked the power to fix this problem, but they thought they knew who could—pediatricians. Pediatricians had the ear of parents and were respected by politicians. The researchers published their findings in the journal *Pediatrics,* where pediatricians would see it, and the use of child car-safety seats increased dramatically. Within 10 years, all 50 states had child-seat laws, and death rates dropped dramatically.

Helpful: Not certain to whom you should assign responsibility for preventing a future problem? Sometimes the best answer is the people who are causing the problem.

Example: A mother and father were frustrated with the nightly battles required to get their kids to bed, so they sat down with those kids and explained why the entire family would benefit if this ongoing issue were resolved. They asked the kids to contribute ideas for preventing future bedtime problems. Their kids helped create a new bedtime system that featured penalties for failing to get to bed on time and rewards for going to bed on time and argument-free. The kids largely adhered to this new system, in part because they had played a role in creating it.

Playing Hard-to-Get Pays Off

Gurit Birnbaum, PhD, associate professor of psychology at Interdisciplinary Center Herzliya, Israel, and leader of a study published in *Journal of Social and Personal Relationships.*

A study of dating behaviors shows that when people present themselves as needing to be won over, prospective partners find them more appealing and invest more effort in the relationship.

Daters: Show initial interest so as not to alienate a potential partner, but keep some cards to yourself. People are less likely to desire what they already have. Building a connection gradually creates a sense of anticipation and a desire to learn more about a potential partner.

Four Hidden Marriage Killers

Michele Weiner-Davis, LCSW, founder of The Divorce Busting Center in Boulder, Colorado. She is a TEDx speaker and best-selling author of eight books including *Healing from Infidelity...The Sex-Starved Marriage...*and *Divorce Busting.* DivorceBusting.com

You're still angry about that? It isn't always a big, obvious misstep such as infidelity or dishonesty that derails a marriage. Some relationships are undone by an event so small or distant that one partner is befuddled about why the other considers it a big deal. Other marriages fail because of misunderstandings or miscommunications that slowly and steadily undermine the partnership. Recently, an added element has exposed how vulnerable many marriages are to stressful irritations. Lawyers say there has been a spike in divorce requests because couples have spent much more time together as they have sheltered in place and because they have faced greater financial challenges.

Here are four seemingly small things that can bring a relationship crashing down...

The Long-Ago Misstep

A wife asked her husband to skip a business trip and stay home to care for her when she felt very sick. He went anyway. Decades later that decision still haunted the relationship. The wife couldn't get past it because, to her, the long-ago business trip was just one example of a larger pattern—she felt her husband was never there for her when she needed him. The event triggered in her a need to constantly monitor her husband's behavior for further evidence that he would disappoint her.

Although there were times throughout their marriage when he took her feelings into consideration, the wife failed to notice these exceptions.

This wife wasn't intentionally being unfair to her husband—she truly believed he kept letting her down. But her belief had less to do with her husband's behavior than it did with human psychology—people tend to seize on evidence that supports their existing beliefs and ignore evidence that refutes it.

What to do: If your partner continually accuses you of a pattern of misbehavior that you do not believe exists, set aside your defensiveness for the sake of the relationship and apologize. Whether or not the accusation is warranted, your partner believes it is. Your relationship will not escape the cycle of blame and defensiveness unless you express contrition and genuine empathy for the pain your partner is feeling. It helps to remember that your partner's pain is real even if the pattern you're being accused of is not. Promise to work hard at correcting the pattern, then go above and beyond to do so. Your promise of change followed by clear evidence of new behavior could convince your partner that a new and positive pattern has begun.

You might be thinking, That's not fair—why should I apologize for something I didn't do? No, it isn't fair. But you have to make a choice—would you rather be right or be happy?

If you are the one who sees a problematic pattern that your partner denies, watch carefully for counterexamples that suggest the pattern is less clear-cut than you believe. Keep a list of these counterexamples to balance the mental list you likely already keep of examples that support the pattern, and then be open to letting go of your negative belief.

Giving Love the Way You Want It

You probably learned the golden rule as a child—treat others as you would want to be treated yourself. Turns out, that's not always good advice for couples.

When people show love for their partners, they tend to express their love in the way that they like to receive love. But the things that make your partner feel loved probably are very different from the things that make you feel loved. Sometimes this is because of gender differences—many women feel most loved when they have deep, meaningful conversations with their partners...while many men feel most loved when they are physically intimate with their partners. But not everyone falls into these gender roles.

There are five broad ways in which people give and receive love to partners, sometimes called "love languages." Some people feel most loved when their partner spends quality one-on-one time with them, doing things together or just listening closely to what they say...or when the couple has sex. Other people feel closest when the partner does things to lighten their load...or provides encouraging words...or gives thoughtful gifts.

When partners speak different love languages, it can leave both of them feeling unloved even when both are genuinely trying to express their love.

What to do: If you have been with your partner for many years, you probably already know which of the five love languages he/she most values. If you don't, it's time to ask. Then express love to your partner this way, no matter your personal preference. Meanwhile, confirm that your partner understands what makes you feel truly loved. Don't get angry if your partner occasionally reverts to showing you love the way that he likes to receive love—it takes time to break habits. When you receive your partner's preferred type of love, remind yourself that your partner is showing you love but in his preferred way.

Seeking Agreement

Many people believe it must be a positive thing for partners to always seek to be on the same page on any given topic. Actually, that thinking can devastate a relationship.

It's not realistic to expect two people to be in agreement on everything, and when couples treat total agreement as a goal, they tend to see their inevitable disagreements as a serious problem—a sign that they're not really right for each other. These problems are exacerbated when one partner squelches disagreements by insisting that the other partner must fall into line and agree.

Example: A man refused to accept that his wife could have different opinions than his own regarding virtually anything, including the state of their marriage. When she suggested that they had begun to drift apart following a relocation to Chicago, he said, "You don't really believe that, right?"

What to do: Remain open to the possibility that two people can have completely different opinions without either of them being wrong. Make it your goal to listen to and understand your partner and to treat her point of view with respect, even if you do not fully agree. Consider differences of opinion as opportunities for engaging in debate or for learning something about your partner—not as arguments or signs of incompatibility.

Feeling Out of Focus

"I love you…but I'm no longer in love with you." When someone says these words, it means that he no longer feels close to his partner but can't point to any big, dramatic reason why. His partner hasn't made any major missteps…the spark is simply gone.

The partner's focus usually is at the root of these feelings. At the beginning of the relationship, you felt like you were your partner's primary focus…but over the years, the focus has shifted to career, kids or other interests. That has left one or both feeling disconnected from the other and wondering, *Is this how I want to spend the rest of my life?*

What to do: Think back to the beginning of your relationship, when you felt passion for each other. What, specifically, did you and your partner do together that made you feel like you were each other's focus? Maybe you had special meals together…or took long walks where you discussed art and movies.

Do those things again, at least once a week. The activities that made a couple feel focused on each other in the past often will do so again in the present. Schedule this together time in advance if life has become too busy to depend on it happening naturally.

Meanwhile, stop keeping score. A partner who feels he is no longer the other's focus probably has been blaming that partner for the lack of closeness for some time. Your feelings of distance are not something that your partner did to you—it's perfectly normal for the passion and focus that existed early in a relationship to be replaced by routine and responsibility as the years pass. If you want that passion and focus back, don't allow your sense of having been hurt or rejected prevent you from doing something positive such as scheduling meaningful time together.

Full House: How to Make It Work

Jane Adams, PhD, a social psychologist based in Seattle who specializes in parent/adult child relationships. She is author of *I'm Still Your Mother: How to Get Along with Your Grown-Up Children for the Rest of Your Life.* JaneAdams.com

Your job was to raise your children and send them off into the world…but what if they come back? As of 2016, about 15 percent of 25-to-35-year-olds lived with their parents, a sharp increase from the

10 percent who did so in 2000, according to a study by Pew Research Center. And the numbers continue to rise, especially with the recent pandemic.

Whether kids are returning home for economic reasons or simply because they are having a hard time cutting the cord, the key is to make the situation successful for all involved. Having a history of getting along is no guarantee that things will go smoothly when adult children move back in. Parent/child relationships change when children become adults (and adults get used to living in their "empty nest"), and it's important to set new ground rules that respect the needs of all involved.

How to create a harmonious home if your adult child asks to move back in…

Setting the Stage for a Successful Return

•**Discuss the potential return with your spouse before responding to the adult child.** When an adult child asks to move back in, the correct reply isn't "yes" or "no"—it's "I'll discuss it with your father/mother."

This is too big of a decision to make without reaching agreement as a couple. Don't assume that you and your partner will be on the same page—it's very common for married people to have different reactions and concerns, in part due to the different roles partners play in the household.

Example: The parent who tends to do most of the housework might react with concern that he/she will have to pick up after this adult child if he moves back in. Or the parent who handles the family finances might be concerned about whether the child's return will affect the parents' retirement plans. If either partner feels forced into this new living arrangement, the household's relationship stresses will rise and things are unlikely to go smoothly. Additionally, it is important to discuss whether this is a healthy choice for the child. Are there any concerns that your adult child is lacking in ambition or afraid to stand on his own two feet?

Often, parental concerns can be overcome by making the child's return contingent on certain agreements—from time-frame goals to monetary concessions (more on these later). But this must be discussed as a couple before the child is given an answer. Be sure to provide a date for a response so that you don't leave your child hanging.

•**Negotiate a set of house rules as you would with any new roommate.** Worried about getting your sleep? A rule limiting noise after 10 pm could be the solution. Worried that the adult child will eat everything in your fridge? There could be a rule that the returning child buys and labels her own food or contributes a certain amount of money to the food budget.

The key is to create these rules together with the adult child—but you have the right to lead the conversation. It's preferable if the rules apply equally to all members of the household. When parents simply impose a set of rules on an adult child, it reinforces the uneven parent/minor child dynamic of the past, which stands in the way of building a successful relationship as adults. If you're thinking, *It's my house and I have every right to set the rules*, you're absolutely correct—you do have that right. But if you make the decision not to take excessive advantage of that right, everyone will benefit. The adult child who is handed a list of rules is likely to feel disrespected and even might respond by reverting to teenager-esque behavior.

Instead, have a sit-down meeting where parents and the adult child propose and discuss potential house rules. Explain why each rule you propose is important to you, then open the rule up for honest discussion. Be willing to modify your proposed rules if the adult child voices valid concerns about them.

Example: You propose a rule that family members must each pick one laundry day per week, so that everyone has a chance to use the washer/dryer. The child points out that sometimes he has to do laundry more often because he works in health care, a reasonable objection. Perhaps the modified rule could be that laundry outside of your designated day cannot go in the wash until after the other person's laundry is done.

Helpful: Check out sample roommate agreement forms. They are free and available from RocketLawyer.com and Nolo.com.

Five Key Topics

There are five topics that need to be discussed and agreed to when parents and their adult children work through the details of the child's return…

• **Money.** If the child is moving in to save money…pay down student debt…or survive a spell of unemployment, it might not be practical to request market-rate rent. Still, adult children who live at home should contribute to the household, even if it's a token amount such as $25 a week.

Exception: If money is extremely tight for the child, you could give him the option of contributing a certain number of hours each week toward household chores in lieu of rent.

Money is especially likely to become a point of contention if an adult child pays very low (or no) rent but splurges on vacations, dinners out with friends and/or excessive clothes. Parents can offer assistance with setting budgets. As time goes on, parents can request an increase in rent if it appears the child is capable of paying more without hardship. It is not appropriate to criticize his spending or demand that it stop. He is an adult who has a right to make his own financial decisions—even if you don't agree with those decisions. But the parents have a right to tell the child he must move out if their goodwill is being abused.

• **Guests.** It is perfectly reasonable for an adult child to have friends over—including romantic friends. But it's also perfectly reasonable for parents to feel a bit uncomfortable about having adult strangers in their house. The best compromise often is to allow guests but set limits. These might include constraining the hours when guests can visit…the days when they can visit (not on weeknights, for example)…the number of days per week/month when guests can visit…and/or that

advance notice be provided when guests will visit. It's certainly reasonable to set a limit on how often romantic friends can sleep over—or even if they can sleep in the same room if it runs counter to your religious or moral beliefs. It's one thing to let your child move back in, but another thing entirely to have his partner virtually living in your home.

• **Curfews.** It is not appropriate to set a curfew for an adult child. If your adult child were living somewhere else, you wouldn't even know she was out late. Some parents struggle with this, lying awake at night worried about the adult child's safety until they finally hear the door open in the wee hours.

It's reasonable to request a text message on nights that she'll be out later than expected. Try presenting this request as a courtesy the adult child could do for you, not an obligation.

Example: "You have every right to stay out late. It's just hard for a parent to get out of that worrying mode, even when their kids are grown. A quick text would really help me."

• **Personal spaces.** Your adult child's room must be treated as his private space. Do not enter the room without permission unless there's some emergency. Do not insist that the child keep his room tidy—that's not your business (within reason, of course…you don't want old food attracting bugs). But you can insist that shared spaces such as bathrooms be kept to your standard of cleanliness. The adult child also should understand that he will be expected to clean up after himself and do his own laundry.

• **Move-out date.** Consider establishing a tentative end date for the child's stay before she moves in.

Examples: Is the child moving in to save money while in grad school? Perhaps the move-out date could be within a few months of graduation. Are you expecting to retire, sell the home and relocate? Share the anticipated sale date with the adult child.

Having a move-out date can decrease the odds of misunderstandings…improve the adult child's motivation to search for a job or pay down debt...and help parents reassure themselves that this is a temporary situation.

Consider the Upside

Having an adult child move back in might feel like a setback—but for many families, it actually turns out very well. This is a chance to build a new relationship with a loved one who previously was your responsibility but who now is something much closer to a peer. You might enjoy having a drink together or trying a new hobby.

Moving back might mean that the adult child will be partially dependent on you longer than expected...but it also means that you can be dependent on this adult child in ways that otherwise might not be possible.

Examples: If you go out of town, he can water the plants and take care of your dog. If you need a ride to the airport, she might drive you.

Remind yourself—and your adult child—that it's perfectly normal for families to be interdependent on each other. Right now, that means you're providing your child with a place to live...but later it might mean that the child is there to help you.

Boost Your Spirits by Helping Others

Bottom Line Personal

Discover rewarding opportunities for volunteering from home. CreatetheGood. AARP.org...VolunteerMatch.org.

Specialized opportunities: Counsel people in crisis—CrisisTextLine.org/become-a-volunteer. Record audiobooks—Librivox.org. Write letters to seniors—LoveForOurElders. org. Transcribe historical documents for the Smithsonian—Transcription.si.edu.

Spread the Love!

Personality and Individual Differences

Studies show that people who have frequent "micro-moments" of connection—even those as fleeting as a kind interaction with a neighbor—tend to have better psychological well-being than those who have fewer.

Helpful: Smartphone reminders may lead to greater awareness of such positive interactions.

Myths Many Older Women Believe About Alcohol Consumption

Women ages 50 to 69 told researchers that their drinking was fine as long as they remained in control, whether or not that amount was above health guidelines. Some also said that positive behaviors, such as exercise, would counteract the effects of alcohol intake—although scientists say that is not true. Current guidelines recommend no more than one drink a day for women.

Study by researchers at Edith Cowan University, Perth, Australia, published in *Sociology of Health & Illness.*

Solve a Recurring Sleep Problem With a Sleep Journal

University of California, *Berkeley Wellness Letter.*

Write down what time you get into bed, how long it takes to fall asleep, when you awaken during the night and when you wake up for the next day and get out of bed. Note how easily you wake up in the morning...the time and length of any daytime naps...sleep disruptions caused by pain, worry, noise or other factors…how rested and tired you feel after awakening…what caffeinated beverages you consume…your tobacco and alcohol use…and any drugs you take. Share your sleep log with your doctor to discuss ways to make nighttime more restful and restorative.

Alcohol-Related Deaths Have Doubled

Study by researchers at Duke University Medical Center, Durham, North Carolina, published in *Alcoholism: Clinical and Experimental Research.*

Alcohol-related deaths doubled between 1999 and 2017 (latest data available). In 2017, about 72,550 people died in the US from liver disease and alcohol-related illnesses. That was more than the 70,000 drug-overdose deaths the same year. Men died from alcohol-related causes more often than women, but the largest increase in deaths was found in white women.

Why Some People Feel Stress More Intensely Than Others

Diego Pizzagalli, PhD, director, Center for Depression, Anxiety and Stress Research and professor of psychiatry, McLean Hospital/Harvard Medical School, Belmont, Massachusetts. He is a coauthor of the study titled, "Distinct Trajectories of Cortisol Response to Prolonged Acute Stress Are Linked to Affective Responses and Hippocampal Gray Matter Volume in Healthy Females," published in *The Journal of Neuroscience.*

Imagine a class full of college students who are about to start their final exam. Some are fairly relaxed…others are nervous but still able to focus…and some are so stressed that they're unable to perform effectively.

What causes these differences has been unclear…until now.

It makes sense that differences in the amount of the stress hormone cortisol a person releases in response to a stressful experience can determine how distressed that person actually feels.

But here's the surprise: Too little cortisol may be just as bad as too much, according to a recent study published in *The Journal of Neuroscience.*

Background: Most stress research in humans has involved inducing a short period of stress and classifying participants as either responders or nonresponders, based on the level of the cortisol in their saliva. In these studies, the average feelings of stress felt by participants in both groups have typically been similar.

Study details: Researchers modified existing lab procedures and induced stress for more than one hour in 79 healthy women. These women were given the Maastricht Acute Stress Test, a test aimed at activating the human stress system by combining physical stress (cold-induced pain) with the stress of being evaluated while doing mental arithmetic tasks.

Surprising: The participants who released either very high or very low amounts of cortisol over time reported feeling more stressed than those who released a moderate amount of cortisol. The high and low responders also had less gray matter in the hippocampus—a brain structure with a large number of cortisol receptors that regulate the stress response—than the moderate responders.

Related result: Another recent study found that individuals with a history of major depression showed reduced cortisol release and higher self-reported feelings of stress. According to Dr. Diego Pizzagalli, director of the Center for Depression, Anxiety and Stress at McLean Hospital/Harvard Medical School and a coauthor of both studies, "This type of data will help us identify individuals at risk for first onset and recurrence of depression."

Bottom line: Experiencing stress and feeling stressed are not the same. Although the link should be investigated further, feelings of stress may be associated with the amount of cortisol you release in response to a stressor or with the amount of gray matter in your hippocampus. These factors are not within your control, but understanding which people are more susceptible to feeling stress or depression—and why—is a step in the right direction toward providing more effective strategies for coping with stress as well as better treatment for those with depression.

7 Tools to Help You Through the Rough Patches

Bruce Feiler, who interviewed hundreds of people in all 50 states and a range of fields—from politics to business to the performing arts—about their life transitions for his most recent book, *Life Is in the Transitions: Mastering Change at Any Age.* His other books include *Walking the Bible* and *Council of Dads,* which was adapted into a series on NBC. BruceFeiler.com

The pandemic time span has been loaded with major transitions for just about everybody. Health threats emerged, jobs were lost, daily routines were altered, and new priorities and plans arose. And although it's rare for the entire planet to undergo a collective life-altering transition, individuals experience major transitions with surprising regularity—few people have one job, one mate and one home for their entire lives. The typical American will experience three to five life-altering disruptions, according to author Bruce Feiler's research, and each will leave him/her unsettled for an average of nearly five years.

Waiting until things "get back to normal" isn't the answer—life rarely returns to the way it was previously. Instead, we must improve our ability to manage life transitions. We asked Feiler to share the seven tools he has uncovered for coping with transitions, based on his interviews with hundreds of people in all 50 states who successfully reinvented their careers, personal lives or other aspects of themselves. *The following tools can be employed in any order. It's best to draw upon as many as possible…*

•**Accept that the transition is happening—and that it will be emotional.** It's natural to resist transitions, even those that are voluntary. We cling to our former lives because that feels safe and comfortable while transitions seem daunting and uncertain.

To accept a transition, we must accept the emotions that it stirs up—even if our natural response to challenges is to push feelings aside—and roll up our sleeves and get to work. Such emotions typically include fear, sadness and/or shame. Guilt and anger also are common.

Some people find that journaling about their emotions helps. Follow-up research from a landmark study done in 1986 at University of Texas at Austin found that 27 percent of people laid off from their jobs who wrote about their thoughts and feelings found new jobs within three months, compared with 5 percent of those who didn't journal.

Whether you journal or not, you should acknowledge what you're feeling and use hard work as a way to overcome these emotions, not as an excuse to ignore them.

Example: Army interrogator Eric Maddox felt fear when he was sent to Iraq—he was trained in Mandarin, not Farsi, and felt ill-equipped for the assignment. Rather than ignore his fear, he told himself, I can turn away because I am scared, or I can go to work and learn how to develop trust in this part of the world through an interpreter. Maddox's interrogations helped track down Saddam Hussein.

•**Create a ritual or tribute to mark the transition.** When people experience a major transition, they often stage some sort of event or activity to commemorate the change. Negative events need closure, while positive events, such as a child's marriage or a new job or relocation, need celebration and acknowledgment to mark the new beginning. These "rituals" take many forms—a memorial service where friends and family members mourn the past or a party to celebrate the future…a good-bye letter written to a deceased partner or former life…a name change, such as a return to a maiden name…cleaning out a home…shaving off a beard or switching to a new hair style…a once-in-a-lifetime activity, such as skydiving…or something else entirely.

A ritual is something you can take control over at a time when much of life feels outside of your control. It also reinforces to you—and to your friends and family—that you are not going back to your old life.

• **Shed old mind-sets, routines, possessions…and even dreams.** To make room for the new self, we must leave behind parts of our former self—possibly even parts that we value. A heart problem might mean that we must give up some favorite foods. A layoff might mean that we have to give up the dream house we were planning. A divorce might mean that we must give up some of the comfortable daily habits we've developed.

It helps to remember that this is a great opportunity to clear away parts of yourself that were not serving you well—decluttering your life to make room for the rewarding life you will create.

Example: When Loretta Parham's daughter died in a car crash, Parham was left to raise her two granddaughters. She discovered that to be a good parent, she had to give up being an indulgent grandparent, a role that she loved. It turned out that, despite the loss of her daughter, the role of parent was tremendously rewarding.

• **Find a creative outlet.** People who find time for a new creative endeavor, such as painting, cooking, dancing or writing, often discover that this helps with their transition. It's more than just a diversion from the long slog and mental strain of a life transition—new creative activities also encourage us to believe that we have it within us to be more than we previously were.

If we can begin baking delicious bread or painting beautiful landscapes, it seems much more plausible that we also can find a new job or new relationship.

Example: Evan Walker-Wells was a student at Yale when he was diagnosed with stage 4 non-Hodgkin's lymphoma. The diagnosis forced him to leave school for six months of chemotherapy and leave behind his youthful sense that he was free to do whatever he wanted. He taught himself to cook and play guitar during this time—he was someone who had the capacity and drive to continue learning and growing under any circumstances. He was recently in his second year at Yale Law School.

• **Seek support from others.** It's probably no surprise that aid from other people is among the most powerful tools to help us through challenging transitions. What is surprising is that different people tend to crave very different types of support—and most of us are not very good at obtaining the type we prefer.

Many people crave comfort during times of transition and so welcome supportive feedback such as, "I love you" or "You can do it." But others want a nudge in the right direction—"I love you, but maybe you should try this." And a smaller percentage want a proverbial kick in the backside—they yearn for someone to say, "Get over yourself—you've had your pity party, now get back to work." People may want different forms of support from different people—a nudge or kick in the rear from a mentor, perhaps, but comfort from a spouse.

The trouble is, the people we go to for support often fail to give us the type we prefer—they give us what they think we need… or what they would want if they were in our position, leaving us frustrated and perhaps deterring us from seeking outside support again.

Solution: Tell people which type of support you hope to obtain and which you don't want…and/or seek support from people who show a tendency to provide specifically what you need.

• **Publicly unveil your new self.** At some point during your transition, a sense of normalcy will return to your life. That's when it's time to make a public statement that you've made a life transition. Tell your friends you're ready to date again…throw a housewarming party for your new home…or update your LinkedIn page to show that you've launched a new career. If the "ritual" described earlier commemorated the end of your old life, this unveiling celebrates your new normal.

Helpful: One way to launch a "new self" is to provide assistance to someone else. Volunteer with a nonprofit, or help a friend in need.

• **Rewrite the story you tell yourself about your life.** When people are in the midst of transitions, they usually think of themselves in terms of what they used to be—I was happily married or I was a successful professional. Rewrite this into a story of overcoming obstacles or of rebirth—I used to be that. I went through a life change. Now I am this.

Example: Chris Waddell, a medal-winning Paralympian, set out to be the first paraplegic to climb 19,000-foot Mount Kilimanjaro—but just 100 feet from the summit, the boulders were too large for his arm-powered four-wheel mountain bike to pass. The other members of the expedition carried him to the summit. Waddell was initially crushed by what he viewed as a failure until he rewrote the story from *I set out to climb a mountain unassisted but failed*…to *Nobody climbs a mountain alone.*

Change Your Mind About How to Change Minds

Jonah Berger, PhD, professor of marketing at The Wharton School of The University of Pennsylvania. He is author of *The Catalyst: How to Change Anyone's Mind.* JonahBerger.com

G o ahead—prod people into accepting your point of view…bury them with evidence that supports your posi-

tion…and carefully recount why a rethink is in their own best interest. Despite your best efforts, much of the time you'll accomplish nothing.

Whether you're trying to convince your spouse to change his/her eating habits or convince consumers to buy a new product, the tactics traditionally employed to change minds usually are ineffective. In fact, sometimes these efforts accidentally push people to dig in their heels even further. Consider all the times you've felt insulted by a manipulative advertisement…or rolled your eyes at political views voiced by someone on the other side of the aisle.

The secret of successfully changing minds often lies not in making a persuasive case but rather in removing the hidden barriers that prevent people from modifying their views. *Three of the biggest barriers and how to overcome them…*

When Pushed, People Push Back

When you try to persuade people of something, their natural reaction is to push back in an attempt to reassure themselves that they remain in control of their own opinions. These people might focus on perceived shortcomings in your argument or voice skepticism about the veracity of your facts, but this may have little to do with the merits of your case and everything to do with the threat that your attempt to convince them poses to their sense of freedom and self-control.

What to do: Rather than try to convince people of what you believe, use strategies that encourage them to convince themselves—people are far more likely to accept ideas that seem to spring from their own minds. *Among the ways to do this…*

• **Provide a carefully selected range of choices.** Offer several options that are all acceptable to you, then let the person you are trying to win over make the final selection from among these.

Example: A wife is bored with the Italian restaurant her husband chooses almost every time the couple eats out. Before their next date night, she asks if he would rather try a Mexican restaurant or a Thai restaurant or a different Italian restaurant. The husband retains control over the final decision, so there's a good chance he won't rebel against his wife's attempt to steer him away from his actual preference.

• **Warn the person that someone is trying to manipulate him/her.** This turns people's natural push-back tendencies to your advantage.

Example: A Florida antismoking campaign found success by warning teens that the tobacco industry was trying to manipulate them with its ads. Rather than push back against the antismoking campaign, as teens tend to do, they pushed back against the tobacco companies and the state's smoking rates among teens declined.

• **Ask questions rather than make challenging statements.** If you suspect that the person already knows he/she is in the wrong, don't tell him this—ask a question that encourages him to say or think it.

Example: The owner of a test-prep company who saw that many would-be business school students weren't putting sufficient hours into studying for the GMATs asked her class, "Why are you here? What's your goal?" The answer, of course, was to get into a top business school. She told the students that 250,000 people take the GMATs every year, and the top 20 MBA programs accept around 10,000 total—only 4 percent make the cut. She then asked how many hours they thought they needed to study not just to do well but to land safely in that top 4 percent.

• **Call attention to a gap between what someone is saying and what the person is doing.** Quote this person's own words back to him—people tend to agree with what they themselves have said.

Example: Your spouse dislikes a local company but does business with it anyway because of its low prices. Rather than say you don't want to work with the company, you could say, "You know, I think you were right when you said, 'These people don't respect their customers.'"

People Stick to Status Quo

One big reason that it's hard to get people to change their minds is that people don't like to change. Most people will go on buying the same brands, voting for the same political party and driving the same route to work rather than investigate other options unless it becomes painfully obvious that their initial selection is lacking. Economists estimate that the potential upside of taking action must be around 2.5 times the potential downside before the average person will make a move.

What to do: Try one of these approaches to stress the benefits of making a change...

• **Expose the hidden costs of not changing.** The costs of change often are more obvious than the costs of keeping things as they are—when we try something new, we often have to learn something new or buy something new, for example. But that doesn't mean the current state of affairs actually has lower costs. Perhaps people have grown so used to the way things are that they no longer notice its costs...or perhaps these costs are hidden because they're not coming out of people's pockets.

Example: Your spouse resists learning how to use a new piece of time-saving consumer technology because he believes his current way of doing things works just fine. Work out how much time he would save whenever he uses the technology, and multiply that by the number of times he would use it each year. If it saves just one minute every day, that's more than six hours a year. Tell him that if saving six hours of effort isn't important to him, then he shouldn't mind spending six hours that weekend doing chores that would normally fall to you.

• **Reframe a change as a return to the way things used to be.** This can overcome people's aversion to doing things that seem new and different.

Example: A husband doesn't want to downsize from a house to an apartment in retirement. His wife could frame the move as a return to the way things were before their first child was born, when they shared a small apartment in the city.

•**Preserve treasured memories.** Sometimes people resist change even when they know that the way things are is less than ideal because it reminds them of earlier, better times. Search for a way to preserve these positive memories yet still change.

Example: A mother doesn't want to transform a child's room into a home gym even though the child is grown and living elsewhere. She could take photos of the child's room, and hang these on the walls of the new exercise room. The photos can preserve the memories, especially since the room will be visited much more often now that it has a new purpose.

People Balk at Extreme Change

A common lament in our politically divided society is that we would have an easier time coming together as a country if everyone would take the time to listen to the opinions of their political opponents, rather than exclusively to media outlets and social media slanted toward the positions they already hold. A 2018 study by a Duke University sociology professor put that theory to the test. For one month, more than 1,500 politically partisan Twitter users read messages expressing views from people on the other side of the aisle.

Results: Republican participants became more conservative, and Democrats became more liberal. Not only had exposure to the other side's opinions not won them over, it had pushed them further away.

The problem isn't that people won't consider ideas different from their own—it's that they won't consider ideas vastly different from their own, at least not with their firmly held beliefs.

What to do: Seek modest progress, not massive shifts, when trying to change minds.

Had that Duke study asked partisans to follow moderate Twitter messages, rather than messages from the other side of the aisle, it might have succeeded in bringing its participants a little closer. View modest change as the first stepping stone on a path to greater change.

Example: An employee is tasked with cutting costs on office supplies, but his boss is reluctant to drop the office's very reliable long-term supplier. The employee convinces the boss to try a new supplier for one small order of supplies. Once the order has arrived quickly and at a lower cost, the employee suggests more and bigger orders from the new supplier.

The Right Way to Help People Who Ask for Your Help

Ellen Van Oosten, PhD, executive coach and co-author of *Helping People Change: Coaching with Compassion for Lifelong Learning and Growth.* She is associate professor at Weatherhead School of Management at Case Western Reserve University, Cleveland, and cofounder of the Coaching Research Lab there. Weatherhead.Case.edu

---

D o you know someone who wants to make a change and is turning to you for help? Most of us have good intentions to help others but go about doing so in the wrong way. Here are four key strategies for helping people—family members, friends or coworkers—achieve their dreams…

Wait for a Coachable Moment

It's natural to want to help people overcome behaviors that are preventing them from achieving their goals and living their best lives. You may notice things they do that are self-sabotaging or misguided—and jump right in with advice. But they may not want your advice. People change their behavior when they want to, not when you want them to.

Problem: Too often we impose our own values and desires on others in an attempt to "fix" them. Your loved one may go along with you out of obligation or respect—if the individual responds at all—but not from inner motivation. As a result, he/she will be unlikely to persist with the effort.

Better: Before you start offering advice, stop and ask the person, "How can I help you now?" If you are invited to proceed, the person will be much more receptive to what you have to say. Seize on these moments when he is willing and able to consider an idea or information that could lead to a shift in his thinking. You could ask questions such as, "Can I share an idea with you?" or "Would you like to know what I am observing?" You need to choose the right time to broach the subject—when the person is willing to listen—and you can plant seeds to help him imagine a desired future and that may help him see how and why he may need to change his behavior. Driven by their own personal reasons for change, people are more likely to adjust their actions and perspectives. Igniting that passion for a long-desired goal—to open a business…lose weight…run in a marathon…leave an abusive relationship—helps people draw energy that will sustain their efforts to change even when the going gets rough.

Be an Active Listener

To facilitate change, you need to first understand what is happening with the individual. Don't assume that you know what another person is feeling or thinking. Make your loved one feel supported by actively listening. Active listening is an art and skill that can be developed by listening deeply with thoughtful attention and positive intention. It takes some effort to be truly focused on the other person and not just be waiting for your turn to speak again. *Here's how to do it…*

TIP #1: **Aim to speak 20 percent of the time,** and allow the person you're talking with to speak 80 percent of the time.

TIP #2: **Remember the acronym WAIT, which stands for "Why Am I Talking?"** to keep the focus on the person you're trying to coach instead of yourself. If you catch yourself telling stories about yourself, stop and shift back to the other person.

TIP #3: **Don't interrupt, challenge or check your phone or computer screen while listening.** Sit near the person speaking to you…give him your full attention…repeat back what is said to you.

Example: Greg, a plastic surgeon, felt dissatisfied with his life. Working 70 to 80 hours a week, he secretly knew he lacked work-life balance, but he wasn't doing anything about it. His coach asked him, "What are things you like about your life?"…"What things would you like to have more time to do?"…"If you could live anywhere, where would you live?"…"What would your ideal job look like?"

Hearing himself answer these questions out loud, a light switched on for Greg. He realized that he wanted to move back to his hometown in Florida to be closer to family and friends, and he wanted to work fewer hours. Soon, he found a new position in Florida and was working part-time and seeing more of his loved ones.

Uncover the Person's True Needs and Desires

As a coach, it's hard to help if you don't know what challenges someone is facing or what drives that person to succeed.

Example: Find out what matters to a friend or family member by asking him to complete an open-ended statement such as, "An ideal day for me is when…" or, "I wish you knew…" *An open-ended sentence may draw responses such as…*

"I would love to have a family dinner once a week."

"I wish you knew how isolated I have felt since my husband died."

Armed with this new information, you can tailor your strategies and be more supportive.

Awaken Positive Emotions

Research at the Coaching Research Lab shows that the key to effective coaching is awakening positive emotions or feelings that help us move forward in life. We call this the Positive Emotional Attractor (PEA). The PEA is anchored in the parasympathetic nervous system, which is where feelings of joy, hope, optimism and engagement are produced. In contrast, the Negative Emotional Attractor (NEA) is linked to the sympathetic nervous system, which is associated with negativity, anger, defensiveness, anxiety and fear. We move between these two states constantly and subconsciously. We need the stress of the NEA to finish projects, juggle multiple demands and stay on task. But the PEA allows us to think creatively, imagine possibilities, demonstrate empathy for others and build relationships. The PEA activates our feelings of hope and helps us move from one step to another—which is why it is so important to awaken it.

Extensive research conducted by our colleagues has shown that spending even 30 minutes talking with someone about a dream, core values or personal vision activates areas of the brain associated with the parasympathetic nervous system—in other words, it ignites positive action and passion.

Try statements or questions that awaken positive emotions in the person you're trying to help. If you won the lottery, how would it affect your life and your work?...If your life were perfect in 10 years, what would it look like? Although these questions seem broad, they can help people work though specific challenges that involve everything from career decisions (Would I be happier in a different job?) to lifestyle issues (Is it time to downsize?).

Avoid negative questions that put people on the defensive like, *Are you keeping up with all of your assignments? Why haven't you put in for a promotion? Why don't you get rid of all this stuff in your cabinets?*

By focusing on supporting, rather than leading or judging, the person you are trying to help, you will be acting out of compassion, helping to ignite the spark of positive change in friends' and family members' lives and encouraging strategies for achieving that change.

Best Ways to Regulate Your Emotions

Roundup of therapists quoted at Self.com.

"Regulating" emotions requires experiencing them head on, not ignoring or avoiding them, which is unhealthy and counterproductive. Getting better at regulating your emotions can mean that you will be less likely to indulge bad habits. Plus, you'll just feel better about yourself in the long run.

Identify your "numbing" behaviors: Do you retreat into video games? TV? After a binge, you may only feel worse. Name what you're feeling: Identifying a negative emotion—without judgment—is the first step toward regulating it.

Ask what the feeling is telling you: What action should you take?

Mindfully express the emotion: Do it however works for you—talk to a friend, write in a journal or have a good cry.

Focus on physical sensations: Take a shower, exercise or get outdoors.

How to Get Beyond Small Talk

Dan Ariely, PhD, the James B. Duke Professor of Psychology and Behavioral Economics at Duke University in Durham, North Carolina, writing in *The Wall Street Journal*.

If the subject matter of your happy hours and other friends and family get-togethers never seems to get any deeper than the weather, it isn't because your colleagues are boring—they likely crave meaningful conversation as much as you do but feel hindered by social convention. Consider using a set of conversation-starter questions such as, "If you had to change one big decision you have made, what would it be?" At a loss for such prompts? Look up online Irrational Labs "No Small Talk" cards and the list of 36 "closeness-generating" questions from psychologist Arthur Aron.

How Not to Be Annoyed by People Who Annoy You

Michele Weiner-Davis, LCSW, founder of The Divorce Busting Center in Boulder, Colorado. She is a TEDx speaker and best-selling author of eight books, including *Healing from Infidelity, The Sex-Starved Marriage* and *Divorce Busting*. DivorceBusting.com

My mother was an amazingly wise, renowned therapist who taught me many important life lessons but none more important than the one encapsulated in the words of a button she gave me: "Never try to teach a cow to sing. It doesn't work, and it annoys the cow."

We all know that cows won't sing. They moo. And because we know this, we allow cows to be cows, which, in turn, avoids irritating them and disappointing ourselves.

Yet, when it comes to our human counterparts, we are not nearly as realistic. No matter how consistently our loved ones moo, we're surprised, disappointed and critical when they aren't singing instead. It makes us miserable. And therein lies the magic formula for happiness in life—let cows be cows.

Not Surprised, Yet Disappointed

In many ways, the people in our lives are fairly predictable. They are who they are. Their behaviors—both desirable and undesirable—show up like clockwork. Your husband's voracious sexual appetite rarely seems to coincide with your interest in being connected physically. Except for wishing

you a happy birthday each year, your sister typically relies on you to initiate contact with her. Your best friend consistently shows up 30 minutes late for everything you plan together. Your relatives get into heated arguments at all family gatherings.

In short, we are well aware of our loved ones' quirks and idiosyncrasies. We know what to expect. Nevertheless, we are oddly taken aback each time a friend or family member moos. We're put off. We're annoyed. We're disappointed.

That's when our little inner voices—the ones that narrate our lives—go on overload. Even after years of experiencing predictable patterns in behavior in the people we love, we find ourselves thinking, I can't believe that _____ (fill in the blank), or I just wish my (friend, family member) would _____ (behave a particular way) rather than _____ (the way they usually act.) *Examples...*

• **I can't believe my sister isn't able to pick up the phone and call me once in a while to say hello!** She has such a sense of entitlement. She takes me for granted.

• **It is so rude that my friend can't meet me at the agreed-upon time.** Obviously, she doesn't care about my feelings. I would never do that to her.

• **It's hard to believe that my family has to ruin every holiday with their obnoxiously heated conversations.** They're so self-centered. They think the world revolves around them.

I think you get the point.

Believe What Is

If you want to find peace in your life and relationships, every time you tell yourself (or those within earshot), I just wish that... I just can't believe that... or Why can't he/she (do this rather than that?), do yourself a favor and start believing what is and stop wishing for what isn't!

If you're thinking, *That's depressing!* It means that people can't change or that I have to live with totally unacceptable behavior, I totally disagree. People can change. They do it all the time—when change becomes important to them. And you shouldn't accept behaviors that violate your own important personal values.

But—and this is a big but—there's probably a good reason the people in your life are in your life. It's not because of their annoying behaviors…it's because of what's good about them. All people are package deals—your family members…friends…your partner. There are lovable, wonderful qualities in all of us, and there are ones that…well…let's just say, aren't so easy to live with.

And we have a choice. We can focus on the exasperating qualities in our loved ones and try to turn moos into songs, or we can shine a light on their endearing qualities instead and allow these qualities to define our relationships.

Acceptance Works!

Here's an example of how I practice acceptance in my own life. I have many fabulous girlfriends. They sustain me. When I stand back and think about how different they are from one another, it truly is remarkable.

One friend—I'll call her Susie—has a need for structure and likes to make plans well in advance of the actual event. She marks it in her calendar in blood. But she loves taking hikes to remote mountainous areas, one of my favorite things to do.

Another friend—I'll call her Jamie—is what I call my "yes friend." She's light-hearted, spontaneous, filled with laughter and always up for the next adventure. She loves last-minute plans and is totally understanding if, for any reason, plans fall through.

Although I find Susie's need for structure and seriousness a bit restrictive at times, I choose to focus on the uplifting, rich time I know we will have together communing with nature. And although Jamie's spontaneity and lust for life has meant that she hasn't always been available, even at times when I've "needed" her—a value that is very important to me—I choose to focus on the laughter and joy I feel when we play together.

I never try to make Susie or Jamie sing when they moo. I'm not surprised or disappointed when they don't sing. I like—no, I love—their moos.

Pay the Right Attention

Ask yourself whether you spend too much time trying to change things that are unchangeable rather than paying more attention to what's good in your life and the people around you.

If it's challenging to find work-arounds for behaviors that bother you, here's one more suggestion—stop making up negative stories about why people behave the way they do. She's spiteful…he's stingy…she doesn't care about my feelings…he's controlling. These stories are just that—stories. They add fuel to the already everlasting fire.

How to Tell If You're the Toxic Person in Your Workplace—and How to Be Better

Inc.com

If you tend to make everything about you—because of insecurity in general or life events that are super-stressful—make an effort to listen more and talk less in group discussions or during virtual meetings. If you give backhanded compliments, ignore coworkers or deliberately exclude certain people, recognize your behavior as anger-driven and find more productive ways to release your feelings, such as exercise before work or frequent breaks during the day. If you are jealous of the success of others, recognize that jealousy is a sign of insecurity—keep your own goals internal and focused, and share in the success of coworkers by recognizing them as a step toward the larger goals of the company.

Beat Loneliness With the Grandkids

Grandparents who help care for their grand-children report feeling less lonely and having a larger social network than those who do not have an active role in their grandkids' lives, according to a recent survey of nearly 4,000 grandparents.

Theory: Helping out with grandkids may boost self-esteem and may also expand one's social circle—an important benefit because limited social interaction increases risk for mental and physical health problems.

Caveat: Too much caregiving may have less benefit, especially if it interferes with the grandparents' other activities.

Eleanor Quirke, researcher, department for health economics and health service research, University Medical Center Hamburg-Eppendorf, Germany.

Steps to Forgiveness

Loren Toussaint, PhD, forgiveness researcher and professor of psychology, Luther College, Decorah, Iowa, quoted at Prevention.com.

Take these steps to forgive someone who hurt you so you can move on: Do not wait for the person to reach out—that gives him/her more power over you. Decide exactly what you want—to let go of bad feelings, to reconnect or something else. Try to see the event as objectively as possible and also from the other person's point of view—try writing out a few descriptions of the event. If you cannot empathize, at least try to sympathize by remembering a time when you did something wrong and were forgiven. Decide whether to tell the other person that you have forgiven him. It is best to do this only if the person has already apologized, taken responsibility or offered to make amends—otherwise he may not agree that he wronged you in the first place. If there has been no apology from the other person, keep your forgiveness to yourself and let it free you from the anger and pain that you have been feeling.

When You Fear You're Not Good Enough

Jessamy Hibberd, DClinPsy, chartered clinical psychologist based in London. She is author of *The Imposter Cure: How to Stop Feeling Like a Fraud and Escape the Mind-Trap of Imposter Syndrome.* DrJessamy.com

Little do they know I don't really belong here…I'm not really qualified…I got lucky—eventually they will find out that I didn't earn my way here.

A recent study of 3,000 people in the UK found that two-thirds of women and more than half of men have felt like frauds at some point. Earlier research in the US concluded that around 70 percent of people will have at least one experience like this in their lives. Known as "imposter syndrome," it often occurs in professional settings but pops up in personal life, too, with individuals secretly fearing that they are not qualified or good enough for the tasks or roles that have been given to them.

Example: I have no business serving on this condo board—I don't know what I'm doing.

Imposter syndrome can trigger anxiety, and when it recurs regularly, it can produce other damaging consequences. It drives some people to overwork, believing that endless effort is the only way they can keep their shortcomings hidden—but such overwork often ruins their personal lives. Others procrastinate, putting off until the last minute tasks that they believe they're unqualified to do—inevitably causing them to perform below their abilities and reinforcing their fears of inadequacy. There also are those who don't seek promotions, positions and relationships because they wrongly believe that they don't deserve them—feeling like a fraud costs these people their chance at success and happiness.

The vast majority of these people actually are perfectly competent. In fact, many are extremely skilled and intelligent. The truth is that they've made it through decades of life getting rewarded and promoted rather than being seen as unqualified by the world. People in creative fields and women are especially likely to fall victim. *Here's a six-step plan for learning to accept your competence and overcoming imposter syndrome…*

1. Reject the voice telling you that you're not qualified. The voice of self-doubt is coming from inside you, but it isn't your conscience or the voice of truth. It's the voice of fear—fear of failure and a heightened awareness of every possible pitfall before you.

Just because the voice of fear is loud does not mean that it's right. In fact, most of the time it is wrong—there's almost never danger lurking in the shadows…just as those footsteps behind you are almost never a mugger. Remind yourself of that fact, and silence the naysayer in your head so you can move forward.

2. Use evidence to challenge your feelings of fraudulence. People who suffer from imposter syndrome tend to remember all of the negative comments and results that they receive but quickly forget the positives to tip the scale in the opposite direction.

Solution: Regularly reread your résumé—it's a helpful reminder of all that you have accomplished professionally. Think about all of the successful, intelligent people you have worked with and for over the years—if you were a fraud, surely those people would have figured it out. Keep a list of all of the compliments you receive and successes you experience, even minor ones, and review this list regularly as well. Save complimentary notes in a file folder.

3. Discuss your imposter feelings with trusted friends. Not only are they likely to reassure you that you're not an imposter… some of them probably will confess that they have felt the same way at times.

One reason you feel like an imposter is that you're comparing the doubt you feel inside your head with the confident exterior everyone else puts on in public. That's not a fair comparison—remember, you're putting on a confident exterior, too. Ask a friend or two if they also sometimes feel like imposters—virtually no one feels fully qualified all the time. And if you do have friends who share this problem, conversations on the subject can be mutually beneficial, reducing your fear that you'll seem needy if you raise the subject again.

When you were a child, you probably looked at adults and imagined that they knew what they were doing. But when you grew up, there was no magic moment when you suddenly felt as if you had mastered adulthood. That doesn't mean you're a fraud—it just means that you made assumptions about those adults when in reality they didn't actually know what they were doing either.

4. Recast your insecurities. When you experience pangs of doubt, instead think to yourself, This is my mind telling me that it's time to review the successes I have had…or confirm that I'm ready to face a new challenge. Review your plans and preparations for whatever it is that has you feeling unsure to reassure yourself that you are indeed on track. If you feel confident of your plans, you can safely set these insecurities aside…if not, it's time to come up with a plan to get back on track. Once you've done this, the feeling of insecurity has served its purpose and you can let it go.

Feelings of insecurity sometimes are a sign that you're pushing yourself outside your comfort zone. That's a positive thing. If you never leave your comfort zone, you'll never grow and improve.

5. Stop treating perfection as the goal. Perfectionists define anything short of 100 percent success as failure—then feel like frauds when the world lauds their 80 percent or 90 percent success rate.

Stop forcing yourself to work absurd hours or berating yourself for the partial win that you're labeling a loss. And accept the fact that there will be some races you don't win. It can help to read the biographies of successful people—these inevitably detail many moments of insecurity endured along the way.

Examples: An editor told a young Walt Disney he lacked imagination…and Oprah Winfrey was fired from her first job in television. Each one might have questioned their abilities or decided that they just weren't good enough to pursue their dreams. Looking at it from the outside, you know that would have been ridiculous. The same is true when doubts come your own way. Moments of negative feedback do not erase your longer-term abilities and successes.

6. Don't attribute your successes to outside forces. Imposter syndrome sufferers often chalk up their victories to luck, teammates or other external forces rather than giving themselves and their abilities the credit. If you were prepared to capitalize on your opportunities or you surrounded yourself with a skilled team, that doesn't mean you're a fortunate fraud—it means you're savvy.

Better Ways to Avoid Loneliness

HealthLetter.MayoClinic.com

Be genuinely interested in other people—ask questions about their lives and pay attention to their responses. Reach out by phone, text message or e-mail to friends you have not been in touch with for a while. Practice making light connections with strangers, such as friendly small talk with a store clerk or restaurant server. Say yes if someone invites you to an event—do not think of all the reasons to avoid going. Get out of your home for religious services, volunteer activities or hobbies. Find your comfort area—some people like one-on-one conversation, while others prefer noisy group activities. Consider animal companions—dogs, cats, reptiles and fish can give you ways to interact and make connections.

Detox Your Relationships

Laurie Steelsmith, ND, LAc, is medical director of Steelsmith Natural Health Center, Honolulu, and co-author of *Great Sex, Naturally.* DrSteelsmith.com

A glance at the statistics demonstrates that relationships, and the entire appeal of them, are essential. As social creatures whose ancestors' survival depended on tribes, we need other people for companionship, friendship and, even to this day, survival—social isolation and loneliness, for one, significantly increase one's risk for premature mortality. For six million years (ancestrally speaking), humans have formed interpersonal relationships, and countless cultural anthropologists can attest to the fact that humans around the globe create systems of social dynamics that allow individuals and groups to thrive.

"Thriving," however, is key here, and can be found only if the dynamics are healthy—it takes more than one person to create and sustain a functional or dysfunctional relationship, after all. And if those dynamics are significantly off, you may experience a range of adverse effects, from depression and anxiety to a propensity to fly off the handle. Indeed, studies show that unhealthy relationships can trigger a host of health problems, including heart disease and even strokes, while the ongoing stress of living with, loving, or working with someone toxic may lead to decreased immunity and a greater chance of anxiety, depression and suicidal ideation.

What Are Toxic Relationships?

Anyone who has ever loved knows this: Relationships can be difficult to navigate at times. Whether that relationship is with your romantic partner or sibling, your parent or your best friend, you know it isn't always sweet. Arguments are normal, and rough patches are common.

But as true as this may be, another sort of relationship experiences more turmoil and distress than those average bumps in the road. Known as a "toxic relationship"—a term communication and psychology expert Dr. Lillian Glass said she coined in her 1995 book, *Toxic People*—this connection is "any relationship (between two people who) don't support each other, where there's conflict and one seeks to undermine the other, where there's competition, where there's disrespect and a lack of cohesiveness." The difference between a toxic relationship and a healthy relationship rests in how—to say nothing of if—those challenges are handled. In a toxic relationship, apologies are rare, one person completely ices out the other after a disagreement, promises are seldom kept, minor differences in opinion turn into major arguments, truths are hidden from each other—and these are just a few examples from a pool of many.

How Do I Know If I'm in a Toxic Relationship?

What I said above may sound familiar. It might also sound like something from which you'd run. But while abusive relationships are clear-cut, toxic relationships are a bit murkier and harder to discern.

A few questions to ask yourself as you contemplate the relationships in your life…

•**Do negative moments outweigh the positive ones?**

•**Are your basic needs being met?**

•**Do you feel that you constantly have to work for approval?**

•**Has the relationship stopped bringing you joy?**

•**Does interacting with the other often leave you feeling drained, sad, angry or anxious?**

•**Do either of you blame each other for your emotions?**

•**Do you feel emotionally safe with the other person, or are you afraid to speak up?**

•**Do you feel manipulated or controlled?**

•**Do you, or the other, maintain a relationship scorecard**—meaning, does one or the other keep track of how many mistakes the other has made and who is more indebted to the other?

•**Do you, or the other, make ultimatums?** For example, does your companion say, "I can't be with someone who is mad at me all of the time" rather than "I feel that you may be angry at me—can we talk?"

•**Have you noticed any harmful shifts in your mental health,** self-esteem, work performance or personality due to relationship dynamics?

•**Have other friends or family members voiced their concerns about your relationship?** Because the signs of a toxic relationship can be subtle, it's important to listen to the worries your other loved ones have.

What Should I Do If I'm in a Toxic Relationship?

First, consider seeing a licensed psychologist. Psychologists can effectively work in the abstract sphere of emotion, where they guide, shape and lead a person to healthier relationships and ultimately a better quality of life.

While everyone's situation is unique, psychologists, I believe, would argue that one principle holds true across the board: You cannot love someone else until you love yourself first. When you think of yourself in derogatory terms—if you criticize and demoralize yourself on a regular basis—there's a good chance that you have normalized such talk to the point that a toxic relationship feels like the status quo. At the same time, if you believe that you are undeserving of genuine love, compassion and respect, you may sell yourself short and remain in a relationship that takes a toll on your capacity to live healthfully and well.

What this means, of course, is that the answer rests in you. The healthier you are psychologically, the healthier your relationships will be. You can neither change nor control other people; you cannot make other people what you wish them to be. You can, however, change yourself. And all change begins with awareness.

The first step towards altering or walking away from a toxic relationship is getting clear about your psychological tendencies and the type of people you tend to attract and accept in your life. Have you historically been around and with people who don't serve your highest good? Are they more depleting than invigorating? Do you have unresolved trauma that is preventing you from being present, and flourishing, in your relationships?

On a more specific level, are you frequently drawn to narcissists (see page 68)? Peer at yourself lovingly but objectively and ask yourself, "do I have symptoms of a codependent personality, such as low self-confidence, hazy boundaries and problems with intimacy?" Are you more of a rescuer and caretaker instead of someone who's enjoyed relationships of mutual support? Or do you take on the characteristics of your partner, family member, friend or colleague? (This is vital to consider. As Henry Cloud, PhD, points out in his article *How to Gracefully End a Bad Relationship*, "when we spend time with people who have bad attitudes, bad habits or chronic bad moods, we dramatically increase the odds that we will suffer from these, too—a phenomenon called 'social contagion.'") Remember, there is no blame here, only the acknowledgement that a particular person or relationship is causing you pain and may no longer suit you.

Next, consider what you do want in a relationship—an exercise that will help you see where yours may be lacking. Do you honor open, clear and consistent communication—inarguably, one of the most fundamental aspects of a healthy relationship? Do you prize affection and generosity? Do you aim for healthy conflict resolution?

Finally, in addition to loving yourself, ask yourself if you adore who you are when you are with this person, for as Anne Tyler sagely wrote in *The Accidental Tourist*, "It is not how much you love someone, but who you are when you are with him." Do they pro-

voke your angrier side? Does interacting with them often lead to self-destructive behavior? Have you adopted damaging habits and behaviors of theirs that have pulled you away from your ideal self and ideal life? The best relationships are those that highlight the best parts of ourselves—empathy, resilience, determination, success, happiness, you name it—and lift us up.

Following this, if you believe that the person with whom you have a toxic relationship is capable of listening to your needs, have a frank, kind, but firm, conversation with him or her. Curate what you want to say ahead of time, and replace accusatory statements ("You did") with "I" statements ("I feel"). A good therapist and counseling can help you create tools and practices that will allow you to move towards a solid, beneficial relationship.

If, however, the toxicity in your relationship is due to a mismatched pairing or, after a careful assessment, is not worth the amount of mental, emotional and physical anguish it has caused you, by all means, give yourself permission to walk away. Whether you choose to let the relationship fade away on its own or to be forthright is wholly up to you. A conversation can help you confront your fears—it can also be cathartic—just as it might help the other realize his or her blind spots. And if the discussion doesn't go well? It's all the more reason to believe that you made the right decision to move on.

Magic Mushrooms Can Relieve Depression

Study of 24 patients with a long-term history of depression by researchers at Johns Hopkins School of Medicine, Baltimore, published in *JAMA Psychiatry*.

Just two doses of psilocybin—the psychedelic compound found in so-called magic mushrooms—brought rapid reductions in depressive symptoms in a study of people with major depression. And half the patients were in remission after four weeks. Psilocybin produces visual and auditory hallucinations and significant changes in consciousness over a period of several hours. It was used along with supportive psychotherapy. The magnitude of the effect was four times larger than the effect of traditional antidepressants, which can take weeks or months to work and may have undesirable side effects. The side effects of using psilocybin were more limited, and its benefits appeared after only one or two uses.

Calming "Monkey Mind"

Carol Krucoff, C-IAYT, E-RYT, Duke Integrative Medicine.

In these stressful times, it's normal to have racing thoughts—sometimes called a "monkey mind." Many people turn to yoga to learn how to calm this mental chatter, quiet the mind, and connect with the spirit.

Too often, people focus on "doing postures" without recognizing that poses are just one part of the yoga toolkit. Breathing and meditation are two other tools that hold the key to quieting your mind. Paying attention to your breath will enhance your mind-body connection and bring you into the present moment. And when you set an intention to stay focused on your breath, you are practicing a form of meditation that trains your mind to become more stable.

Try this simple breath awareness meditation off the mat first: Sit tall and set a timer for one minute. Close your eyes and turn your attention to your breath without trying to change or control it in any way. Just observe it, noticing all the sensations of breathing out and breathing in.

If your mind wanders, notice without judgment that your attention has strayed. Then, kindly and firmly, as if you were guiding a wandering puppy, bring your focus back to your breath. When the timer rings, open your eyes and notice how you feel. Gradually increase the amount of time you're practicing—ideally meditating for at least 10 minutes a day.

Bring this same breath awareness onto your yoga mat during posture practice, and notice how connecting to your breath helps take you out of your head and into your body. Recognize that your attention is like a muscle that can be strengthened with meditation practice. Over time, this can help calm your racing mind.

Chapter 6

FOOD, DIET AND FITNESS

5 Ways to Change Your Attitude and Get Healthy

Maybe you want to lose weight. Maybe you want to create healthier eating habits. Or maybe you want to sleep better at night. If you've been unsuccessful in your efforts in spite of an array of loving, supportive strategies, perhaps some tough-love advice from Oonagh Duncan will do the trick. She is the hilarious and inspiring fitness expert whose unique formula has been helping people ditch the excuses, change their bad habits and get in shape at last.

● **Lose the "all or nothing" approach to eating.** Maybe you eat healthfully all week, forgoing even so much as a sip of wine, and then you go crazy on the weekend. It's a constant pattern of one step forward, two steps back. Or you consciously allow yourself to overeat, promising you will "work it off" later.

Reality check: To burn off an order of French fries, you may have to be on the elliptical for an hour or more.

Instead: Banish thoughts like I'll start over tomorrow or I'll eat healthy next week. This is mental garbage! The idea that you can "work off" a binge with a cleanse is just not the way the body works. You won't see results, but you will do damage to your metabolism. You know that you can't get strong arms by doing 1,000 push-ups in one day, but you can get injured that way. You can get strong only by doing 10 push-ups for 100 days. That's because your body loves consistency and hates extremes.

It's the same way when it comes to food. Many people try to force themselves into strict regimens where certain foods are forbidden. If you try to banish all carbs—or whatever the current "baddy" is—you'll eventually fail because an all-or-nothing approach never works. Instead, go ahead and eat proteins, carbs and fat. Just do it in reasonable amounts.

● **Tame the tiger.** Do you go all out, no matter what you do? Then you're a tiger. Tigers work hard and look very successful, but they tend to go overboard. Because it's hard to sustain their extreme level of effort (showing up at the gym every day at 5 am, for example), they fall off the wagon fast, stop seeing results because they can't keep up

Oonagh Duncan, personal trainer and founder of FitFeelsGood.com. She is author of the best-seller *Healthy as F*ck: The Habits You Need to Get Lean, Stay Healthy, and Kick Ass at Life.*

with such a rigorous plan and end up feeling terrible about themselves.

Instead: Be a turtle. Turtles make one small change at a time. They give themselves the time to get used to each one. Some turtles feel bad because they don't have dramatic weight-loss results. But turtles are so much better than tigers at developing good habits and achieving long-term results. Slow and steady change may make you feel like nothing's happening, but that's what's going to form new habits that will get you lasting results.

• **Remove temptation from your home.** Many people have their daily rituals. They pour themselves a glass of wine or have a bowl of ice cream as a way to make an ordinary day feel special. But that nightly treat has a creep effect. One glass of wine turns into two glasses, and one scoop turns into two…which turns into I might as well finish the whole carton.

Instead: Banish foods from your house that later tend to make you feel awful. Be honest with yourself. If it ended up in your mouth before, it likely will again—even if you claim the cookies are just there for the kids. It's not forever. Those foods and drinks are always there to revisit at the occasional party or in a restaurant.

Go ahead and clean out your cabinets and throw away your trigger foods. Don't feel bad about tossing that half-eaten bag of chips. If you eat it rather than throwing it away, it's still a waste…but it's a waste that can hurt your body and make you feel bad.

• **Get rid of anything in your closet that doesn't make you feel good.** Many people have clothing in three different sizes cluttering their closets (and their lives). They think it's motivating to keep the stuff that once looked great on them. But if those same pants now are cutting into your stomach, you're making life harder than it has to be. You're only going to feel bad about yourself. And no one has ever hated themselves into a body they love. In fact, studies have proven that the more shame you feel about yourself, the more likely you are to gain weight.

Instead: Next time your jeans don't zip, stick with facts, not emotions. Give yourself an honest assessment of how you got here—as in, OK, I've gained weight. My portions have been kind of big, and I've been drinking more than usual. But I'm excited to get fit again and to start reigning in those portions. So yes, they may fit again soon…but for now, get them out of your closet. Stop "futurizing" your life, and concentrate instead on feeling good about yourself now. By building positive thoughts, you are more likely to succeed at your goals.

• **Recognize the weasel words.** Everyone has heard that tempting voice that tells them not to get out of bed when the alarm goes off for gym time. That's because we all are so good at making weasel-y excuses, such as I just don't feel like it today…I'll exercise later, after work…I can skip just one day! The reason that this voice is so seductive is because it helps us postpone the discomfort of change.

Instead: Remember that one of the most important muscles you need to strengthen is the "Do it even when I don't feel like it" muscle. Think about it—you probably also don't really want to pay your phone bill or go to work when it's raining…but you do it! Because you're an adult and know that when you do what's right, it feels good.

Tip: To call yourself out on your excuses, try meditation. It trains your brain to see your thoughts more clearly. And it will stop you from believing in old, unhelpful thought patterns such as, *I must have low metabolism* or *I'm just not good at exercising.* With meditation, you can separate yourself from some of your favorite excuses and look at them from a more detached perspective.

Example: Say to yourself, *There I go… thinking that thought again.*

More from Oonagh Duncan…

Small Wins With Big Payoffs

Think of something that you find hard to do, whether it's going to bed on time or cooking healthy meals at home. Then try to imagine the teeniest, tiniest version of that better habit. Keep thinking smaller until it would be ridiculous to think that you can't do it! Now you are armed and ready for battle. *To get started, here are some examples of "small win" ideas to counter some of the big excuses we all make…*

• I don't have time to make a week's worth of healthy meals in advance!

Could you chop up some veggies to have on hand for snacking?

• I can't handle another salad, and I want something yummy.

Could you throw a few spinach leaves into a blueberry smoothie?

• There's no way I can get seven hours of sleep at night.

Could you go to bed 15 minutes earlier than usual?

• I can't survive on one portion. I'm still hungry!

Could you wait five minutes before getting a second helping?

• I need my glass of wine every night. It's how I relax.

Could you try a half-serving for one night and see how that feels?

Shared Success Stories Help Young Moms Lose Weight, Get Healthier

The study "Mediators of Intervention Effects on Dietary Fat Intake in Low-income Overweight or Obese Women with Young Children," led by researchers at The Ohio State University College of Nursing, Columbus, published in *Appetite*.

Finding the motivation and confidence to make healthy lifestyle changes is a tough hill to climb for most people. For overweight, low-income women with young children, it can be a mountain. When researchers at The Ohio State University College of Nurs-

ing asked these women to identify the type of people they would want to hear from in videos promoting healthy lifestyle changes, the women said they wanted to be inspired by women like themselves. They wanted the truth about what it takes and how it can be done.

The researchers listened and designed a study to fit the wishes of women and recruited participants from the Special Supplemental Nutrition Program for Women, Infants and Children. Women enrolled in the study were low-income mothers who ranged from slightly overweight to just below extreme obesity. These highly stressed women tended to eat high-fat foods.

The researchers enrolled 212 women, ages 18 to 39, into the study. The women were randomly placed into a group that watched videos of women like themselves give tips on meal preparation, managing stress and engaging in physical activity. These videos were designed to motivate the women and give them confidence based on success stories from women they could believe and identify with. In addition to watching 10 videos, the women participated in 10 peer-support teleconferences. The other women were placed into a group that got similar information, but only in the form of print materials.

At the end of the 16-week study, the researchers interviewed the women and asked about their motivation, confidence and diet. They found that the women who were in the video-and-teleconference group reported higher motivation, more confidence and a significant improvement in their diet, with less dietary fat.

Before the start of the study, women told the researchers that they wanted to be better role models for their children, have less stress and maintain healthy family relationships. This study suggests that with a little help from their peers, they can get there.

Lose Your Quarantine Weight Gain

Marjory Abrams, former editor, *Bottom Line Personal* and CCO of Bottom Line Inc.

Weight-gain jokes were flying fast on Facebook when the pandemic started, with all of us suddenly locked at home, spending all day within steps of the pantry and refrigerator. As the country "reopens" and more of us become socially active again, you may be thinking that it's time to make a change. Here are tips from nutritionist Lisa Young, PhD, RDN, author of *Finally Full, Finally Slim*, on how to reverse isolation-induced—or retirement- or work-from-home-induced—weight gain...

• **Plan ahead for all meals and snacks rather than going hunting when you're hungry and grabbing what's convenient and often unhealthy.** Half the time, we don't even like what we're eating! It is better to plan...and portion it out in advance, just as you do when you brown-bag it to work.

• **Serve yourself.** Eating out of the bag is the worst habit for uncontrolled eating because you can't monitor your intake. As soon as you open or cook something, put your current portion into a bowl or on a plate, and put the rest into single-serving containers.

Alpha Lipoic Acid Lowers Body Fat and Weight

Researchers reported that giving people 600 milligrams of this supplement each day for 24 weeks led to a clear loss in body weight and body fat, particularly in women and in the heaviest participants. When taken as a dietary supplement, lipoic acid stimulates glucose metabolism, antioxidant defenses and anti-inflammatory responses.

Gerd Bobe, PhD, associate professor, animal & rangeland sciences, Oregon State University and Oregon Health & Science, Corvalis, Oregon.

• **Eat consciously.** We eat more when we do it while watching television or working at the computer. When you eat, just eat. Chew thoroughly—don't rush. Enjoy the textures and flavors.

• **Be active throughout the day.** Your once-a-day exercise session isn't enough to keep your metabolism revving. Set an alarm every hour to take at least a few minutes for physical activity, be it walking up and down the stairs or some simple exercises such as squats and dips.

Trick to Eat Less

Lisa R. Young, PhD, RDN, author of *Finally Full, Finally Slim: 30 Days to Permanent Weight Loss One Portion at a Time.*

Cut your eight-slice pizza into 16 slices. People tend to eat in units, regardless of size. Works for brownies and other foods, too.

Taste Bud Rehab: Stop Craving Bad Food

David Katz, MD, MPH, founder/CEO of True Health Initiative. His latest book is *How to Eat: All Your Food and Diet Questions Answered,* coauthored with food writer Mark Bittman.

Food makers have packed "bad" foods with sweet, salty and fatty flavors to light up our brains' reward centers.

But you don't have to give in to this fate. With just three weeks of "taste bud rehab," you can create a healthier palate.

Don't believe it? When study participants in the landmark Iowa Women's Health Study adopted a plant-based, lower-fat diet, they actually developed an aversion to unhealthy processed and fast foods within a few months.

To rehab your taste buds, follow these steps (sequentially or concurrently, based on your preference) for three weeks, at which point those unhealthy foods won't be calling your name…

***STEP #1:* Look for added sugar and salt—everywhere—and dial it back.** Whether it's pasta sauce, salad dressing or breakfast cereal, processed foods are easy targets because they are chock-full of un-needed sugar and salt. As your taste buds adjust to lesser amounts, they will become more sensitive to sugar and salt, giving you the same pleasure at lower doses.

Label-reading tips: Keep added sugar to less than 10 percent of total daily calories—or, even better, 5 percent. Be sure to watch out for sneaky forms of sugar, such as sucrose, cane juice, agave and corn syrup. Stick to foods with less than 100 mg of sodium per 100 calories, aiming for a daily total of less than 2,300 mg of sodium.

Also, opt for foods with fewer ingredients—tortilla chips made with just corn, oil and a little salt, for example. Be wary of foods that combine sugar, salt and fat, such as candied nuts or honey-mustard pretzels. This trifecta of ingredients is the hardest to eat in moderation.

Helpful: If you have the time, spare yourself the unwanted ingredients by whipping up a tasty vinaigrette salad dressing from olive oil, balsamic vinegar and fresh herbs.

If that's not your thing, focus on healthier supermarket versions. Once you find a lower-sugar sauce or a lower-sodium dressing you like, stick with it. Consistency helps you stay on track when choosing healthier foods.

***STEP #2:* Think beyond sweet and salty.** Our taste buds also detect sour, bitter and umami (savory) qualities—all found in many nutritious foods. These include bitter vegetables such as kale and broccoli…sour foods such as grapefruit and plain yogurt…and umami-rich foods such as seafood (including seaweed) and mushrooms.

The problem: If we are not exposed much to these flavors, especially as children, our taste buds often reject them.

The solution: Repeated exposure and combining new flavors with those we already love. Children require 10 to 15 samplings of a new flavor to accept it, according to research. But adult taste buds are less sensitive and can be won over with fewer tastings.

For example, you can learn to love beets by pairing them with walnuts and blue cheese in a spinach salad…or add some mushrooms to your stir-fry.

Added tip: Roasting, broiling or grilling can bring out the sweetness in bitter foods, such as brussels sprouts.

***STEP #3:* Manage cravings.** Learning to love kale will not instantly extinguish cravings for chocolate. To minimize cravings, eat a healthy meal or snack every three to four hours. When you get a craving, go for a walk or drink a glass of water. Research shows that many cravings pass within 10 to 15 minutes.

When your sweet tooth demands satisfaction, opt for a contrasting flavor, such as a cup of mint tea…or a food naturally high in sugar, such as fruit.

Your rehabbed taste buds may find it hits the spot!

Guilt-Free Snacks from Top Food Bloggers

Amy Gorin, MS, RDN, owner of Amy Gorin Nutrition in the New York City area. AmyDGorin.com

Ariane Resnick, CNC, Los Angeles–based certified nutritionist, celebrity chef and best-selling author of *Wake/Sleep: What to Eat and Do for More Energy and Better Sleep.* Recipe reproduced by permission of The Countryman Press. All rights reserved. ArianeCooks.com

Tammy Lakatos Shames, RDN, CDN, CFT, and Lyssie Lakatos, RDN, CDN, CFT, aka the Nutrition Twins. Their most recent book is *Nutrition Twins' Veggie Cure.* NutritionTwins.com

Frances Largeman-Roth, RDN, New York City–based nutrition-and-wellness expert and a *New York Times* best-selling author. Her most recent cookbook is *Eating in Color: Delicious, Healthy Recipes for You and Your Family.* FrancesLargemanRoth.com

Lara Field, MS, RD, LDN, founder of FEED Nutrition Consulting in Chicago. FeedNutrition.com

When hunger strikes, your first thought may be to reach for the potato chips. After all, you've been trained to think of snacks as a guilty—and unhealthy—pleasure. But it doesn't have to be that way! We went to top health-food bloggers to find nonguilty snack ideas that are sweet, salty, creamy and colorful.

Amy Gorin, MS, RDN
Amy Gorin Nutrition

Satisfy a Sugar Craving: Choco-Banana "Nice Cream"

Bananas are naturally sweet, and when processed in a food processor or blender, they develop a deliciously creamy texture similar to soft-serve ice cream. One serving of this "nice cream" contains 14 grams of sugar. The cocoa powder adds a strong chocolate flavor and minimal calories. Unsweetened cocoa powder is bitter on its own but sweetens when paired with the natural sugars from the banana. It's all good for you, but it feels so indulgent. Serves two.

2 bananas, sliced and frozen
1 teaspoon unsweetened cocoa powder

Place the bananas and cocoa powder in a food processor or high-speed blender. Process or blend until completely smooth, pausing, if necessary, to push the ingredients toward the bottom of the processor or blender. Serve immediately.

Tip: Have overripe bananas on your countertop? Peel, slice and freeze them, and you'll be ready when your next "nice cream" craving hits.

Ariane Resnick, CNC
ArianeCooks.com

Beat the Afternoon Slump: Matcha Cupcakes

Those bright green lattes at your local café are made with matcha, a powdered Japanese green tea. Each of these pick-me-up cupcakes contains one teaspoon of matcha—the equivalent of more than a half cup of coffee. Yet matcha is less likely than coffee to leave you feeling wired, thanks to a natural abundance of theanine, an amino acid that helps temper the buzz of caffeine. These cupcakes give the energy boost you need without the jitters. Plus, they're low in sugar and have protein from the almond flour. Makes nine cupcakes.

Dry ingredients…
1¼ cups almond flour
¼ cup coconut flour
½ cup Swerve or cane sugar, or a combo
2½ Tablespoons matcha
1 teaspoon baking soda
½ teaspoon salt

Wet ingredients…
½ cup Greek yogurt (dairy or coconut)
2 large eggs or vegan egg-replacer equivalent
½ cup neutral oil, such as avocado or grape
1 teaspoon vanilla extract
⅓ cup almond milk
1 Tablespoon cider vinegar

Preheat the oven to 350°F. In a large bowl, combine all the dry ingredients with a fork or whisk, making sure no lumps of almond or coconut flour remain. Add all the wet ingredients except the vinegar, and stir until uniform in texture. Add the vinegar, and stir well. Pour the batter into nine wells of a cupcake pan (either with liners or greased), filling them nearly all the way, and bake 25 to 30 minutes or until an inserted knife comes out clean.

Tammy Lakatos Shames, RDN, CDN, CFT, and Lyssie Lakatos, RDN, CDN, CFT
NutritionTwins.com

Postworkout Hunger: Avocado Sweet Potato "Toast" with Hummus

Sweet potatoes are packed with slow-burning carbohydrates and beta-carotene, a powerful antioxidant that promotes postexercise recovery by protecting the body against inflammation. They're also rich in magnesium, a natural muscle relaxer that can thwart muscle spasms and cramps. The hummus, made from puréed chickpeas, is an excellent source of protein, which is helpful for repairing muscle damage from exercise. After a workout, this is the snack to grab. Serves four.

1 large sweet potato
2 ounces hummus
Dash cayenne pepper
1 small/medium avocado (3 ounces), sliced
Black pepper
½ lime

Preheat the oven to 400°F. Line a baking sheet with parchment paper. Cut the ends off the sweet potato, and slice lengthwise, one-third- to one-half-inch thick. (Too thin, and they'll be too soft to make a good "toast.")

Place the slices on parchment paper, and bake until they are tender, roughly 20 minutes. When ready, they should be easily pierced with a fork.

Remove the slices from the oven, and allow to cool for two to three minutes. Spread the hummus on potato slices, and garnish with a dash of cayenne. Top with avocado slices, black pepper and a spritz of lime juice.

Note: Refrigerate any unused potato slices in an airtight container.

Frances Largeman-Roth, RDN
FrancesLargemanRoth.com

When Dinner Isn't Ready: Creamy Curried Red Lentil Dip with Raw Veggies and Tortilla Chips

Prepare this go-to dip ahead of time so that you have it on hand when those predinner munchies strike. The combination of fiber and plant-based protein in the lentils fills up that growling hole in your stomach and helps you resist sugary snacks. Lentils and other beans cause your blood sugar to rise slowly and steadily, and the effect continues for hours. Fewer blood sugar swings translate into reduced appetite. Serves eight.

1 cup red lentils, rinsed well
2 teaspoons mild curry powder
1 teaspoon sea salt
1 Tablespoon coconut or olive oil
1 small yellow onion, chopped
Assortment of fresh veggies and whole-grain tortilla chips for dipping

Add the lentils, curry powder, salt and three cups of water to a medium saucepan. Bring to a boil, reduce the heat to a simmer, then cook for 30 minutes, until the lentils are soft and no liquid remains. While the lentils are cooking, add the oil to a sauté pan and sauté the onion for five minutes. Transfer the onions to a blender, along with the cooked lentils. Blend until creamy and smooth. Transfer it to a serving bowl, and add a drizzle of oil on top. Serve with fresh veggies and tortilla chips.

Note: This will keep in the refrigerator for four days, so whip up this dip whenever the urge hits.

Lara Field, MS, RD, LDN
FeedNutrition.com

Movie Night: "Cheesy" Popcorn with Nutritional Yeast

Craving some mindless munching? One serving of this air-popped popcorn is a filling four cups, but it's only about 120 calories—so you can enjoy plenty of guilt-free hand-to-mouth action.

Bonus: Popcorn is a whole grain. Four cups deliver five grams of fiber. Nutritional yeast adds a cheesy, nutty flavor to foods…provides protein (eight grams per quarter cup)…and is incredibly rich in vitamin B-12. Serves one.

¼ cup unpopped popcorn kernels
1 Tablespoon coconut or safflower oil
   (*Note*: If you use the coconut oil, it will add a slight flavor.)
1 Tablespoon nutritional yeast

Place a large, flat pan or popcorn popper on the stove top, and turn heat to medium-high. Add a thin layer of oil to the bottom of the pan. Add in one or two kernels, and cover with a lid until they pop. Then remove those pieces, and add the remaining kernels. Turn the heat down to medium, cover the pot, and wait until the popcorn popping slows. Remove from heat, transfer to a bowl, and add nutritional yeast.

Optional: Mix in one-quarter cup sunflower or pumpkin seeds for a boost of selenium, a brain-boosting mineral that's abundant in nuts and seeds.

Coffee: Drink Up for Less Body Fat

The study "Regular Coffee Consumption Is Associated with Lower Regional Adiposity Measured by DXA Among US Women," led by researchers at Anglia Ruskin University in East Anglia, UK, and published in *The Journal of Nutrition*.

Americans love their coffee. In fact, we drink about 400 million cups each day, making it one of the most popular beverages in the US. That's good news for those who love their cups of joe because there's increasing evidence showing that coffee has lots of health benefits, such as helping to protect against cirrhosis of the liver, to control Parkinson's disease symptoms, to promote heart health and to slow the progress of dementia.

Now: A new study published in *The Journal of Nutrition* has found yet another benefit—coffee drinking is linked to having less body fat.

Study details: The finding was based on 5,000 Americans' responses to the National Health and Nutrition Examination Survey (NHANES), organized by the Centers for Disease Control and Prevention. NHANES asks respondents questions about their nutrition and health and includes measurements of body fat and its distribution using a dual-energy X-ray absorptiometry (DXA) scan. (The scan is also commonly used to measure bone density to diagnose osteoporosis.)

After analyzing the respondents' daily coffee intake and their DXA measurements over a two-year period, the researchers found a link between coffee consumption and body fat in women that varied by their age, while there was less overall effect among the men who were studied. *The specific findings…*

• **Compared with women who did not drink coffee,** women ages 20 to 44 who drank two to three cups per day had 3.4 percent less body fat.

• **Women ages 45 to 69 who drank four or more cups per day** had 4.1 percent less body fat than non-coffee drinkers.

• **Among men, the association between coffee drinking and body fat was less significant…**except for those ages 22 to 44 who drank two to three cups of coffee per day—they had 1.3 percent less body fat and 1.8 percent less trunk fat than men who did not drink coffee.

Interestingly, the benefits were present in those who drank caffeinated or decaffeinated coffee and were not affected by smoking or chronic disease.

"Our research suggests that there may be bioactive compounds in coffee other than caffeine that regulate weight and which could potentially be used as anti-obesity compounds," explained Lee Smith, PhD, senior author of the study and director of research at Anglia Ruskin University's Cambridge Centre for Sport and Exercise Sciences.

At some point, these bioactive compounds could be used as part of an anti-obesity treatment, according to the researchers. For now, however, coffee lovers can rest easy knowing that two to four cups a day could help reduce their overall body fat—and belly fat.

Mainly because of its caffeine content, people with high blood pressure may need to limit their intake of coffee—it can temporarily raise blood pressure in some people. Pregnant women and women who are breast-feeding should talk to their doctors about their consumption of coffee—high intake has been shown to increase risk for miscarriage. The American College of Obstetricians and Gynecologists recommends that pregnant women drink no more than 200 mg of caffeine daily (approximately two cups of caffeinated coffee a day), while research recently published in the *BMJ Evidence-Based Medicine* recommends that they consider avoiding caffeine altogether.

Healthier Coffee Drinking

Unfiltered coffee—such as French press or Turkish coffee—can harm the heart. It contains about 30 times as many lipid-raising substances as filtered coffee—and those substances can increase blood cholesterol, making heart attacks and premature death more likely. Drinking one to four cups of filtered coffee per day is good for health—actually better than not drinking any coffee at all.

Dag S. Thelle, MD, PhD, senior professor, department of public health and community medicine, University of Gothenburg, Sweden, and leader of a 20-year study of more than 500,000 Norwegians, published in *European Journal of Preventive Cardiology*.

Beware the Keto Diet for Weight Loss

Vishwa Deep Dixit, PhD, Waldemar Von Zedtwitz Professor of Comparative Medicine and of Immunobiology, Yale University School of Medicine, New Haven, Connecticut, and leader of a study published in *Nature Metabolism*

In the short term, the super-high-fat, low-carbohydrate diet does trick the body into burning fats instead of carbohydrates, as occurs in a state of starvation—so you lose weight. But in a recent mouse study, after a week, negative effects started to occur. The mice were storing fat as well as burning it, which increased their risk for obesity and diabetes—conditions against which the keto diet is allegedly protective. Long-term clinical studies in humans are needed to confirm the keto diet's most effective time frame. But it does appear that the diet's supposed weight-loss benefits work only when it is used for limited periods of time.

3 Food Myths That Could Hurt You

David L. Katz, MD, MPH, preventive medicine specialist and founder and president of True Health Initiative, based in New Haven, Connecticut. He is CEO and founder of Diet ID, an online diet-assessment and personalization program, and coauthor with renowned food writer Mark Bittman of *How to Eat: All Your Food and Diet Questions Answered.* DavidKatzMD.com

Everyone knows that vegetables are good for you and French fries are not. But we still can't wrap our heads around some of the finer nuances of proper nutrition, such as how much protein to eat and whether we really need to cut our carbohydrate intake… and to even understand what a carb is.

To get a handle on persisting misperceptions about food and healthy eating, we spoke with diet expert and preventive-medicine specialist David L. Katz, MD.

3 Biggest Food Misperceptions

***MISPERCEPTION #1:* You need to eat more protein as you get older.**

Truth: Most adults get more than enough protein to meet their nutritional needs. You would have to have a very unbalanced, quirky diet to be protein-deficient. Government recommendations advise getting 10 percent to 35 percent of calories from protein sources—roughly one-half gram per pound of body weight. Currently in the US, women eat, on average, about 90 grams per day and men eat about 100 grams—more than enough.

It's true that most people begin to lose muscle starting between ages 50 and 60. And it's also true that protein helps you maintain muscle. But it's a myth that eating more protein will help you build muscle. Only exercise enables you to maintain and build muscle. In fact, extra protein above that 35 percent of daily calories will turn into body fat, just as extra calories from fat or carbs do. Too much protein also can stress the kidneys and liver, leading to disease of those organs, as well as weaken your bones.

***MISPERCEPTION #2:* You need to eat animal products to get complete nutrition.**

Truth: A complete protein source delivers all of the essential amino acids (histidine, isoleucine, leucine, lysine, methionine, phenylalanine, threonine, tryptophan and valine) that our bodies can't make but still need to function optimally. Yes, meat provides these essential amino acids in the ideal proportions all at once, but higher intake of meat is associated with higher overall risk for chronic disease and premature death.

Plant foods also deliver all of the essential amino acids, just at lower concentrations. The distribution of amino acids in nuts, grains, legumes, vegetables, fungi and seeds is complementary—if you don't get all the amino acids that your body needs from one type of plant, you'll get it from another. Your body couldn't care less if you get these amino acids—so-called "complete protein"—all at once or from animals or plants. There's no need to worry about food combinations within one meal as long as you get a balance of foods in general.

***MISPERCEPTION #3:* Your diet can be healthy only if you limit carbs.**

Truth: Carbohydrates actually should be the predominant foods in your diet. Whether you are an omnivore, a vegetarian or a vegan, 40 percent to 70 percent of your daily calories should come from complex carbs.

Important: Carbs don't just mean sugar, pasta, bread, grains and other starchy foods. All fruits, vegetables and beans are carbs too. And all of the best diets around the world— "Blue Zone" diets that are associated with health and longevity—are predominantly plant-based and thus carb-based.

Beware: There are plenty of bad processed carbs out there—chips, pizza, candy, white bread, white pasta, cakes, sugary cereals and sugar-sweetened drinks, etc.—all lacking in nutrition and designed to put your appetite into overdrive.

How to Eat

Given what we know, then, how exactly should we be eating? It's actually simple, and it's boring, as you already know. Consume a variety of wholesome, minimally processed foods, including vegetables, fruits, whole— not refined—grains, beans, seeds and nuts. Drink plain water when you're thirsty, as well as coffee, tea, seltzer and mineral water. As you prefer, follow a specific diet plan— from vegetarian to vegan, low-fat, low-carb, Mediterranean, Paleo or flexitarian—but optimize that with plant-based foods.

Best: A vegan diet—no animal products of any kind, including no dairy, eggs or fish— which is good not only for your health but is the kindest diet plan for the environment and animals.

Avoid: A ketogenic diet, such as the Atkins diet, which is too high in saturated fat and meats and too low in carbs.

There never has been a better time to think about improving how you eat. A healthy diet is one of the biggest weapons we have against all types of diseases, including COVID-19. COVID-19 is not an equal opportunity threat. It attacks the elderly and people with inflammatory conditions such as diabetes, obesity and high blood pressure the most severely. That means a low-quality diet that doesn't support your immune health or control your weight will increase your risk for complications if you develop COVID-19.

To assess your diet for free: Visit the website DietID.com (a company I founded) to take a diet quiz and get suggestions on how to boost your immunity through your food choices.

Can You Cheat?

If you follow a healthy diet plan, does that mean you can never eat unhealthy foods such as processed snack foods? Of course not. If you want ice cream, cake, candy or chips, have them—but only occasionally.

Caveat: If you feel like you want to eat these kinds of foods frequently, you're probably not getting your diet right most of the time. Why? Because familiarity with the way a food tastes is a potent determinant of what you'll want to eat.

Example: If you eat a lot of snack foods, sweetened cereals, milk chocolate and foods with artificial sweeteners, you'll crave them. But if you stop eating those foods, your desire for them will decrease within a few weeks. Once you've changed your taste buds, you probably won't want them anymore. They'll taste like the pseudo foods they really are—sickeningly sweet, oversalted or fatty. Junk food will taste like junk.

Better cheats: Whole-grain chips with salsa…homemade oatmeal raisin or dark chocolate chip cookies made with whole-grain flour.

Going Meatless Without Going Hungry

Mark Bittman, author of more than a dozen cookbooks, including the newly revamped version of his classic, *How to Cook Everything,* and *Dinner for Everyone* from which these recipes were taken. He is coauthor of *How to Eat.* MarkBittman.com

The benefits of eating a mostly plant-based diet are well proven. Compared with their meat-eating counterparts, vegetarians are 25 percent less likely to develop heart disease…and they tend to have lower cholesterol and blood pressure levels and a reduced risk for type 2 diabetes. Still, adopting this diet is daunting if you rely on meat and dairy to fill out your meals. Many people worry that they won't feel satisfied without meat. Not true! Famed chef and cookbook author Mark Bittman began this dietary shift more than 15 years ago. *Consider these tips to help you go meatless—without going hungry…*

• **Savor your favorite flavors.** You can keep many of the characteristics of a favorite dish—the spice profile and the sauces—and create a recipe that's just as satisfying as its meaty counterpart. Common sources of plant protein include chickpeas, lentils, peas and tempeh.

• **Aim for variety.** You can have the same dish—beans with a whole grain—every day but use different beans or grains, different spice profiles and different vegetables to add variety. For instance, you can make it Caribbean style with cumin and garlic…or Mediterranean style with garlic, rosemary and lemon.

• **Plan ahead.** Some beans and grains require advance soaking, but you can make a bulk batch of beans or whole grains to use throughout the week so that weeknight cooking is easier. Canned beans can be useful, too, in dishes where you don't mind if they're a little mushy.

• **Change slowly.** Shifting from a meat-focused diet to one with more plants may affect your digestion if you are not used to eating beans and legumes. To minimize possible bloating or indigestion, change slowly. Reduce the portion size of meat at each meal, or cut back from eating meat at 10 meals per week to eating it at eight, then six and so on.

Here are three hearty recipes that are rich in flavor and texture without the meat. Each recipe makes four servings.

Instead of a Sausage Cassoulet, try…

LENTIL CASSOULET
with Lots of Vegetables

Time: 50 minutes.
8 ounces Le Puy lentils, rinsed and picked over
¼ ounce dried porcini mushrooms
1 cup boiling water
¼ cup olive oil
1 leek, trimmed, well rinsed and chopped
1 carrot, chopped
1 small celery root, peeled and chopped
2 Tablespoons chopped garlic
Salt and pepper
¼ cup dry red wine or water
1 14-ounce can diced tomatoes

½ small head green cabbage (about 8 ounces), quartered, cored and cut into thin ribbons
2 Tablespoons chopped fresh parsley
2 Tablespoons chopped fresh thyme, or 2 teaspoons dried
1 bay leaf
⅛ teaspoon cayenne, or to taste

1. Put the lentils in a large pot with enough water to cover by about one inch, and bring to a boil. Once the water boils, cover and turn off the heat. Let the lentils sit.

2. Put the dried mushrooms in a small heat-proof bowl, and cover with the boiling water. The mushrooms will take anywhere from 15 to 30 minutes to soften. When they're ready, lift them from the soaking liquid carefully to leave any grit behind. Chop the mushrooms, and reserve the liquid.

3. Heat the oil in a large skillet over medium heat, add the leek, carrot, celery root, mushrooms and garlic. Sprinkle with salt and pepper. Cook, stirring occasionally until the vegetables soften, five to 10 minutes. Add the wine, and cook, stirring and scraping up any browned bits from the bottom of the pan.

4. Add the vegetable mixture to the lentils along with the tomatoes, cabbage and herbs. Carefully pour in the mushroom soaking liquid, leaving behind the grit in the bottom of the bowl. Stir to combine, and bring to a boil. Reduce the heat so that the mixture bubbles steadily, and cook, stirring occasionally and adding a splash of water if the mixture starts to look dry, until the vegetables are silky and the lentils start to break down and thicken the stew, 25 to 35 minutes. Stir in the cayenne. Remove the bay leaf. Taste, adjust the seasoning, and serve.

Instead of Coq au Vin, try…

ARTICHOKES AND SHELL BEANS
Braised in White Wine

Time: At least 90 minutes.
½ cup fresh lemon juice (from 3 or 4 lemons)
2 cups dry white wine
Salt
1½ pounds baby artichokes, 3 pounds large artichokes or 1 pound defrosted frozen artichoke hearts
3 Tablespoons olive oil
1 large shallot, sliced
1 Tablespoon chopped fresh rosemary, or 1 teaspoon dried
3 cups frozen beans (such as edamame, black-eyed peas, lima beans or green fava beans)
1 Tablespoon drained capers
Pepper
¼ cup chopped fresh parsley, for garnish

1. Put the lemon juice in a bowl with the wine, and sprinkle with a little salt. Trim the tops, bottoms and toughest outer leaves from the artichokes, but leave the stalk and light-colored parts intact. Quarter them, and scrape away the fibrous chokes with a spoon. As you finish each artichoke, toss it with the brine. (For large globes, trim the leaves and feathery chokes from the hearts and slice them. If using frozen, slice them into manageable pieces.)

2. Put the oil in a large skillet over medium-high heat. When it's hot, transfer the artichokes to the pan with a slotted spoon or tongs. Save the liquid in the bowl. Cook, stirring occasionally, until they stop steaming and start sizzling, three to five minutes. Lower the heat to medium, and cook, stirring occasionally with a spatula, until the leaves are tender and crisp all over, 10 to 15 minutes. Transfer to a plate with a slotted spoon.

3. Add the shallot to the pan, and return to medium heat. Cook, stirring, until soft, three to five minutes. Add the rosemary, beans and capers, and strain the wine mixture into the skillet. Bring to a boil.

4. Cook, stirring often, until beans are warmed through and the sauce reduces by about one-third. Return the artichokes to the skillet, toss to coat, taste, and adjust the seasonings, adding some pepper. Garnish with the parsley, and serve.

Instead of Chicken Kebabs, try...

TAMARIND TEMPEH KEBABS

Time: At least three hours, largely unattended.

2 Tablespoons tamarind concentrate
½ cup soy sauce
½ cup mirin
⅓ cup good-quality vegetable oil, plus more for brushing
¼ cup minced fresh ginger
Salt and pepper
1 pound tempeh, cut into 16 pieces
8 long or 16 short wooden or metal skewers
1 large red onion, cut into 1-inch pieces
16 cherry tomatoes
1 broccoli crown, cut into large florets (about 8 ounces)
2 Tablespoons rice wine vinegar
2 teaspoons Dijon mustard

1. Stir tamarind, soy sauce, mirin, oil and ginger in a small bowl, and season with salt and pepper. Reserve one cup in a saucepan, and mix the rest with the tempeh in a shallow dish. Marinate for at least two hours and up to overnight.

2. Heat the oven to 425°F. If you're using wooden skewers, submerge them in hot tap water in a rimmed baking sheet for at least 10 minutes. Drain.

3. Thread a few pieces of onion onto a skewer, then add tomato, broccoli, onion again and tempeh. Repeat on the same stick (or, if using small skewers, start a new one). Repeat with the remaining skewers, and put them on a baking sheet. Brush them all over with oil, and sprinkle with salt and pepper.

4. Roast the skewers until the vegetables soften and the tempeh develops a crust, five to 10 minutes. Turn and roast another five to 10 minutes on the second side. Brush the skewers with the sauce, and return to the oven for five minutes to glaze the tempeh and vegetables. Turn and repeat at least once more, until the skewers are golden brown in spots and the vegetables are crisp-tender, another five to 10 minutes.

5. Add the vinegar, mustard and one-half cup water to the saucepan with the reserved tamarind sauce. Bring to a boil, and cook, stirring often, until slightly reduced and syrupy. Cool slightly, then taste and adjust the seasoning. Serve the kebabs hot or at room temperature, passing the warm sauce at the table.

Reprinted from *Dinner for Everyone*. Copyright © 2019 by Mark Bittman. Published by Clarkson Potter, an imprint of Penguin Random House, LLC.

Lab-Grown Meat Is Coming

TheGuardian.com

Authorities in Singapore have given approval for the first lab-grown meat to be sold for human consumption. The meat is grown in a bioreactor and made from chicken cells and then combined with plant-based ingredients.

Some Foods May Contain Unlisted Ingredients

FDA.gov

The Food and Drug Administration is temporarily allowing manufacturers to substitute alternative ingredients in packaged foods without changing the foods' labels. The rule is in effect because of supply-chain disruptions caused by the pandemic, and no end date for the rule has been set. The FDA says no substitute ingredient can be one of the top eight food allergens unless that substitution is disclosed to consumers. Companies are asked but not required to inform consumers of any temporary formulation changes through their websites or point-of-sale labeling.

Spices May Reduce Risks of a High-Fat, High-Carb Meal

The study "Spices in a High-Saturated-Fat, High-Carbohydrate Meal Reduce Postprandial Proinflammatory Cytokine Secretion in Men with Overweight or Obesity: A 3-Period, Crossover, Randomized Controlled Trial," led by researchers at Pennsylvania State University in University Park and published in the *The Journal of Nutrition*.

If you wonder why 72 percent of the US population is overweight or obese, a good portion of the blame goes to a steady diet of foods that are high in saturated fat and/or refined carbohydrates. Not surprisingly, a regular diet of these same foods also has been linked to chronic inflammation, which increases risk for cardiovascular disease (CVD).

Switching to a diet that's low in saturated fat and refined carbs seems like an obvious solution. But as anyone who's ever tried to stick to such a diet will tell you, that's not always easy. So for those occasional lapses when a person indulges in a high-fat, high-carb meal, could there be a way to blunt the negative health effects?

To explore this question, researchers at Pennsylvania State University devised a study to test how spices might affect the body's response to one of those less-than-healthful meals. The researchers recruited 12 men ages 40 to 65 who were overweight or obese and had at least one CVD risk factor.

Study details: Over the course of three days, the men ate a series of high-fat, high-carb meals and received blood tests before and after the meals to measure their levels of proteins known as cytokines, which serve as markers for inflammation. In random order, participants were given meals that did not have any spices added…had 2 grams (g) of a spice blend added…or had 6 g of the same spice blend added. The spice blend contained basil, bay leaf, black pepper, cinnamon, coriander, cumin, ginger, oregano, parsley, red pepper, rosemary, thyme and turmeric.

The result: After giving blood tests to the study participants hourly for four hours after each meal, the researchers found that the 6 g spice-blended meals significantly reduced cytokine levels compared with the other meals. The 6 g spice blend was roughly equivalent to one teaspoon to one tablespoon, depending on the spice's level of dehydration.

Although this study, which was published in *The Journal of Nutrition*, did not identify which spices work best to lower inflammation, numerous animal and human studies have shown that spices such as turmeric, ginger and cinnamon have anti-inflammatory properties.

Earlier research has shown that meals that are high in fat, carbs and/or sugar lead to spikes in inflammation, known as acute inflammation. It's not known whether these short bursts of inflammation result in chronic inflammation, but the researchers theorize that they do play a role, especially in people who are overweight or obese.

"Ultimately the gold standard would be to get people eating more healthfully and to lose weight and exercise, but those behavior changes are difficult and take time," said Connie J. Rogers, PhD, MPH, lead author of the study and an associate professor of nutritional sciences at Pennsylvania State University. In the interim, the study finding suggests that spices may be an effective and convenient way to at least help reduce the inflammation that results from a high-carb, high-fat meal. Even though this study was small, the researchers hope that larger studies with a more diverse population will support their findings.

Takeaway: The best way to avoid obesity and cardiovascular disease is to exercise, reduce calories and eat a diet that includes lots of vegetables, fruits and whole grains. For that occasional indulgence, adding some spice to your moussaka or lasagna could make your meal both tastier and healthier.

Extraordinary Olives

Dan Flynn, director of the UC Davis Olive Center, dedicated to supporting California olive growers and processors through research, education and other initiatives. OliveCenter.UCDavis.edu

With all the health benefits associated with olive oil, it's easy to overlook olives themselves. But they, too, serve up antioxidant and anti-inflammatory compounds plus add zest to any dish.

Among the important nutrients in olives are oleic acid, a monounsaturated omega-9 fatty acid that helps raise HDL "good" cholesterol and helps eliminate plaque in the arteries, and strong disease fighters called phenols. Oleuropein, its main phenol, is extremely bitter, so most olives are processed, or cured, in one of several ways to "de-bitter" them.

Curing Determines Taste

Olive labels generally do not indicate the curing method, but the approach used definitely affects the flavor.

•**Lye-cured.** Most canned black olives on supermarket shelves are made using a diluted lye bath followed by washing or soaking in water. Lye removes more phenols than other methods and so produces the mildest flavor. You may hear "lye" and think "toxic," but it is thoroughly washed out and poses no danger.

Lye-cured olive to try: The Italian Castelvetrano, which has more taste than most lye-cured olives.

•**Brine-cured.** Sometimes called Sicilian style, brined olives are fermented in a salt-and-water solution, similar to sauerkraut and pickles. With some olives, such as the Greek Kalamata, this often is followed with a red-wine vinegar brine for deeper flavor. "Spanish-style" curing uses lye and then brine, as with the Italian Cerignola.

•**Salt-cured.** Olives dry-cured in salt, such as Throuba Thassos from Greece and Beldi from Morocco, retain the greatest amount of phenol compounds and have the most intense flavor.

Finding New Favorites

Sample both mild and pungent olives by buying small amounts of different varieties from the olive bar at a local supermarket or gourmet shop. You also can find many jarred choices online.

Imported olives come primarily from Mediterranean countries, but a number of varieties are grown in California—farms including McEvoy Ranch and Penna Olives sell direct. Penna and Chaffin Family Orchards even sell fresh raw olives online in the fall that you can cure yourself. The UC Davis Olive Center has an online olive guide at ANRCatalog.ucanr.cdu/pdf/8267.pdf.

Experiment with olives in cooking. Add chopped olives to tuna, egg, pasta and grain-based salads and whole olives to any green salad. The secrets to a true Greek salad are using Kalamata olives and chunks from a fresh slab of feta cheese (not packaged crumbles) and assembling it just as you're ready to eat.

For a tasty accompaniment for grilled fish or chicken, make olive tapenade, a purée easily done in a food processor.

Chunky olive salad, used in the classic Muffaletta sandwich, is a rough chop of olives, pickled vegetables and spices, and on its own makes a great alternative to salsa.

As an ingredient in recipes, olives add complex flavor to Mediterranean dishes, from Moroccan tagines to Italian sauces such as puttanesca.

Hummus and Beans Often Are Contaminated

Alexis Temkin, PhD, is a toxicologist with the Environmental Working Group, Washington, DC. See the full study results at EWG.org.

Hummus and beans often are contaminated with *glyphosate*, the weed killer in Roundup linked to cancer. Investigators tested conventional and organic hummus, beans and lentils purchased online and from major food retailers. Ninety percent of chickpea-based samples had detectable glyphosate, many with quite high levels. Lowest were canned chickpeas from Goya, Hanover and Simple Truth Organic. There also were low hummus samples such as O Organics, The Perfect Pita and Asmar's.

Best: Make your own hummus from organic chickpeas.

Hidden Dangers in Food from China

Tony Corbo, senior government affairs representative at Food & Water Watch, Washington, DC, responsible for food-related legislative and regulatory issues that come before Congress and the Executive Branch. FoodAndWaterWatch.org

---

Regulations that the Chinese government instituted to food-safety laws in December 2019 don't address key problems—heavy metals such as lead, mercury and arsenic in their soil...and the overuse of pesticides, animal antibiotics and additives in food processing. The riskiest foods are fish, shellfish, vegetables and fruits.

Adding to the problem is lack of US oversight. Our agencies don't have the manpower to inspect enough food plants in China or check more than 1 percent or 2 percent of shipments that arrive in the US.

High percentages of the apple juice, processed mushrooms, frozen spinach and tilapia we consume are from China. The USDA has not permitted China to export poultry products from birds raised there to the US until recently. Poultry products have to be cooked, but a hidden provision in the trade act opens the door for fresh poultry to come here in the future.

Our "Country of Origin Labeling" law requires most markets to post where foods, including fresh and frozen chicken, some meats, seafood, fruits and vegetables, come from. So buying whole, fresh foods is safest.

Once a product has been prepared or processed, country-of-origin labeling isn't mandatory. For example, breaded chicken products and dried spices do not have to be labeled. Country of origin usually is marked on the box in which spice containers come to the store, so ask at the customer-service desk.

Note: Other countries that have a high number of food shipments refused by the FDA for contamination are Mexico, primarily for vegetables, and India, notably for spices and farm-raised shrimp. An organic label is not a guarantee or a green light that a product is safe to buy. Recent investigations have found that some foods labeled "organic"—from China and elsewhere—are not.

Beyond the Cucumber: Pickled Vegetables Are a Tangy Treat

Kirsten K. Shockey, coauthor of Fermented Vegetables and Fiery Ferments, from which these recipes are excerpted, and most recently Miso, Tempeh, Natto & Other Tasty Ferments. With her husband, Christopher, she teaches fermentation arts worldwide and hosts workshops on their southern Oregon homestead. Ferment.Works

---

Do you love the taste of a dill pickle... the tang of sauerkraut...or the spicy burn of kimchi? If so, you might be intrigued to know that creating those incredible flavors at home is much easier than you would imagine. All of these tasty treats—and so many more—are fermented, or pickled, foods. Plenty of folks think fermentation is a complicated, mysterious science experiment that requires an advanced degree, but this couldn't be further from the truth.

Making your own pickled vegetables is easy once you know the basics, and the incredible tastes that you'll unlock will keep you pickling for years to come. Plus, it's a great way to use up veggies that you might otherwise be tempted to throw away, which helps reduce waste and can be a good excuse to go a little crazy at the supermarket when your favorite veggies are on sale or in season.

Fermented foods can live up to a year in the refrigerator—you'll never need to worry about being out of veggies at mealtime. They're an instant salad, egg or burger topper…side dish…and great in tacos and almost anything else you're having.

The Basics of Fermentation

Fermentation preserves produce without using heat, so all their lovely vitamins and minerals are retained. In fact, some nutrients become more readily available after fermentation.

Example: Fermentation increases cabbage's levels of vitamin C and adds vitamins B-12 and K-2.

Fun fact: It's believed that Captain Cook minimized scurvy aboard his ships via mandatory servings of sauerkraut.

Making pickles or any pickled vegetables (please note that we're not talking about the common vinegar pickles, but naturally fermented pickles) relies on the lactic bacteria found on the skins of your vegetables. This bacteria will proliferate in the salty environment of the brine and reward you with a good amount of healthful probiotics.

Submerge in Brine, and All Will Be Fine

Dry brining is one of the easiest techniques for fermenting vegetables. It works best for vegetables that are thinly sliced or shredded. In this type of fermentation, you use salt to draw water out of the vegetable's cells, which then creates the brine in which it will soak. Once in the salty brine, the "good" bacteria will start to multiply, and soon you'll have delicious, tangy pickles.

STEP 1: **Salt the veggies.** You can ferment pretty much any vegetable, but the specifics will change a bit whether you're making a sauerkraut with cabbage or pickling whole carrots or daikon (a type of radish). The process starts by adding salt to cut vegetables in a bowl and massaging it in for a few minutes. As you do this, the vegetables begin releasing their juices. This liquid—the brine—provides the optimal anaerobic environment that encourages the good bacteria and discourages any "bad" ones from growing. That's why I say, "Submerge in brine, and all will be fine." Sometimes the vegetables will produce enough liquid to create enough brine, and sometimes you'll have to create your own brine with water and salt, and add that to the vegetables.

Best salt: I recommend a mineral-rich salt free from additives such as Redmond Real Salt ($10.65 for 1.6 pounds, RealSalt.com) or Himalayan Crystal Salt ($29.50 for 2.2 pounds, HimalayanCrystalSalt.com). Do not use table salt with added iodine or, ironically, pickling salt—both contain additives and often produce ferments that have an overwhelming, rather than pleasant, salty taste.

Move the vegetables and brine to a clean, wide-mouthed glass jar. Next, you need to add a weight that keeps the veggies below the level of the brine. An easy way to do this is to use a small, clean, sealable bag filled with water. You also can use a plate that fits the mouth of your jar or even a thoroughly scrubbed, smooth stone.

Keep about an inch or so of space between the top of the vegetables/liquid and the lid of the jar. As the bacteria start to work, they'll create carbon dioxide and the gas will use that space. Make sure to "burp" your glass every day or so. You just need to unscrew the lid until you hear the pssssft of the gas escaping, then retighten. (Don't take off the lid, just loosen it.) You'll know your ferment needs a burp when you see the lid bulging.

STEP 2: **Step back and trust your veggies.** Your work is done. Next, simply move the jar to an area of your kitchen out of direct sunlight, which can cause temperature fluctuations. You'll often hear recommendations to keep ferments in a cool, dark place, but standard room temperature helps the good bacteria to multiply at the right rate, so anything between 60°F and 75°F should be fine. The pickled veggies should be done in about five to seven days, but this will vary based on the temperature in your house. Aside from burping, let the jar be. Once the pickle is sour enough for you, you can remove the weight, put on a lid and store it all in the refrigerator, which will stop the fermentation process.

STEP 3: **Enjoy.** When done, you'll be richly rewarded with deep, complex flavors… punchy tang…healthy probiotics…and the satisfaction of carrying on a magical, ancient tradition.

A Word of Caution

Every now and then, things go wrong, so trust your nose if you're not quite sure about a batch. Pungent and pickle-y, even a little funky scents and tastes are good. Anything that smells like rotting potatoes or compost is not. Also on the throwaway list—veggies that taste slimy or are overly soft.

Two Easy Recipes

These two recipes are ideal for beginners— they're easy but yield delicious results.

Lemon Dill Kraut

> 3 pounds (1 head) green cabbage
> 3 cloves garlic, finely grated
> 1 lemon, juice and zest
> 1½ teaspoons dried dill weed
> 1 Tablespoon salt

Remove any coarse outer leaves of the cabbage. Rinse a few unblemished leaves, and set them aside. Rinse the rest of the cabbage in cold water. Quarter and core the cabbage. Thinly slice, then transfer the cabbage to a large bowl. Add the garlic, lemon juice and zest, and dill. Add the salt, then use your hands to massage the salt into the shreds, then taste. You should taste the salt without it being overwhelming. Add more salt if necessary. The cabbage should quickly start to look wet and limp, and liquid will begin to pool. If not, make sure that there's enough

salt, and let it stand, covered, for 45 minutes and then massage.

Transfer the mixture, bit by bit, to a two-quart glass container with a lid or a wide-mouthed jar. Press down on each portion. Make sure that the brine is covering all the cabbage. Even a small amount of brine is fine as long as it is at the top of the cabbage. If you think you need more liquid, check back in an hour. Often the salt will have pulled more liquid from the cabbage. If not, you can add more lemon juice. Allow two to three inches of headspace. Top the cabbage with one or two of the reserved outer leaves (they should be submerged as well), then top that with a water-filled, sealable plastic bag to keep everything below the level of the brine. Next, tighten the lid. Set aside for five to 10 days. Check daily to ensure that the vegetables are submerged. Using a utensil, you can taste-test the kraut on day five.

You'll know it's ready when it's pleasingly sour, pickle-y tasting without the strong acidity of vinegar…the veggies have softened a bit but retain some crunch…the cabbage is more yellow than green and slightly translucent. When it's finished, toss the top leaves.

Spicy Carrot and Lime Salad

> 1¾ pounds carrots (sliced very thin on a grater or mandolin)
> 3 to 4 Fresno or other hot red peppers, seeded (if you want less heat) and sliced thin, or 1 Tablespoon dried chile flakes
> Zest and juice of 2 limes
> 1 (1-to-2-inch) piece fresh ginger, sliced thin
> 2 teaspoons salt

Combine all the ingredients except the salt in a bowl. Massage the salt into mixture. Pack the mixture into a jar using the method above. Set aside for seven to 10 days. You can taste-test on day seven. When ready, it will have a pleasing acidic smell and taste pickle-y. It also may have a bit of an effervescent zing. A slight cloudiness in the brine is normal.

Prebiotic Foods May Improve Sleep and Reduce Stress

Andrew Rubman, ND, is medical director of South-bury Clinic for Traditional Medicines, Southbury, Connecticut.

Researchers at University of Colorado at Boulder found that rats fed a prebiotic-rich diet had more time in restorative and REM sleep cycles—essential for stress relief. Prebiotics fuel healthy bacteria in the intestine that help produce the hormone serotonin, which regulates sleep-wake cycles. These are fibrous foods such as lentils, cabbage and whole grains. Increase intake gradually to avoid digestive distress as your body adjusts.

Organic Apples Are Better for Gut Health

Study titled "An Apple a Day: Which Bacteria Do We Eat With Organic and Conventional Apples?" by researchers at Institute of Environmental Biotechnology, Graz University, Graz, Austria, published in *Frontiers in Microbiology*.

An apple a day is a good bet for health—especially the health of your gut...and especially if that apple is organic, a recent study has confirmed. The bacteria you consume from eating raw fruits and vegetables support a healthy community of microorganisms (microbiome) of the digestive tract. Raw is the best way to go because cooking kills the healthy microbes that protect your gut.

A balanced and healthy microbiome is key for digestive health and for a healthy immune system. Healthy bacteria—such as *Lactobacillus* found in probiotics—need to balance out harmful bacteria that can cause digestive disorders, such as food poisoning.

The researchers, from the Institute of Environmental Biotechnology at Graz University in Graz, Austria, wanted to see if bacteria in raw fruit differed between organically and conventionally grown fruit. They chose apples because they are among the most common fruits eaten worldwide. Their findings were published in *Frontiers in Microbiology*.

Study details: The researchers picked four organically grown apples and compared their bacterial components with four conventionally grown apples matched for size, color and flawlessness. Although both types of apples had about the same number of bacteria—about 100 million cells—the organic apples had more bacterial variety. The conventional apples had more harmful bacteria, such as E. coli and shigella, which are associated with food poisoning. The organic apples had more probiotic bacteria.

To be labeled as organic, a fruit or vegetable needs to meet certain standards that include avoiding the use of pesticides and chemical fertilizers. The researchers found that although all parts of the apple had bacteria, a large portion of it was found in the seeds and core. To get up to 100 million bacterial cells, you would need to eat the whole apple. Apples provide other health benefits, such as antioxidant flavonoids and heart-healthy fiber from pectin.

Takeaway: This is one more study that points to the importance of including raw fruits and vegetables in your diet. The investigators conclude that organically grown fruit may offer a wider variety and more probiotic types of bacteria that could lead to a healthier, more balanced gut microbiome. And a healthy gut usually means a strong immune system.

Fatty Foods Can Hamper Concentration

Study by Annelise Madison, graduate student in clinical psychology at The Ohio State University, Columbus, published in *American Journal of Clinical Nutrition*.

After eating only one meal high in saturated fat, women who took a test requiring 10 minutes of intense concentration performed 11 percent worse than those who ate a meal high in healthier unsaturated fat. The meals of both groups mimicked fast-food options, and both contained 930 calories. While it's known that, over time, diet can have a detrimental effect on thinking ability, researchers were surprised that this can apparently happen after just a single meal. The study didn't explore why this happens, but previous research has found saturated fat triggers inflammation throughout the body, which may affect brain function.

Using Only Sea Salt or Gourmet Salt Can Lead to Iodine Deficiency

Iodized table salt is the most common source of iodine. Deficiencies can lead to fatigue, weight gain, hair loss and goiter. One-half teaspoon of iodized salt per day meets the daily requirement for iodine. Sea vegetables such as nori, wakame or dulse flakes are another potent source of iodine. Have a modest serving two or three times per week.

Neal D. Barnard, MD, is adjunct associate professor of medicine at George Washington University School of Medicine and Health Sciences in Washington, DC, and president of Physicians Committee for Responsible Medicine. PCRM.org

Don't Throw Away Expired Milk

BonAppetit.com

Just because the expiration date on the carton is past doesn't mean that the milk has to be dumped down the sink (unless, of course, it's curdled). *Pour it.* Use it on sugary cereals, when you make oatmeal porridge, or try it in recipes that call for buttermilk, such as pancakes and waffles. Or if you want to get fancy, look up a Mason-jar ice-cream or panna-cotta recipe. *Bake it.* Using slightly sour milk to make scones, muffins and pretzel knots will help leaven the food and give it a pleasant tang. *Fry it.* Use it when breading and frying cheese, squash, eggplant or green tomatoes. *Make ricotta in your microwave.* Stir the juice of one lemon into two cups of old milk. Microwave until bubbling (about four minutes), then stir until curds form. Scoop curds onto a paper towel-lined strainer, wait five minutes and serve.

How to Cook Safely With Nonstick Pans

LiveScience.com

Generally, Teflon-coated pans are safe to use. However, when heated to high temperatures, these pans release a harmful chemical called perfluorooctanoic acid (PFOA). Since PFOA is linked to many health conditions including cancer and thyroid disease, follow these tips for safe use.

• **Don't overheat it.** Excessive temperatures cause Teflon to release PFOA, so use only medium-to-low heat.

• **Don't overuse it.** Even at lower temperatures, Teflon will break down over time, so avoid scratching the surface with utensils, and keep your pans only for a few years before replacing.

•**Avoid it when pregnant and breast-feeding.** PFOA can disrupt reproductive processes, so don't use it during those crucial times.

•**Consider alternatives.** Teflon isn't the only nonstick material. Anodized aluminum and ceramic work great, and good old cast iron does the job well when treated correctly.

Switch to Sourdough Bread

Andrea Thompson, RDN, registered dietician nutritionist with Penn State Health St. Joseph Hospital, Reading, Pennsylvania.

If commercially baked breads cause intestinal distress even though you do not have celiac disease, switching to sourdough bread made with a homemade starter could help.

Reason: Letting bread dough rise several times before it is baked breaks down hard-to-digest gluten proteins. Most commercial breads now are made using rapid-rise yeasts, and the shorter rising time leaves more gluten proteins intact. The long fermentation required for making sourdough, on the other hand, breaks down more of the gluten, making sourdough easier to digest.

Easy Gluten-Free Sourdough Bread Recipe

Andrea Thompson, RDN, LDN, nutritionist and dietitian with expertise in gluten-free diets, Penn State Health St. Joseph Hospital, Reading, Pennsylvania.
Tricia Thompson, MS, RD, a dietitian specializing in gluten-free nutrition, based in Manchester, Massachusetts and founder of GlutenFreeWatchdog.org.

Sourdough bread not only tastes good, it's good for you! Sourdough is more digestible than other kinds of bread...plus healthy bacteria in the bread boost immunity and your feel-good hormones. And being gluten-free doesn't mean having to be sourdough-free.

What's So Healthy About Traditional Sourdough?

The sourdough method for making bread has been around since the time of the ancient Egyptians. Sourdough is a method for making bread rise, a process called leavening, using only naturally occurring "wild yeast" that is already present in flour and the surrounding air instead of using packaged yeast as is used for other leavened breads. Wild yeast cultivated in flour, such as wheat or rye, and water takes several days to a week to ferment and develop. And making bread with this kind of yeast involves a longer proving process—when the dough rises and develops—than with packaged yeast.

It is this lengthy fermenting and proving that gives sourdough its healthy edge over other kinds of bread.

Improved digestibility: Phytic acid in wheat, rye and other flours used to make bread—including gluten-free flours—inhibits stomach enzymes needed to break down proteins and starch and causes digestive discomfort and bloating for some people. While an enzyme that breaks down phytic acid called *phytase* is released during the making of any yeast-leavened bread, sourdough's longer fermentation time gives the yeast more time to break down phytic acid... helping to make grain's micronutrients more easily absorbed in the gut.

Probiotic edge: Healthy bacteria called *Lactobacillus reuteri* that grow during sourdough fermentation have been shown in laboratory studies to improve immunity, slow weight gain, speed wound healing and even stimulate the brain to release the "feel good" hormone oxytocin.

Celiac vs. Sourdough

While the gluten content may be reduced in sourdough breads compared with other wheat and rye breads, it's still too high for people who need to be gluten-free for celiac disease or other health reasons. The FDA requires foods labeled gluten-free to contain less than 20 parts per million (ppm) of gluten. The Gluten Free Watchdog, which independently tests labeled gluten-free products for gluten contamination, tested three sourdough wheat breads made by artisanal bakeries and found the gluten content could be upwards of 100,000 ppm.

Safe Sourdough!

The good news is that it's easy—and fun!—to make sourdough with flours that do not contain gluten, such as flours made from brown rice, buckwheat, teff, quinoa and sorghum.

Start by searching "gluten free sourdough starter" on the web. While specific directions vary, any sourdough starter is made by stirring together flour and water in a glass jar or ceramic bowl and allowing it to ferment. Once it becomes bubbly, has doubled in volume and smells pleasantly sour, it's ready use—to make bread, pancakes, waffles or whatever your culinary creativity thinks up! You need to refrigerate unused starter…"feed" it once a week or so with additional flour and water…and replace any amount used with an equal amount of flour-and-water mixture.

The process takes some patience and nurturing, but your efforts will be well rewarded!

Immune-Boosting Recipes That Are Bursting With Flavor

Debby Maugans is a food writer based in Asheville, North Carolina, and author of *Farmer & Chef Asheville.* FarmerAndChefSouth.com

Having a healthy immune system helps our bodies to fight back when we're exposed to viruses. One of the best ways to boost your immune system is with a healthy diet full of a broad array of antioxidant-rich fruits, vegetables, herbs and spices.

Flexibility is key, especially if you can't find certain ingredients. If you need to substitute, choose a vegetable or fruit with the same basic texture profile—berry for berry, leaf for leaf, root for root. And if you find fruits and veggies in the fridge that are less than crisp, just add them to a smoothie.

Washing your produce is as important as washing your hands. Rinse them under cold, running water for about 30 seconds right before you use them.

Chicken Almond Satay Wraps

You can substitute two medium carrots, shredded, for the cucumber…and one cup of thinly sliced sugar snap peas for the red bell pepper strips.

¼ cup red miso
3 Tablespoons honey
3 Tablespoons low-sodium soy sauce
2 Tablespoons minced fresh ginger
3 cloves garlic, minced
¼ cup smooth almond butter
3 Tablespoons water
1 pound skinless chicken cutlets
12 water-soaked 6-inch wooden skewers
12 medium-size lacinato kale or romaine lettuce leaves
1 medium seedless cucumber, diced (about 1½ cups)
1 large red bell pepper, very thinly sliced into strips

Combine the miso, honey, soy sauce, ginger and garlic in a medium bowl. Measure out two tablespoons of this mixture, and place in a small bowl. Add the almond butter and water to the small bowl, and stir well. Reserve for serving.

Place the chicken cutlets between two pieces of wax paper. Lightly pound until they are an even thickness. Slice the chicken cutlets crosswise into one-quarter-inch-thick strips.

Add to the remaining miso mixture, and toss until well-coated. Thread onto wooden skewers, and arrange on a baking sheet.

Position the oven rack at the top level, then preheat oven on broil. Broil chicken one to two minutes on each side or until browned and cooked through.

To serve, place each chicken skewer on a kale leaf and remove the skewer. Top with cucumber and bell pepper. Drizzle each with about two teaspoons of the miso–almond butter mixture. *Yield:* Four servings.

Roasted Sweet Potato and Kale Quinoa Bowl

You can substitute spinach for the kale if needed, and cooked brown rice or farro for the quinoa.

- ¼ cup pure maple syrup
- 2 Tablespoons fresh lemon juice
- 2 Tablespoons butter, melted
- ½ teaspoon kosher salt
- ¼ teaspoon pepper
- 2 pounds (3 large) unpeeled sweet potatoes, cut into ½-inch dice
- 8 ounces cremini mushrooms, sliced
- 1 bunch lacinato or curly kale, stems removed and cut into 1-inch slices
- 1 cup dry quinoa, cooked according to package directions
- ½ cup chopped unsalted roasted almonds
- ¼ cup pomegranate seeds
- Garlic Lemon Yogurt Topping (recipe follows)

Preheat oven to 400°F. Position rack in bottom third of the oven. Place a large, rimmed baking sheet on the rack while the oven heats. Tear off a piece of foil that will fit over the baking pan.

Combine the maple syrup, lemon juice, butter, salt and pepper in a large bowl. Stir to blend well. Add the sweet potatoes, and toss to coat well.

When the oven is hot, remove the baking sheet from the oven. Pour the sweet potatoes onto it, and spread into a single layer. Bake until just fork-tender, about 20 minutes, turning once.

Remove the baking sheet from the oven, and move the sweet potatoes to one-half of the pan. Add the mushrooms to the other half of the baking sheet. Return to the oven, baking 10 minutes.

Remove the baking sheet from the oven and scatter the kale over the sweet potatoes and mushrooms. Return pan to the oven, and bake five minutes or until wilted.

To serve, spoon hot quinoa into four serving bowls. Spoon sweet potatoes, mushrooms and kale over quinoa, dividing evenly. Sprinkle each serving with two tablespoons of almonds, one tablespoon of pomegranate seeds and two tablespoons of Garlic Lemon Yogurt Topping.

Garlic Lemon Yogurt Topping

- ⅛ teaspoon kosher salt
- 1 clove garlic
- ½ cup 2 percent low-fat plain yogurt
- 1 Tablespoon fresh lemon juice

Crush the garlic with the salt in a mortar with a pestle, or place the garlic and salt on a cutting board and crush with the flat of a knife. Place the yogurt and lemon juice in a small bowl, and stir in the garlic mixture until blended. Makes about one-half cup.

Roast Cod with Fennel and Tomatoes

If fennel is unavailable, substitute a large onion, sliced. Any white fish will work, such as haddock and tilapia.

- ¼ cup extra-virgin olive oil
- 3 cloves garlic, minced
- Grated zest and juice from 2 lemons
- ½ teaspoon kosher salt
- ¼ teaspoon freshly ground pepper
- 4 (5- to 6-ounce) cod fillets
- 1 fennel bulb
- 1 pint cherry or grape tomatoes

Combine the olive oil, garlic, lemon zest and lemon juice, salt and pepper in a small bowl. Place fish on a plate. Spoon and spread one tablespoon of the mixture on the fish, and turn to coat all sides.

Preheat oven to 400°F.

Arrange fennel slices in a shallow one-and-a-half-quart baking dish. Top with tomatoes. Bake 20 to 25 minutes or until fennel is just tender. Arrange cod over fennel and tomatoes. Drizzle with remaining marinade. Bake seven to eight minutes or until fish just flakes with a fork.

To serve, use a spatula to lift fennel and fish slices onto serving plates. Spoon tomatoes and juices over fish. *Yield:* Four servings

Zesty Papaya Salsa

Papaya's buttery texture and lightly sweet taste pairs well with spicy dishes as well as simple baked pork, chicken or fish. If you can't find papaya, substitute avocado or mango.

2 cups seeded and diced (½-inch dice) from one large papaya (about 2 pounds)

¼ cup pomegranate seeds or wild blueberries

3 Tablespoons minced fresh cilantro

2 Tablespoons finely chopped green onion (white and light green parts)

2 Tablespoons fresh lime juice (1 lime)

⅛ teaspoon kosher salt

4 bell peppers, seeded and cut into 8 wedges

Combine the papaya, pomegranate seeds, cilantro, green onion, lime juice and salt in a small mixing bowl. Toss to combine. Serve with bell pepper strips, spooning a heaping teaspoon of salsa on the end of each pepper strip. The salsa can be made up to one day ahead and refrigerated in an airtight container. *Yield:* Two cups

Super Spinach Hummus

You actually can use any green vegetables, herbs or colored bell peppers that are beyond their peak in this recipe instead of spinach.

1 (15-ounce) can chickpeas, drained and rinsed

¼ cup water

¼ cup packed fresh parsley sprigs

3 Tablespoons lemon juice (1½ to 2 lemons)

2 Tablespoons well-stirred tahini

2 cloves garlic, minced

1 Tablespoon minced fresh ginger

½ teaspoon kosher salt

¼ teaspoon pepper

1½ cups packed fresh spinach leaves

Place the chickpeas, water, parsley, lemon juice, tahini, garlic, ginger, salt and pepper in a food processor. Process until smooth, scraping the food processor bowl as needed. Add the spinach to the food processor bowl, and process just until the mixture is bright green and smooth, scraping the bowl as needed. Spoon into an airtight container. Cover and refrigerate one hour or up to two days. *Yield:* About two cups.

Unsweetened Dried Fruit

Study by researchers at Pennsylvania State University, State College, published in *Journal of the Academy of Nutrition and Dietetics.*

Unsweetened dried fruit is a good alternative to fresh fruit—it is portable, shelf-stable and often less expensive than fresh fruit. Try eating it as a snack instead of junk foods. Just be careful to reduce the portion size—a serving of dried fruit seems much smaller because the water has been removed.

Homemade Fruit Leather

SkinnyTaste.com

Homemade fruit leather is better for you than the store-bought kind and has less added sugar. And it is easy to make, with only three ingredients and five minutes of preparation. Preheat the oven to 150°F, and line a sheet pan with a silicone baking mat. Peel and chop a large mango, put it in a blender or food processor, blend until smooth, and set aside. Then put six ounces of fresh strawberries and two tablespoons of sugar in the blender or food processor, and blend until smooth. Put small amounts of the purées on the pan, and spread evenly with a small spatula. Bake for two-and-a-half to three hours, rotating the baking sheet every hour. Remove when the fruit is tacky but not too sticky or wet...let cool...remove from the mat...and place on wax paper. Cut the cooled fruit and wax paper into strips with scissors, and roll the strips with paper side out. Store in a sealed container at room temperature for up to a week.

Skip the Soda

Fill ice cube trays with juice or blended fruits. Add these juice/fruit cubes to your sparkling water to create a great soda substitute.

Lisa R. Young, PhD, RDN, author of *Finally Full, Finally Slim: 30 Days to Permanent Weight Loss One Portion at a Time.*

Foods to Wash—and Not Wash

WebMD.com

Do not wash raw chicken, red meat or fish—washing spreads bacteria around the sink and can cross-contaminate other foods. Kill bacteria by cooking poultry, meat and fish to recommended internal temperatures. Do wash cantaloupe and other melons, whose skins can trap bacteria that can be moved into the flesh by cutting...and avocado, whose skin can also carry bacteria that can transfer inside. It is not necessary to wash foods that are dusty when they come out of the bag, such as dried beans, farro and quinoa.

The Sweetener Stevia Could Disrupt Your Gut

Karina Golberg, PhD, is an expert of biotechnology engineering at Ben-Gurion University of the Negev, Be'er Sheva, Israel, and leader of a study published in *Molecules.*

Although stevia, the low-calorie natural alternative to sugar, generally is considered safe, new research suggests that it inhibits communication between different bacteria in the gut microbiome, which could lead to a number of gastrointestinal health issues, including irritable bowel and obesity. While more research is needed to confirm the finding, you might want to limit the use of stevia if you find that it triggers digestive problems.

Calcium: The Rest of the Story

Nicole Avena, PhD, a nutrition and diet expert and assistant professor of neuroscience at Mount Sinai Icahn School of Medicine in New York City. Dr. Avena is the author of *Why Diets Fail* and other nutrition-related books. Her research is focused on appetite and brain mechanisms that regulate food intake throughout the lifespan. DrNicoleAvena.com

It has been drilled into us for decades that calcium is crucial for the health of our bones and teeth. When we hit age 50, we hear the refrain even more loudly—don't slight your calcium intake, since bone-thinning osteoporosis affects one in four women and about one in 20 men in later life. Calcium even helps us keep our teeth as we grow older.

So you might have missed the rest of the story on calcium—that your muscles, heart, immune system...indeed, your very well-being ...are linked to this mineral, which comes from what we eat and drink rather than occurring naturally in our bodies.

And even though calcium is often pigeon-holed as something mainly older women need to worry about, virtually every cell in every person's body, throughout one's lifespan, depends on this nutrient to work properly. *What you need to know about calcium—and the levels you need to stay healthy…*

Too Little Can Be Too Late

At a fundamental level, calcium serves as a link between cells throughout the body. *Among the key body functions that involve calcium…*

•**Muscle contraction.** All the muscles in your body rely on calcium to trigger contraction by reacting with certain proteins in muscles that regulate movement. Without enough calcium, muscle contraction can be impaired, leading to muscle spasms.

•**Heart rate.** The heart is a muscle, of course, and its ability to pump relies heavily on calcium. Without it, a dangerously irregular heartbeat (arrhythmia) can develop.

•**Brain health.** For communication between our neurons to occur, we need calcium. Calcium is known as an intracellular messenger and plays many roles in the brain's ability to function properly.

•**Blood clotting.** Calcium contributes to the essential ability of blood to clot—for example, to stop the bleeding if you cut yourself. (This is different from life-threatening blood clots such as occur with atrial fibrillation, when the heart beats irregularly and/or quivers, causing blood to pool and form clots in the heart's chambers.)

•**Immune response.** Calcium is vital to the cell communication that helps regulate how well our immune system fights off germs and other invaders. Low levels of the mineral can lead to disruptions in the production of infection-fighting white blood cells.

•**Skin and other connective tissue.** Since our bodies are constantly creating new cells—a process that's key to the skin's elasticity—low calcium levels can contribute to sagging skin. The nutrient also helps support ligaments, tendons and other connective tissues.

The Testing Conundrum

Unfortunately, there is no good way to determine whether someone is running low on calcium. Technically, a simple blood test can measure your level of calcium. But because the body pulls calcium from the bones and teeth to make sure there is enough in the blood for critical body functions, the blood test isn't a reliable gauge.

Even if the blood level were consistent, this alone cannot reveal how well your body absorbs calcium. You may be consuming "enough," but what's most important is how well your body is using the mineral. Certain dietary habits, such as consuming a lot of salt, can interfere with calcium absorption.

Bone-density testing presents a catch-22. This type of test is able to deduce whether you're low on calcium by revealing problems such as osteopenia or osteoporosis after it's already developed…or worsened.

By then, the body has leached too much calcium from the bones—its calcium "bank"—and the only option is damage control to help prevent further bone loss since it's too late to completely shore up a weakened skeletal system.

Osteoporosis drugs can help slow further bone breakdown, but they can't reverse it. Some studies suggest that strength training can help to rebuild muscle strength and bone, which are related, but the mechanisms through which this occurs aren't well understood.

Nutritional Teamwork

Since our bodies don't produce calcium, our stores depend on what we consume in our diets. But the process is more complicated than simply downing calcium-rich foods.

Notice how a carton of milk might say, "Fortified with calcium and vitamin D"? Certain other nutrients (known as synergists) interact with calcium, boosting the mineral's ability to be more fully absorbed. This is why so many foods, such as dairy products, orange juice and cereals, are fortified with calcium and vitamin D. Another significant synergist is vitamin K, which is rich in vegetables such as cabbage, watercress, broccoli and asparagus.

Magnesium is also important to calcium functioning. It converts vitamin D into its active form so that it can help with calcium absorption. Other minerals, such as potassium, also play a role in calcium absorption.

It's not that difficult to fulfill your daily calcium requirements with a healthful diet. Ideally, look for fortified versions of dairy products such as yogurt, milk and cheese...and eat plenty of dark-green, leafy vegetables such as kale, collard greens and broccoli, which are also rich in vitamin K. Fish with edible, soft bones, such as sardines and canned salmon, are also calcium-rich and good sources of vitamin D.

The task gets more challenging for people who forgo dairy products. Fortunately, Lactaid, a lactose-free milk, and almond and other nondairy milk alternatives come in calcium-fortified versions. You can also double up on dark-green, leafy veggies and add other calcium-rich foods to your diet, including beans (such as kidney, navy and Garbanzo) and fruit (such as oranges, figs, apricots, kiwi and papayas).

To make sure you're getting enough calcium, aim for these daily levels through your diet and/or supplements (see below): For women age 19 to 50, the recommended dietary allowance (RDA) is 1,000 mg per day...and 1,200 mg daily after age 50. For men age 19 to 70, the RDA is 1,000 mg daily...and 1,200 mg thereafter.

Helpful: To make sure you are consuming enough calcium each day, you can use an app to log your food intake, which will show how much calcium you are getting.

Since excess caffeine intake, certain medications, renal disorders or diets rich in foods that contain phytic acid or oxalic acid (such as whole grains, rhubarb and spinach) may cause a decrease in calcium absorption, ask your doctor whether it's wise to consume a bit more, considering your age and any health conditions. This may be especially important if you have pancreatitis, celiac disease or inflammatory bowel disease.

How to Use Supplements Safely

Even though the foods described above—which offer multiple nutrients—are the preferred source of calcium, supplements can be used to ensure that you're getting enough of this vital mineral. While calcium supplements are available in many forms, calcium citrate is typically best absorbed. Look for a sublingual (under-the-tongue) version, which dissolves faster...and without sugar.

Proceed With Caution

Of course, too much of anything is bad, and that's true for calcium as well. People who are predisposed to kidney stones face a greater risk for these nasty visitors if they consume more than the RDA of calcium, since the kidneys can't reliably filter out calcium that's not readily used by the body.

Some research also has linked the use of calcium supplements (without adequate levels of vitamin D) to cardiovascular disease. And calcium supplements may be associated with increased risk for dementia in older women who have had a stroke, according to research.

To help with bone health, research shows that it may require taking a vitamin D supplement (800 IU daily). Also, certain medications, such as H2 blockers and proton pump inhibitors for reflux or tetracycline antibiotics, can affect the efficacy of some calcium supplements. If you use one of these drugs, talk to your doctor before taking a calcium supplement.

The Vitamin Deficiency You Don't Know You Have

Sheldon B. Zablow, MD, assistant professor, department of psychiatry, UC San Diego School of Medicine, and author of *Your Vitamins Are Obsolete: The Vitamer Revolution.* https://sheldonzablowmd.com/author

Few vitamins are as misunderstood as B12. Considered by patients and doctors alike to be plentiful in the body and a concern only for vegetarians, deficiency in this crucial vitamin, along with its partner folate, is responsible for a vast array of seemingly unrelated—and often misdiagnosed—issues.

People with low levels of B12 and folate (B12/F) have been erroneously treated for multiple sclerosis, Alzheimer's disease, fibromyalgia, Parkinson's disease, dementia and depression, while their B12/F deficiencies go unnoticed.

Consequences of Deficiency

The most well-known sign of B12 deficiency is anemia, but it can also lead to memory problems, fatigue, depression, muscle weakness, poor balance and permanent nerve damage. Low folate levels have been associated with a poor response to antidepressants, forgetfulness, difficulty concentrating, irritability, depression, behavioral changes and memory loss.

If the body doesn't have enough B12/F, other vitamins and even medical interventions are less effective. For example, you could have plenty of vitamin D and calcium, but if you don't have enough B12/F, you can still develop osteoporosis. Having ample supplies of B12/F helps reduce inflammation and plays an essential role in DNA formation, reducing the damage caused by toxins. Studies show that low levels of B12/F are linked to various forms of cancer.

Causes of Deficiencies

Deficiencies in B12/F are common. Consider that only 30 to 40 percent of people have enough of the enzyme that efficiently converts the folic acid found in supplements and grain products into folate, the bioactive form used by the body. Similarly, there is plenty of B12 and folate in red meat, but 50 percent of people over the age of 50 can't manufacture enough stomach acid to break down the protein to release these vitamins. Vegetarians are commonly deficient.

A long list of medications can induce deficiency or block enzymatic reactions needed to convert common supplements into usable B12/F, including antacids, anti-inflammatories such as prednisone, nonsteroidal anti-inflammatory drugs like ibuprofen, antibiotics, anticonvulsants, estrogen and estrogen substitutes, nitrous oxide anesthesia, and drugs to treat diabetes, asthma, hypertension and high cholesterol.

Vitamin vs. Vitamer

In theory, supplementation should be a simple way to boost and maintain optimal levels of B12/F, but in reality, they often don't help. That's because vitamins come in many forms, and those found in supplements are not necessarily the kind the body uses. Most vitamins are made from inexpensive artificial compounds that are manipulated to improve their shelf life. But before the body can use these compounds, it has to convert them into biologically active structures called vitamers.

The B12 molecule exists in four configurations.

Two are vitamers: *Adenosylcobalamin* (A-B12), found in the body's cells, plays a vital role in providing the energy for reproduction, cell maintenance, and fighting off infection. It also prevents the buildup of a molecule called methylmalonyl acid, which can damage the protective myelin sheath that covers the nerves.

Methylcobalamin (M-B12) circulates in the bloodstream until it's needed. When it's pulled into the cells, it works with folate to convert a waste product called homocysteine into S-adenosyl methionine (SAMe). When M-B12 is lacking, homocysteine accumulates in the bloodstream, where it has toxic effects on blood vessels in the heart and brain, increasing the risk of heart attacks, strokes, and dementia.

Taken orally, A-B12 and M-B12 are absorbed quickly and reach all cells in the body. (Your doctor may also give you B12 injections.) The two other forms of B12 have to be converted through a multi-step process before the body can use them. Hydroxocobalamin (H-B12) is manufactured by bacteria and cyanocobalamin (C-B12) is made in a lab.

If you take a B12 supplement, you most likely take C-B12: It's found in 99 percent of all supplements in the United States. C-B12 requires a multistage conversion process to become usable—a process that can be disrupted by aging, infection, medications, toxins, or drinking alcohol. Because the vitamin is absorbed by passive diffusion, you use only about 1 percent of what the bottle advertises.

Folate

Folate (B9) is B12's partner vitamer. They rely on each other to complete a wide variety of cellular tasks. There are several causes of folate deficiency, including medications, alcohol consumption, celiac disease, and obesity. You may consume inadequate amounts via your diet, or your body might absorb the vitamin poorly. If you are fortunate, your body absorbs about 50 percent of the folate you eat, depending on the food (dark leafy greens, peanuts, and liver are good sources), its freshness, and how it is processed, stored, and prepared.

Supplementation: Buyer Beware

Supplementation can improve levels of both folate and B12—if you take the right product. Unfortunately, the labels on many supplement bottles do not accurately reflect what's inside the pills.

• **Folate.** While many supplements claim they contain folate, they actually contain folic acid, which is the synthetic form of folate used in food fortification and dietary supplements. As with C-B12, the body must convert the artificial folic acid into folate. The conversion process is genetically impaired in more than 50 percent of the population; therefore, many people don't use sufficient amounts of folate even though they're consuming large amounts of folic acid via fortified foods and vitamin pills.

The U.S. Food and Drug Administration notes that 1 milligram (mg) is the maximum recommended dose of over-the-counter folate, but it turns out that number is probably the minimal optimal daily dose of L-methylfolate for most people. The recommended dose of L-methylfolate is at least 1,000 mg per day, but the hard part is finding a good source. The best bet (for any supplement) is to buy a brand from a reputable manufacturer that you have researched. Consumer Lab (ConsumerLab.com) is a reliable, independent source that tests supplements taken off the shelf in stores, rather than bottles provided by the manufacturer.

• **B12.** When it comes to B12, choose a supplement in the vitamer form, either as A-B12 and/or M-B12 in a total dose of at least 2 mg per day (such as Jarrow Formulas Methyl B12 or Global Healing Center's Sublingal B12). Avoid C-B12. You often have to read labels and ingredient lists carefully to tease out what form of B12 the supplement contains.

Taking Your Vitamer Supplements

Always make sure your physicians know about all supplementation used, to avoid any contraindications with other medications. Once you get the go-ahead, take B12 and folate together on an empty stomach, with 4 ounces of water. The 4 ounces are necessary to fully dissolve the tablet and dilute the ingredients for efficient absorption. Vitamers are sensitive to the presence of other vitamins and minerals (iron), so take them without other supplements or food.

The first thing you may notice is thicker nails and hair as well as skin injuries that heal more quickly. You may have subtle positive changes in your mood, speech and memory. If you don't notice any benefits after three months, stop taking the supplements for three to four weeks. Sometimes you don't realize how much a supplement has helped until you stop.

You Can Have Confidence in Vitamin C Supplements

Tod Cooperman, MD, is president and editor-in-chief of ConsumerLab.com.

All 17 common brands tested by ConsumerLab.com contained the amount of C advertised, were free of contaminants and broke down correctly—so don't stress about brands. Pills or powders are better than gummies, which cost more, stick to teeth, add calories and are too easy to consume like candy.

Vitamin C Is Associated With Higher Muscle Mass

Ailsa Welch, PhD, is professor of nutritional epidemiology at University of East Anglia, Norwich, UK, and leader of a study of 13,000 adults ages 42 to 82, published in *The Journal of Nutrition*.

Women with sufficient levels of vitamin C in their blood had about 4 percent more fat-free muscle mass than women with insufficient levels...men, nearly 2 percent more. After age 50, we lose 0.5 percent to 1 percent of muscle mass per year, contributing to health problems and earlier death.

Best: Obtain vitamin C from a range of vegetables and fruits.

Strength Training After 50

Brad Schoenfeld, PhD, associate professor of exercise science at Lehman College in Bronx, New York, and a certified strength and conditioning specialist (CSCS). He is the author of numerous fitness books including *Women's Home Workout Bible*. Brad Schoenfeld.com

Have you been shying away from weights? You're not alone. Less than 15 percent of older adults regularly do strength training, according to a study published in *Clinical Interventions in Aging*.

Yes, cardio is a must for heart health, and those tai chi classes are terrific for mind-body wellness and balance. But when it comes to building up the muscles that will help you be independent and flexible, strength training is the ticket.

Unexpected bonuses: In addition to improving key biomarkers, such as blood sugar and blood fats, research shows that strength training even improves executive functioning and memory.

With all those benefits, what's stopping you? While it's easy to lace up your walking shoes, many people just don't know how to get started with a strength-training regimen.

The good news is, it's never too late to start—and strength training can be easy to do. However, if you're new to strength training, it's wise to book an appointment with a personal trainer, who can assess your abilities, show you proper form and customize a routine for you with body-weight, free-weight and/or machine exercises.

It takes only about 10 to 15 minutes two or three times a week to obtain benefits in health and functional capacity with a strength-training workout. To gain muscle strength, you need to do as many repetitions (reps) as it takes to reach exhaustion. One set (eight to 12 reps) of each exercise usually does the trick if the weight is heavy enough. To continually challenge your muscles, add weight and/or reps as you progress.

To get started, here's a simple strength-training program...*

Get Strong With These 6 Simple Exercises

• **Squat.**

Target: Quads (front of thighs), glutes (buttocks) and hamstrings (back of thighs).

What to do: While standing with your feet shoulder-width apart and slightly turned out, contract your core (abdominal and back) muscles and slowly lower your body as though sitting down in a chair until your thighs are parallel to the floor. Once you reach the "seated" position (or as low as you can safely go with proper form), straighten your legs to return to start.

Goal: When you're just beginning, do the exercise without hand weights and work up to using weights that challenge your muscles.

Good rule of thumb: If you aren't struggling on the last repetition, then the weight is too light.

• **Front plank.**

Target: Core.

What to do: Lie on your stomach with your forearms on the floor and feet together. While keeping your spine straight, lift your body off the floor, balancing on your forearms and toes and contracting your core muscles. Hold for up to 60 seconds.

Goal: To make the exercise more challenging, work up to balancing on your hands instead of your forearms.

• **Chest press.**

Target: Pectorals (upper chest).

What to do: Lie face up on a bench with your legs on either side, feet flat on the floor and holding a hand weight in each hand.

*As with any new exercise program, consult your doctor before starting.

Bring the weights to your shoulders, palms facing away and upper arms pressed to your sides. Then extend your arms straight up, bringing both weights together until they touch when your arms are fully extended.

Alternative: If you don't have a bench, you can lie on the floor when performing this exercise—but it will limit your range of motion and somewhat lessen the results.

• **Lateral raise.**

Target: Deltoids (shoulder).

What to do: While standing with your feet shoulder-width apart, grasp a hand weight in each hand, palms facing your body and arms at your sides. Keeping your elbows slightly bent, raise your arms out to the sides and lift the weights to shoulder level. Be sure not to raise your shoulders as you lift the weights.

• **Single-arm row.**

Target: Back.

What to do: Place your left hand and left knee on a flat bench with your right foot firmly on floor. Grasp a hand weight in your right hand, palm facing your body and arm at your side. Raise the weight straight up until it's just below your armpit. Contract the muscles in your upper back as you lower the arm back down. Complete reps on one side, then repeat on the other side.

Alternative: If you don't have a bench, you can grasp any secure object. If it's a chair, be sure that it's very sturdy to avoid injury.

• **Calf raise.**

Target: Calves.

What to do: While steadying yourself with a handrail, stand on a stair tread with your weight on the balls of your feet, heels hanging off and below the stair. Rise up as high as you can onto your toes until your ankles are fully extended. Contract your calves, and then slowly return to starting position.

Beat the Heat: Five Surprising Ways to Keep Cool

Tom Holland, exercise physiologist and certified strength and conditioning specialist and CEO and founder of TeamHolland, LLC, a fitness consulting company, Darien, Connecticut. He is author of *The Micro-Workout Plan: Get the Body You Want Without the Gym in 15 Minutes or Less a Day.* TeamHolland.com

Do hot days leave you feeling listless? There's a reason—in the sweltering heat, your body must devote much of its energy reserves to maintaining a safe internal temperature, leaving you with little left in the tank for other activities.

Beyond placing yourself in front of the air conditioner, there are several surprising ways to maintain your energy levels when the mercury climbs...

• **Eat smaller amounts more often.** Hot-day dining poses a challenge from an energy perspective. If you eat hefty meals, you will feel tired as your body must devote much of its already heat-drained energy resources to digestion. If you consume fewer calories than you need, the resulting hunger will leave you feeling spent as well. Meals should be comprised of mostly slow-releasing complex carbs such as vegetables and whole grains with a little protein—roughly a 3:1 or 4:1 ratio of carbs to protein.

It is best, therefore, to eat small amounts throughout hot days rather than big stomach-filling meals. Or reduce the size of your meals to two-thirds their normal size, for example, and eat healthy snacks in between to make up for the missing calories. *Two smart hot-weather snacking options...*

• **Fruit is a great hot-weather snack because it helps you stay hydrated.** Not only are most fruits full of hydrating fluid, they're also high in carbohydrates, which boost glycogen levels. Glycogen improves your body's ability to retain water. Fruits that are particularly high in carbs include apples, bananas, pineapples, mangoes, watermelon and cherries.

• **"Energy gels"**—carbohydrate-rich products often consumed by endurance athletes during draining events—provide a hydration- helping glycogen boost, too. And unlike fruit, these small one- to one-and-a-half-ounce packets can be stowed safely for months in pockets, purses and glove compartments, so you can always have one handy when you feel spent on a summer day and need a quick energy fix.

Examples: GU Energy Gels ($32.97 for 24) and PowerBar PowerGel ($36.99 for 24 packs). Each is available in a range of flavors.

Other good options: Honey sticks and honey-sweetened snacks from Honey Stinger.

• **Cool your neck and the inside of your wrists.** Cooling your blood is one of the major energy-draining challenges your body faces on hot days. Your blood circulates right under your skin on your neck and inside your wrists—that's why you can take your pulse there. When you cool these areas, it makes this chore less demanding, preserving your energy.

One way to cool these areas is to soak a bandana and wristbands in cold water, then tie the bandana around your neck and put the wristbands on your wrists before heading out into the heat.

For a deeper, more lasting chill, freeze the wet bandana and wristbands before donning them. Or use items specifically designed to hold the cold, such as the Mission Lockdown Cooling Headband ($14.99) and the 12-in-1 Adult Cooling Gaiter ($14.99), Mission.com. Instant-cold packs also are helpful to keep in your bag.

If you're stuck out in the heat without these items, buy a cold beverage in a can or bottle and hold it against your neck and/or the insides of your wrists before drinking. This helps maintain your energy in two ways—the cold container cools your blood...then consuming the drink helps you stay hydrated. As you probably already know, dehydration is a common cause of energy depletion on sweaty days.

Helpful: If a cold sports drink such as Gatorade or Powerade is available, choose that. If you've been sweating, the carbs and electrolytes that it provides truly will help your body restore its hydration and energy levels—that isn't just empty marketing. For people who want to avoid sugar, a good choice is mineral water, which naturally contains electrolytes, instead of sugary drinks. Or you can eat a piece of fruit.

Don't worry about whether you drink caffeinated or noncaffeinated beverages—caffeine ingestion during exercise does not have the diuretic effect commonly believed. But don't overdo it with caffeinated drinks on hot days either. Soda, iced tea and iced coffee can be tempting beverage options, but excessive caffeine consumption after the morning hours can make it hard to fall asleep.

• **Cover up with breathable, sweat-wicking fabrics.** People tend to show skin when it's hot, donning tees, tanks, skirts and shorts that leave their limbs exposed. But even if you use sunscreen responsibly and avoid sunburn, the sun's heat on that exposed skin can drain your energy over the course of the day.

If you're going to be in direct sunlight for a significant amount of time on a hot day, it's better to cover your limbs with loose-fitting, light-colored garments made from sophisticated synthetic fabrics that are designed to allow heat to escape and wick sweat away from the body.

Examples: Under Armour Iso-Chill, Arctic Cool and Nike Dri-FIT make garments for men and women. For professional wear, there's Rhone's Commuter Dress Shirts for men ($118) and Long Sleeve Delta Pique Polo for men ($68). Lululemon offers Everlux garments for women, such as In Movement leggings ($98).

Also, wear a visor or a brimmed hat made from a breathable, sweat-wicking fabric. This will keep you cool by keeping sunlight off your face and won't trap heat around your head.

Example: Under Armour Airvent Iso-Chill Fish Cap, $28.

• **Keep cool at night to boost energy levels during the day.** One reason people lack energy on hot days is that they failed to get sufficient sleep the previous night because of the oppressive heat. If you don't have air-conditioning throughout your home, consider getting a window air conditioner for your bedroom. At a minimum, run a fan in the room while you sleep.

• **Exercise indoors with fans pointed directly at you.** Outdoor workouts are unnecessarily dangerous on hot days. Extended exertion in such steamy conditions could lead to heat stroke, which can cause permanent damage to the brain, heart and/or kidneys—and it even can be fatal.

On hot days, exercise inside, using equipment such as a treadmill, elliptical machine or stationary bike…or with simple exercises you can do anywhere, such as squats, push-ups and planks. But before starting these indoor exercises, set up one or more fans aimed at the spot where you will be doing your workout and set them to high speed. (Be sure to do this even if your home is air-conditioned.) The breeze will allow your sweat to evaporate, which will cool your skin.

If you don't want to skip your outdoor exercise on a hot day, at least schedule it for early in the morning or late evening, when temperatures are cooler.

Warning: If you experience potential symptoms of heat stroke, such as faintness, dizziness, confusion, rapid heartbeat or rapid breathing, seek hydration right away…bring your body temperature down as quickly as possible with ice packs, cold drinks and/or cool showers…and seek medical attention immediately.

The Beauty of Winter Hiking

Philip Werner, former New Hampshire wilderness guide and founder and editor of the hiking website SectionHiker.com.

A coating of snow can make a hiking trail breathtakingly scenic and blissfully uncrowded. But safe winter hiking requires some additional planning and equipment. *Here's what you need to know...*

Winter Hiking Gear

Warmth and waterproof are the two key features to keep you safe and comfortable on cold, snowy or icy winter hikes...

•**Winter hiking boots are waterproof and much more heavily insulated than other hiking boots.** Many manufacturers also claim that their winter boots have soles that grip especially well on ice, but don't put too much faith in those claims—even the best soles will slip on ice. Fortunately, most winter boots also are designed to be compatible with aids such as microspikes and snowshoes that can dramatically improve traction (see below). Just three decades ago, they tended to be big and bulky, like military surplus gear, but advances in fabrics and insulation mean they're now lightweight, comfortable and breathable. Some are designed to protect hikers in remarkably cold temperatures, as low as –40°F, but a boot rated to –20°F or below should be more than sufficient for most day hikes.

Recommended: Oboz Bridger nine-inch Women's Insulated Boot, $199*...and Salomon Toundra Pro CSWP Snow Boot for men or women, $200.

•**Microspikes are like tire chains for the feet.** They typically attach to hiking boots with strong rubber or elastic straps, positioning

*All prices in this article reflect recent prices from major online sellers.

metal chains and small spikes underfoot to dramatically reduce the odds of slipping on ice. The marketing materials of many winter hiking boots claim their soles grip well on ice, but don't believe it—no rubber sole grips anywhere near as well as metal spikes. Most products are relatively easy to put on and take off, so you can adjust depending on the ground conditions. They're most useful when the trail is icy, which is especially likely when earlier hikers have tamped down all the snow.

Recommended: Kahtoola MICROspikes Traction System, $70/pair...Hillsound Trail Crampons, $65/pair. Both fit a wide range of winter footwear and rarely slip off, a chronic problem with lesser products.

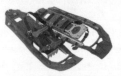

•**Snowshoes are like portable platforms that strap onto your boots,** preventing your feet from sinking deeply into soft snow. Without snowshoes, walking in snow that's deeper than a few inches quickly becomes a tiring and unpleasant battle. Snowshoes also have metal teeth underneath to provide grip on icy surfaces.

You don't wear microspikes and snowshoes at the same time, but unless you're certain about trail conditions, it's worth having both with you so that you can switch between them as needed. Snowshoes are too bulky to fit in the typical backpack, but they can be strapped to it. They should be worn with winter hiking boots.

Recommended: Atlas Serrate, available in versions for men, $265, and women, $203... MSR Evo Ascent, $200. Snowshoes come in many different sizes, shapes and styles, however, so before buying consider trying out a few different models to determine what feels best to you. Many ski centers and REI locations rent snowshoes.

Helpful: Walking in snowshoes is awkward at first, and novices sometimes trip. Using ski poles can greatly help with balance. Walk with a slightly wider gait than normal, as if riding a horse, to reduce the odds that you'll step one snowshoe onto the other. Don't attempt to step backward or turn around quickly while wearing snowshoes—walk instead in a tight circle.

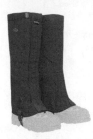

•**Gaiters strap onto your lower legs over the pants and boot tops to prevent snow from getting into boots when hiking or snowshoeing.** "High" gaiters, which come up almost to the knee, are best when there's more than a few inches of snow on the ground. These typically have a strap that goes under the sole of the boot. Confirm that the boots you select have a gap or arch in the sole that is sufficiently wide enough to fit the strap of the gaiters you intend to purchase. Otherwise this strap would wear against the ground.

Recommended: Outdoor Research Crocodile Gaiters, available in men's and women's versions, are thick and insulating, providing an extra layer of warmth for the lower legs, around $90 for most sizes and styles...REI Backpacker Gaiters, $55, are waterproof but lightweight and breathable...as are Outdoor Research Rocky Mountain High Gaiters, available in versions for men and women, $49.

•**Socks worn while winter hiking should be wool or synthetic,** never cotton, which absorbs moisture and will leave your feet cold and uncomfortable.

Recommended: Darn Tough Mountaineering Socks, available in men's and women's versions, $30.

•**Water bottles should have a mouth nearly as wide as the bottle itself**—wide-mouth bottles are less likely to freeze shut on frigid hikes than are narrow-mouth bottles.

Recommended: Nalgene 32-ounce Wide Mouth Water Bottle, $9.

Store water bottles upside down in your backpack—after confirming that they don't leak—to further reduce the odds that the mouth will freeze shut. Wrapping bottles inside insulted gear such as a spare shirt or sock inside your backpack also reduces freezing risk. There also are insulators that keep your bottle somewhat protected from cold temps even when clipped to the outside of your backpack, saving you from having to dig through your backpack each time you want a drink.

Recommended: Outdoor Research Water Bottle Parka, $42.

Naturally, you'll also need other cold-weather clothing such as jackets, hats and gloves, but the winter gear you already own for activities such as shoveling snow or skiing might suffice. Wear multiple layers that you can remove and stow in your backpack as needed. If you hike or snowshoe aggressively, your body is likely to generate so much heat that you find yourself removing layers even though it's cold out, but it's still vital to have enough layers with you that you would be safe and comfortable if you stopped moving—whether that's to take a break and enjoy the scenery or because you're injured and must wait for help. Avoid cotton, which provides little insulation when it gets wet, and choose moisture-wicking base layers.

Pack multiple pairs of socks and gloves so that you can change these if they become wet from sweat or snow.

Remember to wear sunglasses and sunscreen. Sunlight can be as punishing to the skin and eyes in winter as in summer.

Winter Hiking Strategy

Hike with a partner or group. Also let a friend who isn't coming on the hike know where you'll be hiking and when to call the authorities if you fail to report in. Naturally, you should bring your phone on the hike so you can call for help if necessary, but don't depend entirely on a phone for safety—hiking trails often are in areas with poor cell reception, and cold temperatures reduce battery life, which means your phone might run out of power sooner than expected. A whistle is a simple and effective winter-hiking safety tool, calling help to your location if you get lost or hurt. If your phone battery life isn't great, it's worth bringing a portable battery pack and cord to recharge it as well.

Your first few winter hikes should be relatively modest distances—half the distance or less that you could comfortably hike during warmer months. Hiking requires more effort and energy per mile in snow, especially deep snow that requires snowshoe use.

Carry a printed map of the trail system even if the trail is well marked and/or you can access a trail map on your phone's GPS. Some trail markings might be obscured by snow, and GPS can be deceiving at a walking pace—the GPS might misinterpret which direction you're traveling and point you the wrong way, for example. Also, your phone's GPS can't help you if the battery runs down. Hiking on trails you already have traversed during warm months also reduces the odds that you'll get lost, though trails can look very different under a layer of snow.

Drink water before beginning a winter hike—as much as a liter. It's easy to become dangerously dehydrated on winter hikes, because you're not only sweating, you're also expelling moisture with each breath in the dry air. If you hydrate immediately before the hike, you're much less likely to become dehydrated on the trail.

Make Money When You Walk

MoneyTalksNews.com

Several smartphone apps pay users to take walks. At StepBet, you keep yourself motivated by putting your own money down as a bet that you will hit your fitness goals. If you reach those goals, you split the pot—and get a bit of profit—with everyone else who met their goals. MyWalgreens provides points—redeemable for store coupons—if you work toward weekly health challenges, including walking. LifeCoin tracks your steps and awards points redeemable for gift cards. Rover pays you for walking other people's dogs, and so does the similar app Wag!

Build Muscle With This 'Rubber Band" Workout

Stephanie Mansour, certified personal trainer, Certified yoga and pilates instructor, and host of *Step It Up with Steph* on PBS. StepItUpWithSteph.com

If your image of a powerful muscle workout includes a lot of shiny and expensive equipment at an expensive health club, think again. You can get a full-body workout with a set of rubber resistance bands that costs less than $20 and can be stashed in a drawer when not in use or even packed in a suitcase when you go on vacation.

Rather than using weight, these stretchy tools use resistance that you must move against to strengthen your muscles.

Bands actually can be more effective than hand weights in terms of toning and injury prevention because their constant tension engages multiple muscles simultaneously through the range of motion, particularly the smaller, stabilizing muscles in the back, hips, quads and glutes. And resistance bands can be used to work your leg muscles as well. Try doing that with a dumbbell!

Resistance bands are available in various forms, such as flat strips and tubes with handles on the ends. But your safest bet are minibands—circular rubber bands that loop around the arms and legs. You don't need to worry about losing your grip...or about strips flying out of closed doorjambs and snapping you in the face...and you can purchase them in multipacks for varied resistance, changing them out as your fitness level advances.

Bands come in bright colors. The resistance tends to increase as the color gets darker.

Example: A light green band offers less resistance than a blue band. *Two brands that I like...*

Gaiam Restore Mini Band Kit: $9.98 for a set of three bands.

4KOR Fitness Resistance Loop Mini Band Set: $23.45 for a set of four bands.

Resistance Band Workout

The following six moves will work all the major muscle groups in your body. Turn them into a circuit workout by performing them in the order listed, repeating the entire sequence three times. It takes 20 minutes or less, depending on the number of reps.

Do the exercises at least three times per week for maximum benefit. Start with 10 reps per exercise. As you gain strength, increase to 15 reps. Once this becomes simple—probably in two weeks—move on to a higher-resistance band level.

• Half Squat

Muscles worked: Quads, hamstrings, gluteus (buttock) medius, stabilizing muscles around the ankles.

Get ready: Step into the miniband, positioning it a few inches above both knees. Stand with toes forward, feet hip-width apart, creating a bit of tension around the band. Place your hands on your hips to help with balance.

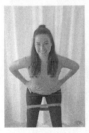

Go: Begin squatting down as if you were about to sit in a chair, but stop midway. As you lower down, contract your abdominal muscles by pulling your navel toward your spine, and gaze downward to ensure your knees are aligned with your second toes, which will keep your hips, thighs, knees and ankles in proper alignment and ensure that the correct muscles are being activated.

Once you are halfway through the squat, press down through your heels to stand up, squeezing your glutes at the top. Be sure to stand fully upright at the top of each rep looking straight ahead with shoulders relaxed and glutes engaged. Strive to maintain outward tension on the band throughout the exercise.

Step it up: Squat all the way down, with knees bent at a 90-degree angle, as if tapping your butt in the imaginary chair.

• Side Step

Muscles worked: Quads, gluteus medius, gluteus maximus, stabilizing muscles around the ankles.

Get ready: Begin in the half-squat position as above with the band a little above the knee. Place your hands on your hips to help with balance.

Go: Step your right foot about six inches to the right (band tension will increase), then step your left foot to the right the same amount (band tension will decrease a bit but should never go slack). Complete 10 steps to the right, then repeat the sequence to the left. Your navel should stay pulled in, abdominals contracted, as if you're steeling yourself for a punch to the stomach. Doing this will help protect your low back throughout the move. If you do experience low-back discomfort, stand up and try the Side Step with just a very slight bend in the knees.

Step it up: You can grab some dumbbells and do bicep curls as you step to the side to work your arms…or reach your arms up to the ceiling without weights to challenge your balance.

• Lying Down Bridge

Muscles worked: Transverse abdominis (the deepest layer of front abdominal muscles—beneath your "six-pack" muscles), rectus abdominis core (the more superficial abdominal muscles—the ones that form the six pack), glutes. If you perform the advanced version, you also will work the gluteus medius, which is notoriously weak in many people and critical for stability when

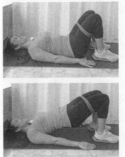

you move, such as walking and climbing stairs, and keeping the body in proper alignment to prevent hip and knee problems.

Get ready: Sitting on the ground, position the miniband a few inches above both knees as in the exercises above. Lie down, bending your knees so feet are flat on the ground, hip-width apart, and heels are positioned so that when you lay your arms by your sides and reach along the ground toward your heels, your fingertips touch or almost touch your heels. Strive to maintain tension in the band throughout the exercise.

Go: Inhale deeply, filling your stomach with air. As you exhale, tilt your pelvis up, pressing your low back into the ground. Now, press down through your heels and lift your tailbone off the ground, followed by your low back and middle back, squeezing your butt tightly at the top. Your butt will be a few inches off of the ground.

Hold for two or three counts before slowly returning down, starting with the middle back, then the low back and finally the tailbone. Rest for a count, then press back up until you complete all reps.

Step it up: At the top of each bridge, open your thighs out and in three times, pushing against the band's resistance.

• Banded crunch

Muscles worked: Transverse abdominus, rectus abdominis.

Get ready: Assume the same starting position as in the Lying Down Bridge, miniband above your knees, knees bent, heels close enough to your butt that you can touch (or almost touch) them with your fingertips. Tilt your pelvis so your low back presses into ground.

Go: Place your hands behind your head, and lift your head and neck a few inches 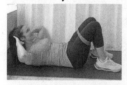 off the ground. Pulse up and down through your repetitions without resting on the ground in between. Keep your elbows out, and avoid pulling on your head. Maintain tension on the band throughout.

• Shoulder Blade Squeeze

Muscles worked: Shoulders, upper back.

Get ready: Standing with feet hip-width apart, place the miniband around your forearms and extend your arms in front of you at shoulder height, palms facing in but pulling apart from one another to create tension in the band.

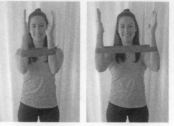

Go: Concentrate on keeping your shoulder blades back and down, as if you are squeezing a ball between them. Then spread your arms apart as far as you can. (Depending on your band's resistance, you'll be able to move them six inches to one foot apart.) Return to the starting position, not allowing the band to collapse as you continue through all repetitions.

• Modified Banded Lat Pull Down

Muscles worked: Lats, core, biceps.

Get ready: Choose a looser band for this exercise. Standing with feet hip-width apart, knees softly bent, place the miniband around your forearms and extend your arms 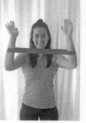 overhead, palms facing in but pulling apart from one another to create tension in the band. Avoid hunching your shoulders as you do this move, and keep your ribcage still throughout rather than bobbing up and down.

Go: Pull your navel in toward your spine, and contract your abdominals as you pull your elbows down to the sides and slightly behind you—almost like cactus arms—as if you were performing lat pulls down at the gym. Return to the starting position. Repeat for all reps.

Free Ways to Do Workouts at Home

MoneyTalksNews.com

Download the free FitOn app, specify your fitness goals and stream videos on your TV, computer or smartphone. Go to Orangetheory's YouTube channel for a new workout every day—you do not have to be a member. If you have exercise bands, use them—perform exercises as you usually would, but keep tension on the band at all times for a better workout. For weight-based training, use common household items, such as canned food or drinks for bicep curls. Do interval training with the stairs in your home by moving up them as quickly as possible, then walking slowly back down to catch your breath, and repeating several times.

Cutting-Edge Athletic Shoes to Up Your Performance

Pete McCall, MS, CSCS, independent exercise physiologist and consultant and American Council on Exercise–certified personal trainer based in San Diego. He is author of *Smarter Workouts: The Science of Exercise Made Simple* and host of the *All About Fitness* podcast. PeteMcCallFitness.com

Nike's new Vaporfly running shoes are so good that they were nearly banned from the Olympics. These super-performance shoes aren't the only new sneakers that might deserve a place in your closet. *Here's a look at innovative shoes for a range of activities…*

Running: Nike ZoomX Vaporfly Next%2. Vaporflys are a source of debate in the competitive track world. They boost running speeds by 4 percent to 5 percent, which critics consider an unfair advantage. But if your goal is to run faster or farther, there's no debate—they're the best running shoes on the market.

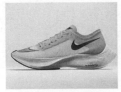

Vaporflys have a carbon fiber plate hidden inside the thick foam padding underfoot. This acts like a catapult, springing the runner forward subtly with each stride, increasing speeds while reducing leg fatigue. $250. Nike.com

Cross-training: Vivobarefoot Primus III. The growing consensus among fitness pros is that less is more with cross-training shoes. Less foam underfoot and a relatively flat base means more stability thanks to better sensory feedback from the nerves and joints of the feet.

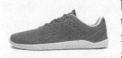

A less constraining "toe box" lets the toes spread out, further improving balance. Vivobarefoot is the "minimalist" shoe expert—the ultra-flexible Stealth IIIs are like gloves for the feet. $145. Vivobarefoot.com

Walking: Nike Free RN 2018 Current thinking is that walking shoes should find a middle ground between minimalist footwear and thick-soled running shoes. These Nikes, which the company calls a running shoe, are a well-made example of that. They're a reasonable choice for short runs, too. $65 to $85. Nike.com

Off-road running: La Sportiva Wildcat. Like off-road tires for your feet, these trail-running shoes have thick, grippy treads for traction on dirt, grass and gravel—without the weight and limited ankle flexibility of hiking boots. The sole provides both cushioning and stability. They are great for light hikes, too. $110. Sportiva.com

Biking: Vans Old Skool. Unlike the other shoes on this list, these Vans are not new and innovative—they're named "Old Skool" for a reason. What's new is that these venerable sneakers are increasingly popular for casual bike rides. Originally designed for skateboarders, their wide, level, grippy, stiff soles are ideal for maintaining control of bike pedals. Unlike cycling cleats, they're comfortable for walking when you get off the bike. $60. Vans.com

Exercise Outside

American Heart Association

Researchers have discovered that people who spend more time around trees, grass, and other green spaces have a lower risk of dying from heart disease. In their study, for every 0.10 unit increase in greenness, deaths from heart diseases decreased by 13 per 100,000 adults. The relationship is likely linked to lower air pollution in green spaces.

Too Busy to Exercise? "Fidget-cisers" Can Help Anytime, Anywhere

Denise Austin, host of the longest-running TV fitness show in history. She is author of 12 books on fitness and creator of more than 100 workout videos and DVDs as well as the magazine *Denise Austin's Fit Over 50*. DeniseAustin.com

---

If you think exercise is too time-consuming, think again. You can improve your fitness and muscle tone in just a few minutes at a time in the middle of everyday activities.

I call these quick movement sessions fidget-cisers because they are almost as easy and convenient as fidgeting.

Benefits: They increase circulation...improve flexibility...strengthen muscles, including the deep abdominal (or "core") muscles that protect the back... and give you an infusion of energy.

Ideally, fidget-cisers should complement—not substitute for—more vigorous, extended cardiovascular exercise. But even a little movement can improve your health and mood. How often should you do a fidget-ciser? Anytime you think of it! A good way to start is to do one of these exercises once an hour. Set an alarm on your phone.

Important: Don't overdo the intensity on any of these. You should feel a stretch but no pain.

In the Kitchen

While your dinner is simmering or the coffee is brewing...

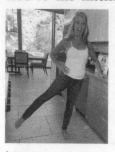

•**Leg lifts.** This exercise is like what ballet dancers do at the barre. Stand with your side to the kitchen counter, and place your hand lightly on the counter for balance. Tense your stomach muscles, and slowly raise the opposite leg in front of you, keeping your raised leg and your back straight. Pointing your toe will make it easier to keep your leg straight. It's more important to control the movement going up and down than to raise your leg high. Hold the position for one second, then slowly lower your leg. Now raise your leg to the side and hold for one second, then lower and raise it toward the back for one second. Do three repetitions on that side, then turn and do three repetitions on the other side.

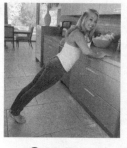

•**Countertop push-ups.** Stand facing the counter, a few feet away. Place both hands on the countertop, and do 10 slow push-ups, taking two full seconds going down and two seconds going back up.

•**Countertop squats.** Face the counter, feet shoulder-width apart, toes forward. With your hands on the counter for balance and your back straight, bend both knees a few inches while sitting back slightly, weight in your heels. Then squeeze your buttock muscles as you slowly push through your heels to come back up. To protect your knees, don't go down too far—I do mini-squats, just bending slightly as I sit back. It's the coming up that works your butt. Start with five to 10 squats, and work up to 30 at a time.

On Your Couch

While you're watching TV, talking on the phone or reading...

•**Bicep curls.** Keep a three- to five-pound hand-held weight nearby for this exercise. You can do it seated or standing. Sit up or stand straight, and tighten your abdominal

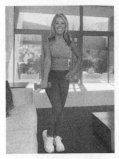

muscles to protect your back. Pick up the weight in one hand, and position your arm down at your side, with the inside of your elbow facing front. Slowly bend your arm at the elbow until your forearm is perpendicular to the floor. Repeat with one arm for a total of five times, then do five repetitions with the other arm.

Be sure to lift and lower slowly so that your muscles are doing the work rather than relying on momentum.

●**Tricep dips.** Sit at the edge of your couch, feet far enough away from the couch

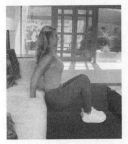

so that your lower legs are perpendicular to the floor. With arms at your sides, place palms on the couch, fingers facing forward. Keeping feet and knees together, press the heels of your hands into the couch to support yourself, and scoot your rear slightly forward so that it's just in front of the couch. Bend your elbows, and slowly lower your rear toward the floor, then straighten your elbows to lift back up. You should feel the backs of your arms working hard. Start with five repetitions, and gradually increase to 15.

●**Invisible Hula-Hoop.** Stand up and swivel your hips a few times in one direction, then the other, as though you are keeping a Hula-Hoop in motion. This movement works all the muscles in the torso. Keep going for 30 seconds, and work up to one minute.

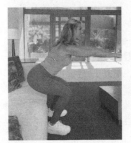

●**Rear and hamstring toner.** Stand in front of the couch, and face away from it, feet hip-width apart, arms at your sides. Keeping your buttock muscles tight, lower your rear until it briefly taps the couch, and at the same time, raise your arms in front of you to shoulder height, palms facing the floor. Return to standing as you lower your arms to the sides. Think of the seat tap and the return to standing as one fluid motion. Work up to 15 repetitions.

●**Reverse lunge.** This fidget-ciser particularly works the front thighs as well as the hip flexors. Stand a few inches in front of the couch, facing out at a 45-degree angle, with your right leg closer to the couch and your hands on your hips. Lift your left leg, point the toe and stretch the leg behind you so that the top of the left foot rests on the couch. You should be standing up straight with your weight on the front leg, like a ballerina doing an arabesque. Keeping your head level and your torso straight, tighten your abdominal muscles and bend your right knee (your left knee will bend, too), then come back up.

Do 10 lunges on one side, then turn to the other side, and do 10 with the other leg.

Standing Around

While waiting on the checkout line at a store…on the phone with a friend…or while your dog does his business…

●**Rear toner.** Squeeze your buttock muscles as you pull in your abdomen. Hold for five seconds, and repeat three times.

●**Calf toner.** Slowly rise onto the balls of your feet, and hold that position for five seconds. Slowly lower your heels back toward the floor. Repeat three times. If keeping your balance is a concern, then be sure to do this exercise only when you have a cart or something else to hold onto.

●**Invisible balance beam.** This exercise tones your leg and core muscles, improves balance and even works your brain. Place one foot directly in front of the other. Engage your abdominal muscles, and stay in that position with feet flat and legs straight for up to 10 seconds. Then put the other foot in front. This is harder than you might think—try it next to a railing, wall or counter for stability until you get the hang of it. Over time, increase the distance between the front and back foot.

It's Time to Get Back On a Bike

Gabe Mirkin, MD, wellness expert, retired sports-medicine physician and author of 16 books including *The Healthy Heart Miracle: Your Roadmap to Lifelong Health.* DrMirkin.com

---

You say you haven't been on a bike since you were a kid? Don't despair. Even if you think you're too out of shape, too old or too busy coping with aches and pains due to arthritis or some other chronic health problem, cycling is one of the best forms of exercise…and popular electric bikes and three-wheelers make it accessible for everyone. *Here's the lowdown…*

Why Cycling Gets the Nod

Especially as we get older, cycling is much easier on our bodies than a high-impact cardio exercise, such as jogging. When you jog, your foot hits the ground with a force that can break bones and tear muscles. When you cycle, you pedal with a smooth rotary motion that is gentle on your joints while effectively working your muscles—including your heart.

My path to cycling: I used to be an international marathon runner and now, at age 84, I can no longer run…but I do ride my bike seven days a week for a total of 150 to 180 miles.

Note: If you have any medical problems or disabilities, always check with your doctor before biking.

Get Pedaling!

Though it's said that you never forget how to ride a bike, you may be worried about your balance or the safety of riding outdoors. If your coordination or balance is questionable—or if you need greater protection against injury because of a condition such as osteoporosis or other medical problems—try a recumbent three-wheel bicycle that is low to the ground.

If you're not comfortable riding on roads, try a stationary bike in your home or gym. You can get all the health benefits from a stationary bike, and it will also strengthen your muscles and coordination so that you will be more comfortable if you decide later to ride outdoors. However, if your balance is so compromised that you are in danger of falling off a stationary bike, it may be safer for you not to ride at all.

To determine the length of your cycling sessions, listen to your body instead of relying on other measures such as tracking your distance or time. If you're out of shape or have arthritis pain, you may be able to pedal a stationary bike for only a few minutes or less at first—I've had patients who could do only five or 10 seconds before they felt pain in their leg muscles, joints, shoulders or back, but in a few weeks, they were up to 20 minutes or more of comfortable riding.

If you experience pain anywhere in your body that does not go away when you stop pedaling, you should end your workout immediately and try again the next day. If the pain goes away but returns when you resume pedaling, also call it a day. You can expect to be injured if you do not listen to your body.

The Right Bike for You

The wide range of bike styles for the road means that there's a design for just about everyone and for every budget. *Among the newer options…*

A recumbent three-wheeler is designed for easier mounting and dismounting because the center bar is just one foot off the ground. But this is not a kid's trike—some of today's fastest riders are using three-wheelers. Prices range from $200 up to $2,000.

An electric-assist or e-bike works well if you're out of shape, have weak muscle tone or simply want to be able to ride with faster riders for longer periods of time than you could on your own. Even though an e-bike has an electric motor, it doesn't mean you aren't working out—you can pedal with or without the assistance of the motor so your muscles and heart still get a great workout.

Most e-bikes can reach speeds of 18 mph with the motor alone to 28 mph with pedaling. E-bikes are available in two- and three-wheel models in both upright and recumbent styles. Prices of e-bikes start at around $1,000 and top out at $5,500 or more.

A stationary bike can be a recumbent, upright or spin version. Stationary bikes also are available with an Internet-connected screen that displays trails around the world or puts you in virtual classes led by a trainer. Prices range from $400 to $2,000 or more. For Internet-connected classes, popular options include Peloton, NordicTrack and Echelon. Compare prices, monthly fees and the number of live and prerecorded classes offered.

Put Safety First!

If you're biking outdoors, dedicated bike trails (check local and state parks) are safer than riding in bike lanes on the street. Scenic and historic bike trails can be found in many parts of the US via the Great American Rail-Trail (RailsToTrails.org).

To avoid head injuries, you must wear a helmet.

Helpful: When you open your mouth as wide as you can, the helmet should press against the top of your head. If the strap feels tight on the bottom of your chin, it is too tight and should be loosened a bit. *Also…*

•**Never ride without lights, even in the daytime.** Outfit your bike with a white light in front and a red light in back. Use 1,000 lumens lights, which give the best visibility—both to be seen and to see what's ahead.

•**Wear a jersey in a bright color like yellow.** Most accidents involving cars are due to driver distraction, so grab drivers' attention with a bright color.

•**Consider using shoe cleats or toe clips.** Your feet are far less likely to slip off the pedals if you use shoe cleats or toe clips.

However, if you have to dismount suddenly for a traffic stop or emergency, you may not be able to disengage your foot from the pedal and you can fall. Ask a qualified bike specialist for advice.

•**Practice the ABC check before every ride—air, brakes and chain.** Squeeze the tires to make sure there's adequate tire pressure…make sure the brakes work…and check that the chain moves smoothly.

Then start biking!

Bicycles That Won't Break the Bank

Michael Yozell, former gear editor of *Bicycling Magazine.* He is a professional bike mechanic based in Emmaus, Pennsylvania, with more than 30 years of experience, and a bike consultant to consumers and the industry.

It's easy to get sticker shock in a bike shop—some stellar bicycles cost $3,000 to $10,000. But excellent bikes for casual cyclists, with lightweight aluminum or alloy frames rather than featherweight carbon-fiber frames, can be had for $700 to $1,000. Late summer through autumn is a great time to find bargains, although pandemic-related supply interruptions and increased demand have made that more difficult.

Here are some of the best reasonably priced bikes for assorted types of road surfaces, all of which have aluminum or alloy frames and weigh 30 pounds or less—except the last one…

Best for comfortable rides around town: Linus Rover 9 is ideal for easy trips on paved paths and neighborhood roads. Its upright riding position and comfortable seat let riders take in the scenery, while its 1.75-inch-wide tires provide a soft, stable ride—the

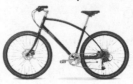

wider the tire, the larger the cushion of air under the bike and the greater traction. Many bikes in this "beach cruiser" class have just one to five gears, but the 28-pound Rover 9 features a nine-speed gear system, which helps riders handle hills. $789.

Best for travel on unpaved and paved surfaces: Co-op Cycles CTY 2.1, sold by REI, is a "gravel" or "hybrid" bike—a middle ground between a road bike and a mountain bike. With 24 speeds and large wheels, it's fairly fast on pavement…but its relatively wide 1.57-inch tires and durable construction mean that it's very capable on gravel and dirt paths, 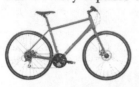 too. The 30-pound CTY 12.1 has straight handlebars that create a fairly upright riding position. $799.

Best for biking adventures: Salsa Journeyman Claris 700 is capable on paved and unpaved surfaces and has a comfortable, relatively upright riding position like the gravel bike mentioned previously. But the durable 16-gear, 26-pound Journeyman also has abundant mounts for bags, luggage racks and water bottles, making it appropriate for camping trips. And this versatile bike's standard 700c wheels can be swapped out for 2.2-inch-wide 650b wheels with mountain bike tires to convert the Claris 700 into an even more capable off-roader. $949.

Best road bike: Giant Contend 3 provides everything you need in a road bike for hundreds of dollars less than comparable offerings. Giant is the biggest bike manufacturer in the world, and its economies of scale let it undersell its competition. The Contend 3 is smooth, fast, comfortable and durable. At 23 pounds, the 16-speed bike is impressively light and agile compared with other bikes in its price range. $775.

Best carbon-frame road bike bargain: Cervélo R-Series costs considerably more than other bikes on this list…but considerably less than other carbon-fiber-frame 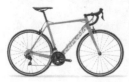 bikes in its class. Carbon-fiber frames are extremely lightweight yet still strong. This stylish, nimble and very fast

bike will fit right in with the $10,000 bikes in competitive races…or lined up in front of the snootiest coffee shop in town. It weighs 17 or 18 pounds—and the R2 features highly regarded Shimano 105 components. $2,500.

Create a "Peloton" Experience for Less

Louis Mazzante, test director for Hearst Enthusiast Group, which includes *Bicycling* magazine, Center Valley, Pennsylvania. Bicycling.com

The popular Peloton indoor exercise bikes provide remote access to fitness-club spin classes from the safety of home. But the $1,895 price (down from $2,245) plus the $39 monthly subscription fee is a lot to pay to pedal a stationary bike. The newest model, the Bike+, will cost even more—$2,495. But it's possible to create an engrossing indoor riding experience and stay in shape for a lot less, especially if you already own a stationary bike or a conventional outdoor bike. *Here's how…*

Subscribe to an App

There are a number of indoor-cycling apps that offer benefits similar to the Peloton membership for a lot less—simply position a digital device running one of these apps in front of a stationary bike. You can use the screen-mirroring function available on some phones and tablets or a screen-casting device such as Google Chromecast to display the phone or laptop screen on a smart-TV screen.

Zwift lets you pedal your indoor bike on a wide array of virtual outdoor rides—cross deserts, climb volcanos, explore a futuristic version of New York City and much more. You can ride with friends, compete in races or join classes with coaches and—if you have compatible equipment (see next page)—Zwift will track performance data such as your speed, distance and heart rate. You also can use Zwift while running on a treadmill. $14.99/month. Zwift.com

The Sufferfest uses licensed footage from past events such as the Tour de France to put you right in the middle of world-class races. With compatible equipment, it will track your performance, including basics such as heart rate and speed plus advanced measurements such as neuromuscular power and anaerobic capacity. It also offers on-screen coaching tips. Strength-training and yoga classes are available on the app as well. $14.99/month. TheSufferfest.com

Peloton Digital offers access to the exact same celebrity instructor–led spin classes and vibrant virtual biking community that Peloton owners receive through their memberships—but for less than one-third of the monthly membership price. In addition to spin classes, there are yoga and strength-training classes and more. But unlike with full Peloton membership—or with either of the previous apps—the Peloton Digital app won't communicate with your exercise equipment to provide onscreen performance stats such as your speed and distance covered, and the instructor won't be able to monitor your performance. $12.99/month. OnePeloton.com/app

Convert a Bike to Indoor Use

A "trainer" converts an outdoor bicycle into an indoor stationary bike by holding the rear end of the bike off the ground and providing resistance. If your goal is to create a Peloton-like experience, purchase a "smart" trainer, which connects wirelessly to a bike-training app on your phone, tablet or other digital device. Two types worth considering, both are compatible with apps including Zwift and The Sufferfest…

With a "direct drive" smart trainer, the bike's rear wheel is removed. By pedaling, you spin a flywheel that's part of the trainer. These systems usually are quiet and can adjust resistance levels

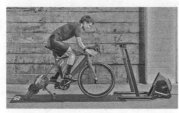

automatically when a rider pedals up or down virtual hills in a compatible indoor-cycling app or when your workout calls for more effort. They cost much less than the Peloton, but they're not inexpensive.

Recommended: Wahoo Fitness KICKR Core Bike Trainer, $900.

With a "friction" smart trainer, the rear wheel remains on the bike and turns a resistance-providing cylinder. These tend to be affordable but loud. The rider must shift gears to adjust resistance levels—this won't happen automatically when there's a virtual hill in a biking app.

Recommended: Kinetic Road Machine Smart 2 Bike Trainer, $299.

A Few More Details

To complete the experience…

•**Point a fan at the bike.** Aim it so the airflow is directed at your torso as you ride. It keeps you from overheating.

How to Spot-Train Your Butt

The idea of targeting one specific body part to shed fat is a myth. But you can certainly target a specific area for muscle growth and toning.

Here's how to train your glutes: First, learn to activate your glutes through resistance-band or body-weight exercises such as kickbacks, air squats and unweighted lunges. Once you have successfully mastered contracting one butt-cheek at a time, you're ready for weighted lifts. Deadlifts, sumo squats, barbell glute bridges, reverse lunges, curtsy lunges and weighted step-ups work the glutes from all angles and make your butt perkier, rounder, fuller and firmer. (YouTube is a good resource for how to perform each one properly or to find a premade booty workout.)

Roundup of personal trainers reported at Health. com.

• **Put a yoga mat under the bike.** This will absorb some of the bike's noise and keep sweat off the floor.

• **Wear a heart-rate monitor.** These wirelessly track your heart rate through a biking app.

Recommended: Wahoo Tickr, $50, is comfortable and compatible with Zwift, The Sufferfest and Peloton apps. Or if you own a watch or other wearable device that tracks your heart rate, use that instead.

Raising the Barre

Kristen Gasnick, PT, a doctor of physical therapy at Excel Orthopedic Physical Therapy, Livingston, New Jersey.

Don't let the dance origin of barre exercise scare you off. This popular workout focuses on simple movements that people of any ability can do to build strength, increase flexibility, improve balance, and optimize posture and core stability.

Barre is low impact, so it puts less pressure on the body's joints that activities like running. It employs a combination of bodyweight movements and light weights for resistance training as well as high repetitions of very small movements called isometric exercises.

What a Workout Looks Like

Barre workout should incorporate both upper and lower body movements as well as exercises that target balance and core strength. If you take a class, you'll use a ballet barre for balance. At home, you can use a sturdy chair. *Here are four exercises to try...*

• **Backward lunge.** Stand upright and take a large step back with one foot. Lower your body until the opposite thigh is parallel with the floor. Keep your front knee over your front ankle. Return to a full standing position and switch sides. Do three sets of 10 repetitions. When you are in the lowered position, try adding in a set of pulses where you move up an inch up and down an inch 10 times.

This movement targets the gluteus muscles unilaterally, ensuring that both sides of the body are being worked equally, and improves balance when transitioning between starting and ending positions.

• **Lateral leg lifts.** Lift your leg to the side and slowly raise it to hip height or as far as is comfortable, and lower it back down. Do three sets of 10 repetitions. You can also add in pulses when your leg is lifted.

This movement targets the gluteus medius, a hip muscle that is key for providing stability to the pelvis and maintaining balance.

• **Arm sweeps.** Sweep your arms out to the side while rotating your palms toward the front of the room. You can do this exercise with or without hand weights. The lifting motion targets the shoulder muscles (deltoids), while rotating the palms forward encourages external rotation and activation of the rotator cuff musculature that stabilizes the shoulder. Bring the arms all the way back down and complete three sets of 15 repetitions. A set of pulses can be added at the top of the movement.

• **Seated core.** Sit on the ground with your knees bent and your feet flat in front of you. Lean back so that your torso is at about a 45-degree angle. Holding this position for five to 30 seconds without using your hands to touch the ground or hold onto your legs for support will get the core muscles firing. When holding this position becomes easy, increase the challenge by adding dynamic arm movements, such as alternating arm lifts, or by rotating the arms and trunk from side to side.

Challenges

While anyone can benefit from barre exercises, people with poor balance need to be careful. Many instructors, whether in a studio or through an online video, provide modifications for different fitness levels.

Chapter 7

GET THE CARE YOU NEED

Women Need More Attention in Medical Research

It's been a long-standing tradition that most medical studies have focused only on Caucasian males because researchers feared that hormonal differences in women would skew the findings. The problem is, that approach ignores how various diseases and medications can affect the sexes differently.

Without distinguishing between the sexes, research would not have revealed that heart disease, for example, affects men and women differently...or that certain drugs, such as the widely prescribed sleeping pill *zolpidem* (Ambien), are metabolized at different rates, potentially affecting dosage recommendations.

After the shortcomings of sex-biased medical research began to receive more attention, researchers set out in 2009 to see whether more women were finally being represented in medical studies. The results were disappointing—only 28 percent of the studies reviewed that year included women.

As concerns grew around biased medical research methods, the National Institutes of Health (NIH), the largest public funder of clinical trials in the US, implemented a 2016 policy requiring researchers to consider sex as a biological variable, which involves comparing research results between men and women.

Latest development: To find out whether more females are now being represented in medical studies, a team of researchers conducted a 10-year follow-up on sex-biased research by looking at a body of scientific literature published in 2019. The meta-analysis, which was published in *eLife,* included studies that focused on both laboratory animals and humans in clinical research.

In the review, researchers looked at more than 700 studies that covered nine biological fields. The results were a mixed bag. While the number of studies that included females grew from 28 percent in 2009 to 49 percent a decade later, there was no increase in the number of studies that broke down the findings by sex. In fact, in the field of pharmacology, the percentage of research that included

Study titled "Meta-Research: A 10-Year Follow-Up Study of Sex Inclusion in the Biological Sciences," by researchers at Northwestern University Feinberg School of Medicine, Chicago, and Smith College, Northampton, Massachusetts, published in *eLife.*

female sex as a biological variable fell from 33 percent to 29 percent.

Meanwhile, approximately one-third of the studies that included both male and female subjects did not quantify the sample size by sex. This practice occurred most often in the fields of neuroscience, immunology and general biology—the same areas that showed the greatest increases in the use of female study participants.

Takeaway: When sex differences are ignored in medical research, the development of effective disease prevention and treatment strategies for all individuals is significantly hampered. For this reason, the authors of the follow-up meta-analysis call on medical researchers to provide a rationale for not including women in future studies. Along with that, the study authors encourage journal publishers and medical schools, universities and institutions that give research grants to advocate for sex-based research.

Don't Let Medical Care Take Over Your Life

Mary Tinetti, MD, professor of medicine and public health and chief of geriatrics at Yale University School of Medicine in New Haven, Connecticut. She is the author of more than 200 peer-reviewed papers, a MacArthur Foundation Fellow and a leader of the Patient Priorities Care initiative, which conducts research into and disseminates information about Patient Priorities Care. PatientPrioritiesCare.org

If you've got a chronic illness such as heart disease, diabetes, cancer or arthritis, staying on top of your medical care is essential. But the truth is, it also can take a lot out of you.

A trip to the doctor or lab can take up to half a day when you include transportation and waiting time. Medications can sap your energy and cloud your thinking, while special diets and exercises can put a crimp in your lifestyle.

If you have more than one chronic condition—as do 67 percent of adults age 65 and older—you can double, triple or quadruple your doctor visits, tests and medications. It's no small wonder that many patients feel overburdened by their medical care.

Your health is precious to you, because it allows you to live your life the way you want—to do activities that bring you pleasure and to connect with people you love and give meaning to your life. If you must sacrifice whatever makes life worth living, you may wonder what's the point of that health care?

In an ideal world, medical care would fix our health problems and allow us to have full, rewarding lives without any hassle or discomfort. But in reality, trade-offs are almost always necessary. We must decide what's truly important to us and what we're willing to give up for the sake of our health.

Better way: A new approach looks at the way a person's medical care fits with his/her life priorities so that smart choices can be made by patients and their doctors. *Here's how...*

What Are Your Priorities?

Everyone's priorities are different. For one person, it means being free enough from pain to be able to walk more. Another wants to keep a clear head and remain alert enough to drive—even at the price of some discomfort.

While you are the expert in what matters most and what you're willing to do or give up in a trade-off, your doctors are experts in how to achieve your goals. That's why you need to work together. Helping people do that is the idea behind "Patient Priorities Care," a program designed and developed by a research team that includes patients, doctors and scientists at Yale University, New York University and Baylor College of Medicine.

In a pilot study, the research team showed that this approach, which incorporates the patient's assessment of how his/her life priorities fit into treatment decisions, can work in a busy medical practice. A member of the health-care team can help patients identify their health priorities—what they want to focus on in their health care while clinicians can learn how to align their care with these priorities—all without much extra time. Patients and clinicians report liking this approach.

Based on the program's principles, The American Geriatrics Society has recommended that doctors put these ideas into action when working with older adults who have multiple medical conditions. And the research group is working to expand the program into the health-care community at large.

Putting Patients First

When using this program, patients are guided by a nurse or other health-care professional through a systematic process to specify their personal health outcome goals and identify the aspects of their medical care that they feel either advance these goals or are too difficult, burdensome or unhelpful.

Participants begin by identifying their "core values" that don't change as life circumstances and health change—things that mean the most to them, such as relationships, independence, longevity and physical and mental capacity. They then pinpoint specific, achievable activities linked to their core values. For one person, it may be seeing her grandchildren every week...for another, it may be a desire to be strong and clear-headed enough to travel.

Doctors and other health-care professionals are trained to elicit and respond to patients' concerns...and to tailor treatment to what they value. Communication in both directions—patients getting their needs and values across, and doctors making it clear what goals are realistic and what trade-offs will be involved—is essential.

Try This at Home

Even though Patient Priorities Care was designed for use with professional guidance, you can gain many of the same benefits on your own.

STEP 1: **Start by creating a road map of your own priorities by considering what aspects of life you value most.**

For example, ask yourself...

●**What relationships mean the most to you?**

●**What gives you particular pleasure?**

●**What aspects of function do you value most highly**—for example, independence... keeping your mind sharp...maintaining physical abilities...and/or learning new things?

●**What do you most want from medical care?** For example, is a long life or highest quality of life more important? What about freedom from pain?

STEP 2: **Consider three specific, realistic activities that allow you to realize these core values—ones that you'd hate to give up.**

Examples: Walking to the park daily to see friends...driving yourself to your weekly poker or bridge game...traveling abroad with a loved one.

STEP 3: **Consider what aspects of your health care help you achieve these goals**—for example, medication that relieves pain so you can walk or regular exercise that boosts your mood.

STEP 4: **Consider three aspects of your health care** (for example, medications, health-care visits, tests or procedures or self-management tasks) that get in the way of achieving your goals or that you find too difficult or burdensome. Examples might include drugs that make you too tired to socialize...or a prescribed diet that forbids your favorite foods.

STEP 5: **Once you have identified your personal priorities, work with your doctor—or doctors—to align your health-care goals with them.** Your task is to make your doctor understand that even though optimal results for each of your diseases are desired, other things also matter—maybe even more—to you.

These conversations may be challenging. Doctors are trained to focus on diagnosing diseases and then choosing effective treatments for them. But if you say very explicitly what you care about, they will find it hard to ignore.

Be simple and direct: "I really want to focus on being able to visit my family regularly, so what should we work on to enable me to do this?"

Also, share what aspects of your health care you think make it hard to achieve your goals. The more information the doctor has, the better you can work out trade-offs with acceptable risks and optimal benefits. For example, if you have diabetes, you may be willing to stick to a diet that helps stabilize your blood sugar but want to forgo taking insulin shots because of the inconvenience of the shots and difficulty that you have self-administering them. You are willing to consider oral medications that help control your blood sugar.

Another trade-off might be to reduce blood pressure medications that make you too tired or dizzy to complete your desired exercise routine even if it means a small increase in your risk of having a stroke down the road.

It's an ongoing process. Whenever the doctor prescribes new medication or orders tests, ask, for example, "Staying physically active is what really matters to me. Is this treatment/test likely to help me do it better?" Keep your goals flexible, too. A change in your condition, such as a stroke or worsening of arthritis, may alter what you can realistically expect to achieve.

The Best Way to Advocate for Your Health: Ask the Right Questions

Dr. Suzanne Steinbaum is a cardiologist who has devoted her career to the treatment of heart disease through early detection, education and prevention. She is author of *Dr. Suzanne Steinbaum's Heart Book: Every Woman's Guide to a Heart Healthy Life.* DrSuzanneSteinbaum.com

Questions are interesting: They are not facts. They aren't necessarily based on anything tangible. And they often mean much more than the literal meaning of the words used to form them.

As a doctor, I have discovered over many years that questions can reveal as much about a patient's condition as lab tests. Doctors get a lot of questions, and these are worth paying attention to because they are a window into what someone is thinking and how someone is feeling.

A perfect example of this is a simple question I often hear from patients: "Am I going to be on this medication forever?" This seems like a direct question at first. They want to know if there is an end point to their prescription. *But this question can also mean many other things, such as...*

Am I ever going to get better?

Am I always going to feel sick without this medication?

Is this medication a cure or just a cover for my symptoms?

Will I have to budget for a lifetime of this medication? Can I afford that?

Has my life changed irreparably?

Ultimately, what they are really asking is: "Am I going to die?"

Questions like this are gifts. They are a gesture of true intimacy from patient to doctor. If the doctor really listens, she or he can respond in kind, addressing that intimacy by continuing the conversation and offering real information rather than platitudes. But that takes vulnerability on the part of the patient and a willingness to really listen on the part of the physician.

On the other hand, all too often, patients don't ask the burning question. They may not think their question is important enough to bother their doctor about. They may believe their question doesn't matter or is "stupid." Sometimes, they don't know how to ask the question the right way, so they don't try. And in many cases, they don't really want to know the answer.

A new patient recently came in to see me for a second opinion. I looked in her chart and saw that she had been deemed "non-compliant" by another doctor. She had atrial fibrillation but was not taking the blood thinner that doctor had prescribed for her. When the patients don't follow this direction, the chart often gives the reason why. But there was no reason in this chart. Why was she "noncompliant"? I couldn't tell. The doctor had noted that she wanted a second opinion, so I could only guess that she wanted to know if she actually needed a blood thinner. Maybe she wanted to know if it would cure her, and if not, she wasn't interested? Was she completely uninterested in taking care of herself? I couldn't know without asking a question.

But when I met her, I decided not to wait for her to ask me a question. I opened the conversation with an open-ended question: "How can I help you?"

I could have said other things. I could have been judgmental or given her a lecture. I could have asked, "Do you realize the danger in not taking your blood thinner?" But this kind of question takes the power away from the patient. It implies that the doctor doesn't care about the patient's feelings or respect that she may have a reason for what she is doing. I could have asked, "Why wouldn't you take a blood thinner, if you knew you could get a stroke?" That kind of question is scary and intimidating. Instead, I asked a question that opened the door for her to direct the conversation, and her answer revealed to me that this was the right choice.

As much as I have talked in the past about the doctor-patient relationship and the need for communication, I continue to see this connection disintegrating. As we head full steam into a world increasingly governed by technology, including doctor visits over the Internet or even over text, through apps, or via e-mail, the opportunity to take advantage of the nuances of these subtle exchanges gets lost in the digital shuffle. Everyone wants to move faster, get things done more efficiently, and move on to the next thing, but with a quick-and-dirty question like, "No meds? You are noncompliant!" the subtext

gets stamped out. There is no room and no time for the question, "Why?"

The more you know people, the more you understand who they are and the greater chance you have to discover what they really need. What could be more important for a physician? But one of the most important qualities this kind of exchange requires is empathy. Without this ability to understand how someone else is feeling, asking questions is like throwing rocks into the ocean. It's a longshot whether or not you'll hit on anything important.

But back to my "second opinion" patient. As it turned out, she was a lovely woman and not "noncompliant" at all. Her insurance company had changed her blood thinner to a new drug that she was not familiar with, and she was concerned to take it because of all the side effects she had read about in the materials that accompanied the medication. This is a sensible and natural response from a patient who is not willing to take a new medication blindly. She had opted not to take the medication until she could speak to her doctor, but when she tried to talk to her doctor (more than once), she got only the question: "Are you taking your medication?" When she answered, "No," the doctor documented it and labeled her in a way that made me, the next doctor down the line, question her motivation to take care of herself because she was not following her doctor's recommendations.

You can see where this communication broke down, resulting in the mislabeling of a patient who had all the best intentions. Words have power, but even more dangerous than words is the inability to listen to the words of another—the inability to ask the right questions and to receive and listen to the answers with an open mind and an empathetic heart.

You won't always have a doctor who is good at this, but I suggest that you find one if you want the best care. A good doctor will not expect your questions to be perfect or exactly on target or even obviously relevant to your condition. A good doctor will listen and get to the bottom of the "why."

Considering all of this, here are some guidelines for communicating with your doctor…

• **Don't be afraid to ask your questions.** They are critically important!

• **To get your thoughts fully together, write down your questions before your doctor's visit.** If your doctor tells you not to read the list and just ask your questions, explain that you are nervous and don't want to forget what's important for you to understand.

• **Doctors sometimes fear that patients will have an extremely long list of questions.** They prefer to deal with issues one at a time, so keep your questions focused on the reason for your visit. For other issues, make a separate appointment. However, don't be afraid to bring up issues you think might be related to your primary issue, even if you aren't sure.

• **If the answers you get to your questions are not direct enough or you don't get the answers you need, ask again in a different way.** You can always say that you aren't sure you fully understand. Don't be afraid to continue a conversation after a short and insufficient answer.

• **Sometimes your doctor might be busy, overwhelmed, or have another patient who might be on her/his mind.** Give your doctor the benefit of the doubt and ask again. Doctors get distracted sometimes, but they should never be rude.

• **If you have a question that's hard to ask, say so, but then get up the courage to ask exactly what you need to know.** Even if it is embarrassing!

• **Bring someone with you for moral support if it will help you to stay focused and be braver.**

• **Know that you are not alone.** Your doctor has probably heard your questions many times before. Humanity is funny like that, so ask away! Your doctor probably has good guidance for you, once you understand each other.

• **Finally, you must advocate for yourself always, and asking questions is where this begins.** It is essential, so don't be afraid to do it! This takes some bravery, I know, but your doctor works for you and is there to help you. Questions are the perfect way to get the help you need and to foster a healthy doctor-patient relationship. And that's one of the most important ways to achieve wellness.

What a Health Coach Can Do for You

Leigh-Ann Webster, NBC-HWC, executive director for the National Board for Health & Wellness Coaching (NBHWC.org), a nonprofit organization that has created a professional standard for health and wellness coaching. She is a certified personal trainer and founder of 52 Healthy Weeks, a virtual studio that provides personal training, nutrition education and health and wellness coaching services. 52Healthy Weeks.com

It's a form of lifestyle failure that we're all familiar with. You decide that you want to be healthier—exercise more, eat better, lose weight, feel less stressed or get a health problem under control. You set a health goal, such as walking 30 minutes every day—and for a while you manage to stick with your new habit. But before you know it, you've reverted to your old ways.

Where most people get tripped up: Just deciding that you want to be healthier doesn't work—if it did, we'd all be healthier! What does work is connecting with your deepest inner wants and needs—with a motivation that can compel you to make and sustain a lifestyle change. That's where a health coach comes in.

A health coach is trained to ask the type of "open-ended" questions that will help you connect with your inner motivations for change—the real drivers of your day-to-day behavior. Their nonjudgmental questions get you to think deeply about your goals in life and why you are motivated to achieve them. A close-ended question such as "Did you have a successful week?" allows you to answer "yes" or "no." An open-ended question such as, "What about last week made it successful?" provokes thought and reflection. And once the questions are asked, health coaches know how to listen in attentive, companionable silence, letting you think and talk about what you really want.

Example: A 60-year-old woman with type 2 diabetes knew she had to eat better and lose weight to control her disease and stay alive—but she kept failing at doing it. Through in-depth conversation with her health coach, she pin-pointed a reason to live a longer life: to spend time with her grandchildren. Once she identified that as her inner motivation, she was able to make permanent changes to her diet.

Another common scenario is that a person thinks he/she has one reason for seeing a health coach—but discovers that he really has another.

Example: A man hired a health coach to become more fit. Through working with the coach, he discovered that he is overcommitted in his work and social life—and has no time for himself, including time to exercise. So first, the coach and the client focus on prioritizing self-care and time management—and "exercising" the right to say no.

Studies show that working with a health coach can help individuals achieve and maintain an impressive array of better-health benefits—including fewer hospitalizations and better lung capacity in patients with chronic heart failure…better adherence to a medication regimen…and a reduced number of emergency room visits among "super-utilizers" of emergency care. In cancer patients, health coaching has been proven to have particularly strong psychological benefits.

Even for people without life-threatening illnesses, a health coach can help make lasting changes. Health coaches work with people who would like to better manage their stress, improve their eating habits, increase their cardio fitness, improve their sleep, reduce the time they spend sitting and more. In addition, health coaches help clients find creative solutions for situations in their lives that are impacting their well-being.

What you need to know about working with a health coach…

Stages of Behavior Change

Most health coaches use a science-supported and widely accepted model of behavior change called The Transtheoretical Model of Change, which addresses six distinct stages of change…

Precontemplation: You don't even know that you want to change, but you know something isn't right, such as always feeling tired.

Contemplation: You're thinking about change but haven't made a commitment to act and are researching pathways to change—such as seeing a health coach.

Preparation: You decide to act, and you gather information and plan. Most people skip this stage when they try to make changes on their own often leading to failure after a few weeks.

Action: You begin to change your behavior and lifestyle.

Maintenance: You've sustained the change for at least six months.

Termination: The change is permanent. You're no longer tempted by your former behavior.

Example: The client's "contemplation" is to eat more fruits and vegetables. The health coach helps the client prepare to reach his goal—perhaps by looking at his current consumption of these healthy foods, understanding what's keeping him from eating them and then helping him figure out how to eat one more serving per day for the next two weeks—that is a realistic and achievable goal.

Next, the coach helps create a plan of action—such as planning a weekly visit to the grocery store's produce department and finding enticing, yet easy recipes.

New topics or ideas tend to surface over time as the level of trust and rapport between the client and the coach deepens, and the client spends more time reflecting on his life and well-being to figure out the drivers to change.

Finding a Health Coach

The best place to start is at the website of the National Board for Health & Wellness Coaching (NBHWC.org). This organization collaborates with the National Board of Medical Examiners to provide a rigorous board-certification examination. Health and wellness coaches who hold the National Board Certified Health & Wellness Coach (NBC-HWC) credential have had a minimum of 75 hours of training and education. In addition, they have passed a 4.5-hour exam that is provided in partnership with the National Board of Medical Examiners, and they have completed at least 200 hours of coaching sessions.

There are other resources to help you find a health coach. Many doctors work with them, and many employee-wellness programs offer access to one.

Or try your hospital, health system or insurance company. Gyms and fitness facilities such as the YMCA or Life Time also offer health and wellness coaching.

Choosing a Health Coach

Interview at least two or three coaches, and choose the one with whom you feel the most rapport—someone with whom you'll feel comfortable sharing your deepest thoughts about your life and your need for improvement. You want a coach who really listens and doesn't dominate the conversation.

Be sure to ask where the person received his/her training—and confirm that it's a program approved by NBC-HWC. A list of approved programs is on its website.

Before you hire a health coach, you also should be sure of what services are offered. Personal trainers and nutritionists are very directive—if you want to run a 10K, for example, a personal trainer tells you exactly what to do…a nutritionist will tell you what to eat. A health coach, on the other hand, is trained to partner with you on many different aspects of your life, including your diet,

exercise, stress, mood, relationships, work and spirituality.

Health-Coaching Sessions

Most people meet with a health coach virtually—this was so even before the pandemic. Sessions typically are 50 to 60 minutes, held weekly or every other week, reviewing the previous week (or two) and setting goals for the next time period. This encourages you to be accountable—another key step in achieving goals.

Many coaches offer a six-month program—that's the amount of time it takes to establish and master a new life skill. The cost per session tends to range from $50 to $150.

More from Leigh-Ann Webster, NBC-HWC…

E-Coaching: Your Virtual Guide

Most health and wellness coaching is face-to-face, in conversation, even if it's via a video call. But there's also e-coaching—no face-to-face interaction or ongoing relationship but only interaction through an app, chat, text or e-mail.

Noom is a psychology-based platform that empowers users to make healthier choices. It offers individual and group coaching included in the $59/month fee. Fitbit Care—a health and wellness program available to employees through their employers—uses an app but has no face-to-face interaction.

Banish Physician Phobia

David Yusko, PsyD, a psychologist and co-founder of the Center for Anxiety & Behavior Therapy, in Bryn Mawr, Pennsylvania. Dr. Yusko specializes in the treatment of anxiety disorders, with a focus on obsessive compulsive disorder, panic disorder, social phobia, generalized anxiety disorder, and specific phobias.

Imagine this: You get a message reminding you that it's time for your regular check-up. Your doctor's office would like you to call for an appointment.

If the thought of making that call makes your heart race and your blood pressure rise, you may have iatrophobia: fear of doctors and medical care.

It's a very real problem that causes real harm, including potentially dangerous delays in medical care. Think of the cancer that's found too late, the high cholesterol that goes untreated, the minor infection that spreads.

Understanding Phobias

Data suggest that 12 percent of adults suffer from a phobia some time in their lives. Medical phobias, which can include fear of hospitals, dentists, blood, needles or anyone wearing a white coat, are among the most common.

All phobias are forms of anxiety, but they differ from generalized anxiety disorder, a broader kind of persistent and excessive worry. Here, the fear is triggered by something specific.

Once that trigger is pulled, the symptoms can be intense. Physical symptoms may include increased heart rate, fast, shallow breathing, spikes in blood pressure, sweating, nausea and feeling faint. Emotional symptoms may include fear and thoughts of impending doom and disaster.

In the grips of such strong feelings, which are rooted in the fight or flight responses our ancestors relied upon for life-threatening emergencies, people typically respond in one of two ways.

The first response is often avoidance. In the short term, avoidance can feel great, but it's a trap: The sense of relief you feel over canceling one medical appointment makes you even more likely to cancel another. Some people end up going years without care.

People with phobias also may engage in safety behaviors, things they feel they must do to make a threatening situation endurable. A person with a medical phobia might go for a check-up only if they take a sedative first.

How to Reduce the Fear

While such crutches might help ease anxiety in the short term, they don't solve the underlying problem. In fact, they can make it worse because they reinforce the idea that going to see your doctor is a scary situation.

So how do you make it less scary? If your symptoms are fairly mild, you might be able to break the cycle of fear one uneventful appointment at a time.

But if your symptoms are more severe—especially if they are causing you to skip needed care—you may need assistance from a psychologist trained in cognitive behavioral therapy, a kind of talk therapy. If possible, you should see someone specializing in anxiety and phobias.

Exposure Therapy

At your first appointment or two, the therapist will learn about how your fear of medical care affects your life and which situations trigger your symptoms. Then, you will likely begin something called exposure therapy.

The idea is to expose you, in a safe, supportive setting, to a carefully selected series of images and experiences, presented in order from the least to the most threatening. At each step, you will likely feel some anxiety. But if you stick with each exposure long enough for the anxiety to subside, you will gain the experience of facing your fears and getting past them.

An early session might involve looking at pictures of a red cross then a stethoscope. You might move on to pictures of an ambulance, a doctor's waiting room, and a doctor in a white coat. Next, you might watch videos, starting perhaps with a funny cartoon followed by a scene from a medical drama and then a scene of a real doctor at work. Finally, you may work through the steps of a real medical encounter, including a visit to the doctor's parking lot, then the waiting room, and then the exam or consultation room. Some therapists may invite a doctor to participate in the session via video conferencing.

The process typically takes eight to 12 sessions. Most people who complete it will overcome their fears and find a doctor's office to be a truly safe space.

How to Survive the Hospital Now

David Sherer, MD, an anesthesiologist now retired from clinical practice whose career spanned 40 years. He is author of the newly updated *Hospital Survival Guide: The Patient Handbook to Getting Better and Getting Out* and the Bottom Line blog, "What Your Doctor Isn't Telling You" at BottomLineInc.com.

With or without a pandemic, hospitals are a scary labyrinth of bureaucracy and dangers. New systems such as electronic health records and "hospitalists" theoretically improve things but are far from infallible. *Steps to take whether you are going for a planned surgery or other procedure...*

Presurgery/Preprocedure Consult

This crucial meeting gives your doctor information about you and your medical history to help your procedure go well and informs you about how to best prepare for it. It typically is held about one week before...but schedule it farther out if you have a serious medical problem, such as COPD or uncontrolled blood pressure or blood sugar. *At this meeting...*

• **Review the hospital's electronic health record (EHR),** updating your current medication and supplement list as well as filling in missing information, such as an omitted specialist, dietary restrictions and emergency contacts.

• **Bring a written snapshot of your medical history.** This information may not be in your EHR if the doctor doing the surgery or procedure, the hospital/surgical center and your primary medical doctor are not all in the same network. *Include...*

•Current supplements and medications with product name, dosage, frequency and the name of the prescribing doctor.

•Contact info for all your doctors and what each treats you for.

•Other critical facts such as food or latex allergies...medications that have caused negative reactions...past hospital difficulty, such as with intubation or anesthesia...artificial implants, pins or other foreign objects in your body.

Smart: Also bring copies of this snapshot to the hospital for your anesthesiologist and other medical personnel.

Ask these key questions at this procedure consult...

• **Can I have an early-morning time slot?** The operating staff will be fresher, and you'll have less time to feel hungry or anxious. Also, avoid scheduling surgery in July, when new med-school grads begin their hands-on hospital learning.

• **Which medications and supplements should I take the morning of my procedure?** And how far in advance should I stop others, such as low-dose aspirin, blood thinners or fish oil, due to bleeding concerns? Don't start anything new to avoid potential interactions with medications you'll be given at the hospital.

• **Should I donate blood in case I need a blood transfusion?** This will depend on whether you're healthy enough to do so and the potential for blood loss.

• **What will my recovery be like?** Ask for an honest assessment of the healing process... whether you'll need special rehab or equipment at home...and any likely side effects.

• **Am I a candidate for *bupivacaine* (Exparel)?** This local, time-released anesthetic injection now is approved for use during many surgical procedures. It may eliminate the need for post-op opioids.

• **What is the hospital/facility policy regarding patient advocates or companions?** Having someone with you is ideal, and fortunately, more facilities are allowing patients to have companions as the pandemic wanes.

Getting Ready

You know not to drink alcohol the night before a surgery and often you can't eat after midnight. It's also important not to overeat. You don't want bloating and discomfort to spoil your sleep. Your stress levels will be much higher if you don't rest well the night before.

•**Skip all cosmetics and skin-care products the morning of the procedure.** Make-up could get on the surgical team's gloves and into your body. Nail polish could prevent a fingertip pulse oximeter from accurately measuring the oxygen in your blood. Body lotion could keep surgical tape from adhering.

Note: If your skin is thin or frail, ask that paper tape be used.

•**Pack smart.** For better sleep—thereby better healing—bring eyeshades, ear plugs, your favorite pillow and a white-noise machine. Personal items, from body wash and lip balm to a tablet computer loaded with books and other diversions, can make the hospital stay less unpleasant. Bring throat lozenges to soothe any soreness from the breathing tube during sedation. Many people feel nauseated after surgery, so consider a wearable antinausea device such as Relief Band or ginger supplements (get the doctor's OK before using).

At the Hospital

During check-in, review your EHR again. Yes, it's redundant but still worthwhile.

When you meet with your anesthesiologist before your procedure, alert him/her to reactions you've had to narcotics such as sedatives, your typical pain threshold and any allergies. The more information you provide, the better he can tailor your anesthesia. Ask about possible side effects and how to get relief. Make him aware of loose teeth, crowns and other dental work, and if you're used to sleeping with your head on two or more pillows—lying flat for a long time could cause breathing difficulties.

After Your Procedure

Answering the same questions every time a staff member enters your room is tedious but helps avoid mistakes, including administering wrong tests and medications. *To stay on top of your care…*

•**Get to know your care givers.** Hospitalists are doctors who work exclusively for the hospital and may be responsible for your post-op care rather than your primary doctor. Chances are you won't meet the hospitalist until you're in your hospital room. Some hospitals rotate hospitalists, so you may have more than one. Engage doctors and staff in pleasant conversation so that they relate to you as a person rather than by your ailment.

There are more staffing shortages than ever before, and some tasks may have been offloaded to untrained nurse assistants—their badges might read "patient care associate" or "patient care partner." Make sure that only qualified nurses insert IVs, catheters and gastric tubes, change sterile dressings, treat damaged skin and give injections.

•**Don't be shy.** When an unfamiliar staffer enters your room, check his/her badge and ask about his credentials and why he's there. If you have a legitimate concern, politely but firmly say, "I'd like to speak with my doctor first to be sure this is something I'm supposed to have."

•**Confirm that you're getting the right doses of the right meds**—generics of your daily medications can look different from what you take at home. Any time you're given a medication, ask what it is and why. Also, remind the doctor or nurse about any allergies. Write down the drug name, dosage and frequency for your records.

If many doctors are involved in your care, when one orders a major procedure or changes your treatment, make sure the hospitalist(s) and your own doctor are notified.

•**Watch when your dressings are changed** so you'll know how to care for yourself at home.

•**Ask if telemedicine can be used to contact specialists at other institutions** if your case needs an expert consult and also for your follow-up visits.

•**Transition to recovery at home as soon as you can.** Even before COVID-19, hospitals were hotbeds of germs. A silver lining of the pandemic is that many safety practices, such as frequent handwashing, single-use gloves, gowns and face masks or shields are now standard, but ask all staff to follow these measures if they aren't.

Don't Be Misdiagnosed

David E. Newman-Toker, MD, a professor of neurology, ophthalmology, and otolaryngology at the Johns Hopkins University School of Medicine in Baltimore. He is also the director of the Armstrong Institute Center for Diagnostic Excellence at Johns Hopkins, and the president of the Society to Improve Diagnosis in Medicine.

An 83-year-old woman had diarrhea, which her doctor said was a side effect of her diabetes medication. She was treated with a change in medication and diet but received no further tests. Several years later, she was diagnosed with incurable metastatic colon cancer.

A 36-year-old man suffering from fatigue and lethargy was diagnosed by different doctors with depression and anemia. Months later, an examination showed he had endocarditis, a bacterial infection that had destroyed one wall and two valves of his heart.

A nurse had a severe headache that radiated to her shoulders and waistline. A doctor diagnosed her with a tension headache and prescribed pain medication. She collapsed several days later, after which doctors discovered she had a ruptured blood vessel in her brain.

Defining Misdiagnosis

These are true stories of misdiagnosis, or diagnostic error. In general, there are two types of misdiagnoses: Doctors miss the opportunity to treat a dangerous disease, or they mistakenly treat a person for a disease or health problem they don't have. Most diagnostic errors occur in primary care, though some happen at the hospital. And they're very common. Experts say most people will experience at least one diagnostic error in their lifetime.

Different Types of Harm

Yearly, an estimated 500,000 to 1 million people suffer permanent disability or death because of a misdiagnosis. Millions more aren't disabled or killed, but they are permanently harmed. Others endure serious short-term suffering, such as ending up in an intensive-care unit for weeks on end. Still others deal with lower levels of suffering for longer periods. For example, a patient of mine suffered from near-constant dizziness. She had seen two neurologists, two ear-nose-and-throat specialists, and two psychiatrists, all of whom concluded that she had psychological problems. But I was able to diagnose her with vestibular migraine, an unusual form of migraine that may cause dizziness without headaches.

There's also psychological harm. As with my patient, many misdiagnosed patients have been told they are imagining it or their problem is all in their head—an insensitive comment that can cause psychological trauma. Patients may lose faith in doctors and the health-care system.

The Big Three

Health problems that affect tens of millions of people, such as fractures and high blood pressure, are commonly misdiagnosed. But some rare problems are misdiagnosed, too, such as spinal abscess, with 20,000 to 30,000 yearly cases and a misdiagnosis rate of 65 percent; and aortic dissection, with 50,000 to 100,000 yearly cases and a misdiagnosis rate of 25 to 35 percent.

New research by my colleagues at the John Hopkins University School of Medicine and I show that diagnostic errors in three categories of illness generate 50 percent of all disability and death from misdiagnoses. *In fact, just 15 diseases in those three categories are the main causes of serious, permanent harm…*

• **Vascular events,** including stroke, heart attack, venous and arterial thromboembolism (blood clots in the legs, feet, arms, or groin), and aortic aneurysm and dissection (a bulge or tear in an arterial lining);

• **Infections,** including sepsis, meningitis, encephalitis, spinal abscess, pneumonia, and endocarditis; and

• **Cancer,** including lung cancer, breast cancer, colorectal cancer, prostate cancer, and melanoma.

Before, During and After

Avoiding misdiagnoses in these three categories could save 100,000 lives every year, including your own. *And you can help your doctor do it by taking three steps…*

• **Come prepared.** Before your primary care visit, put together a one-page, easy-to-read list of your symptoms and the timeline during which they occurred. This helps you avoid a common mistake: talking about what previous doctors have said. The executive summary also saves precious time. Instead of the doctor spending 10 to 15 minutes finding out about your symptoms, he or she can spend that time thinking about what caused your problem.

• **Ask this key question.** As a patient, you have to guide the doctor in giving you a detailed explanation about what he or she thinks is going on. To do that, ask this question: "What is the worst problem this could be and why is it not that problem?"

This forces the doctor to give you specific information. For instance, if your major symptom is dizziness, you're hoping to hear something like this: "The pattern of my findings is consistent with vestibular neuritis, an inflammation of a nerve in your ear, which causes dizziness. The problem I'm most worried about is stroke, but there is substantial evidence that my findings in this exam confirm your problem is vestibular neuritis."

This shows that the doctor is thinking clearly and systematically about the problem and can articulate the rationale for the diagnosis. It also shows that he or she is thinking about making sure you don't get harmed by a diagnostic error.

However, if the doctor says something like, "You don't need to worry about that," or "I see a lot of this, and it is very common," you should immediately find another doctor or at least get a second opinion. Research from the Mayo Clinic shows that 87 percent of patients who seek a second opinion leave with a refined or changed diagnosis (66 percent refined, 21 percent changed, and 12 percent confirmed).

• **Stay vigilant.** During your visit, your doctor will give you a treatment plan, such as, "This problem should go away by itself in a week," or "Take this pill, which should solve the problem." However, when things don't go according to plan, patients tend to think they have received the wrong treatment. If you've been given a pill, you might think you need a higher dose or a different medication. But you may not have the wrong treatment for the right disease: You might have the right treatment for the wrong disease.

If you're not getting better, it's time to make sure your diagnosis is correct and to keep the possibility of diagnostic error on the physician's radar by giving the office a call.

Lead Shielding Does Not Protect During X-rays

Roundup of experts on lead shielding and X-rays, reported at KaiserHealthNews.org.

It has been recommended since the 1950s to guard patients' ovaries (and testicles in men). But new studies show shielding has unintended negative effects. Shields are hard to position properly and often miss the areas they are meant to protect. Even when placed correctly, they can obscure the areas doctors need to see…they can cause machines' automatic exposure controls to increase radiation in an attempt to see through the shield…and they do not protect against radiation scatter, in which radiation ricochets inside the body and ends up affecting internal tissues. The amount of radiation needed for a modern X-ray is about one-twentieth what it was in the 1950s, and no measurable harm from it has been found after a search through decades of data. Several physicians' groups now recommend that shielding be discontinued as a routine practice.

Before You Say "Yes" to Outpatient Surgery

David Sherer, MD, retired anesthesiologist, is author of *Hospital Survival Guide: The Patient Handbook to Getting Better and Getting Out.*

Before you say "yes" to outpatient surgery, make sure the facility has medications for anesthesia-induced complications on hand and the health-care providers know how to use them. *Dantrolene* treats malignant hyperthermia, a reaction to general anesthesia. *Intralipid* treats reactions to local anesthetics. Such dangerous reactions are rare, but patients have died when doctors were not properly trained in the use of these medications… or when the meds were expired or not on hand at the facility.

Virtual Post-Op Visits Work

Study titled "The Value of Time: Analysis of Surgical Post-Discharge Virtual vs. In-Person Visits," by researchers at Atrium Health, Charlotte, North Carolina, presented at the virtual American College of Surgeons Clinical Congress 2020.

If you visited your doctor during the COVID-19 pandemic, you may have seen him/her virtually on your computer screen. Two-way audio and visual communications are called telehealth or telemedicine, and it's not surprising that they can take a lot less overall time than an in-person appointment. Recent research also confirms that videos are efficient…and satisfying, especially for patients after surgery.

Important recent finding: A new study presented at the 2020 virtual American College of Surgeons Clinical Congress finds that virtual visits are working well for both doctors and patients following certain surgical procedures. This was one of the first studies to look at a comparison of how much time virtual visits save and how much actual time patients spend one-on-one with their surgical care providers.

Study details: For the research, surgeons randomly assigned more than 400 patients to either a virtual or in-person follow-up visit after minimally invasive surgeries (either a laparoscopic gallbladder removal or appendectomy). They recorded the overall time spent for the visit, the actual time spent with the surgical caregiver and patient satisfaction with the visit. *Key findings included…*

• **Overall time for in-person visits averaged 58 minutes compared with 19 minutes for virtual visits.**

• **Patients spent 80 percent less time checking in and waiting for virtual visits than in-person visits.**

• **Actual time spent with the surgical care provider was the same for both visits, just over eight minutes.**

• **Patient satisfaction was similar for both types of visits, 94 percent versus 98 percent.**

The surgeons said that they were able to check the patient's incisions visually, answer patient questions and plan additional care as needed during the virtual follow-up visits. Patients were able to save on travel time and do their visits with minimal interruption to their work or need for child care.

Bottom line: The researchers concluded that for certain types of surgical procedures, follow-up virtual visits compare favorably to face-to-face visits.

Make the Most of Video Visits with Your Doctor

John L. Bender, MD, family medicine physician and senior partner at Miramont Wellness Center in the Fort Collins, Colorado area, past president of the Colorado Medical Society and a pioneer in the implementation of telemedicine in his state. He has written various pieces of legislation governing telemedicine. Miramont.us

Telemedicine technology has been ramping up for some time, but the need for health-care alternatives in the face of the coronavirus pandemic has led to it being adopted at warp speed. Even some injuries can be managed by video chat.

Whether your telemedicine visit is with one of your existing providers or via a telehealth-service doctor you have never met, here are the steps to take before and during your appointment to get the most out of it.

•**Test out the software.** Health systems and medical practices have various telemedicine applications to choose from, so unless all your specialists belong to the same network, the software may be different from one provider to another. You may need to install a mobile app—some software works only on a tablet or a smartphone rather than on a computer—or sign up for an online account with a telemedicine platform.

Once an appointment has been made, you may receive a text or an e-mail with a link and directions for you to test the system and fill out forms. Don't wait until the last minute in case you need time to troubleshoot. You'll be guided through a few screens to make sure your camera and speakers can be accessed…that you can see and hear the doctor…and that you can be seen and heard by him/her.

In order for some telemedicine programs to work correctly, you may be prompted to exit other programs or close out of other websites. If your home Internet connection is spotty, you might try running the test on your various devices to see if the platform works better on one than on another.

•**Take your vital signs.** With a few moderate-cost devices, you can perform many of the health checks a nurse would do in the office and report them to your provider. *Depending on the nature of your call, these can be very helpful…*

- Thermometer
- Bathroom scale
- Blood pressure cuff (you may have a lower reading at home because you're more relaxed).

You can take your pulse on many gadgets and track atrial fibrillation on an Apple Watch.

If you're managing a chronic condition and haven't invested in monitoring tools—such as an advanced blood glucose monitor for diabetes that can store and relay information to your doctor's office or a fingertip pulse oximeter for measuring blood oxygen if you have COPD—now may be the time. Some or all may be covered by insurance. Getting these readings from you in advance helps the doctor prepare for your appointment.

•**Create a script of your symptoms and concerns.** This will help you stay focused and ensure that you don't omit any details or questions, especially if it feels awkward to communicate through a screen. State your list of concerns at the beginning of the appointment so that issues can be prioritized, and the time will be well-managed from the start. If you have a visible issue, such as a swollen joint or a rash, take clear, straight-on photos and send them to the doctor as a text or e-mail attachment. This is usually a lot easier than trying to find the right angle at which to hold the affected area up to your device's camera during the appointment.

•**Have a written health history to refer to.** Of course, this is essential if you're talking to a telemedicine-service doctor you've never met, but even if you're meeting with a member of your existing medical team, be prepared to succinctly communicate the pertinent parts of your medical history as a reminder for your provider. While all of this information should be in your doctor's records on you, reviewing it all helps prevent errors. It should include a detailed medication list with product names, dosages and frequency and the names of the prescribing doctors...any allergies (this will help to prevent drug interactions if the telemedicine doctor e-prescribes a new drug)...a list of significant hospital stays and surgeries... and any other information that could be pertinent to why you're being seen. If there's a chat box, you can use it to type in complex drug names.

• **Be patient.** As in a real office, you might experience a wait time.

• **Get past any self-consciousness.** As surprising as this sounds, even when sick, some people suddenly worry about how they look when they see their face on the screen. One of my patients actually aimed the camera at her feet! Remember that we've seen it all before and we want to see you— eye contact and nonverbal cues assist in making a diagnosis.

• **Have your care advocate with you.** Just as your spouse or another loved one—or your caregiver—might accompany you to an office visit, he/she can be on the virtual visit, too, whether to describe symptoms, provide tech help or take notes.

• **Take and read back notes.** This is important because you can't just turn to the nurse for clarification after the doctor leaves the examination room as you might if you were in the office. Ask if any instructions can be e-mailed to you.

• **Clarify the follow-up.** A virtual visit might lead to an in-person checkup if your condition doesn't improve or if your problem needs a physical examination. If it is a check-in to see how you're managing a chronic condition, you may be able to schedule your next visit virtually as well. If your next step is a lab test, ask whether the script will be sent to you or straight to the lab and how the results will be communicated to you.

As telemedicine technology continues to advance and as patients and doctors get better at using it, it will become even easier to access care without leaving your home.

Best Health-Monitoring Devices to Have at Home

Andrea Chymiy, MD, MPH, a family physician in private practice in Poulsbo, Washington. She is a Medical Reserve Corps coordinator, an Urban Search & Rescue team physician and an emergency-preparedness blogger. LeftyPrepperMom.com

When it comes to routine health care these days, you're more likely than ever to meet virtually with your doctor. Having the right home health devices can help you provide necessary data to your doctor. *What everyone should have...*

Heart-Rate App

Why own one: A suddenly elevated or reduced pulse may signal a severe medical problem. And while phone apps lack the accuracy of professional equipment, they can give you a close idea.

What to look for: A highly rated app with an easy-to-use interface that works off your phone's camera—it takes pictures of your fingertip to calculate your heart's rhythm.

Top pick: For iOS, Cardiograph Classic ($0.99, App Store). For Android, Instant Heart Rate (free to use for heart-rate monitoring, but other features cost $9.99 per month, Google Play).

Pulse Oximeter

Why own one: Normally you wouldn't need this fingertip blood-oxygen–measuring device unless you had a lung disease. But low blood oxygen has been linked with COVID-19, so pulse oximeters have been flying off shelves.

What to look for: Easy use (single button)...large display.

Top pick: ClinicalGuard CMS-50DL Finger Pulse Oximeter ($11.45, widely available).

Blood Pressure Monitor

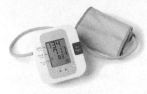

Why own one: Blood pressure is an important statistic in medical emergencies as well as routine virtual visits.

What to look for: One-touch operation, a clear display and mobile/cloud data storage and sharing. Get a cuff that goes over your bicep, not your wrist, and choose an established brand with a track record of reliability.

Top pick: Omron 7 Series ($89.99, Omron HealthCare.com).

Bathroom Scale

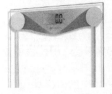

Why own one: Sudden weight gain or loss can indicate serious illness. Weight change of 5 percent or more up or down in less than a week, assuming you're not trying to lose weight, should be discussed with your doctor. Measure your weight weekly to know your baseline and so you don't miss dramatic changes.

What to look for: Simplicity, sturdiness and a backlit display.

Top pick: Etekcity Digital Body Weight Bathroom Scale ($19.99, widely available).

Thermometer

Why own one: To diagnose fever. A temperature greater than 100.4°F is considered a fever.

What to look for: Something practical and easy to use. The general consensus among doctors is that oral thermometers are most accurate. If you prefer something faster, go for an in-ear or on-forehead, also called temporal, model. All are accurate, but in-ear temperature usually is 0.5°F higher than oral, and forehead temperature is usually 0.5°F lower.

Top picks (all widely available): For an oral thermometer, iProven Digital Thermo-

meter ($8.99). For in-ear measurements, Braun ThermoScan 7 ($48.59). For a forehead thermometer, iHealth Non Contact Infrared Thermometer ($19.99).

Otoscope

Why own one: This device is recommended for parents of young children and for adults who are prone to ear infections. A quick YouTube search for an explanatory video will give you enough know-how to discern between healthy ear tissue and infection.

What to look for: 5X magnification and a glass lens for greater clarity.

Top pick: Dr. Mom 4th Generation LED Pocket Otoscope ($28.92, DrMomOtoscope.com).

Images: GettyImages

Owning a Pulse Oximeter

Owning a pulse oximeter can help if you contract COVID-19. While most patients are able to recover at home, individuals should go to the hospital when serious warning signs emerge, such as trouble breathing, persistent pain or pressure in the chest and bluish lips or face. This device, which clips over the fingertip, measures oxygen saturation levels and can provide an early warning sign that breathing difficulties may take a turn for the worse. Normal readings are in the 95-to-100 range. Anything below 90 is low, and the person should head to the hospital.

Laurie Steelsmith, ND, LAc, licensed naturopathic physician and acupuncturist in private practice in Honolulu. She writes Bottom Line's "Natural Healing Secrets for Women" blog and is coauthor of *Natural Choices for Women's Health* and *Growing Younger Every Day.* DrSteelsmith.com

Trusted Health Resources

NIH.gov

Directory of hotlines for help with Alzheimer's disease, arthritis, burns, stroke and many other medical topics. From the National Institutes of Health. NIH.gov/health-information/health-info-lines

The Right Way to Measure Your Blood Oxygen

Timothy Connolly, MD, medical director of respiratory care services at Houston Methodist Hospital. HoustonMethodist.org

Pulse oximeters, which use infrared light to painlessly measure blood-oxygen levels, have become popular during the pandemic, since some COVID-19 sufferers experience dramatic—and dangerous— drops in blood oxygen without realizing it. *Here's what you need to know about using this device…*

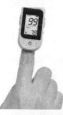

•**Pulse oximeters can't diagnose COVID-19.** A normal reading is not evidence that you don't have COVID-19. The majority of people who are infected never see any change in their blood-oxygen levels. But if you have been diagnosed with COVID-19, low blood-oxygen levels could be a sign that the infection has led to a potentially dangerous pneumonia and that you should contact your doctor to see if you should head to the hospital.

•**Some people have low blood-oxygen levels all the time.** That's especially common among people suffering from chronic lung diseases such as COPD, pulmonary fibrosis and congestive heart failure. If you consistently get readings below 94, mention it to your doctor and ask him/her what pulse oximeter reading you should consider problematic, especially following a COVID diagnosis.

To ensure an accurate reading, take your blood-oxygen levels at least a few times when you're healthy to establish your normal level. Before you put the device on your finger, spend a few minutes moving around to get your blood pumping…and warm up your hand, such as by putting it under your armpit—cold hands are a common cause of inaccurate, low readings. Which finger you use doesn't matter.

Warning: Fake fingernails or dark nail polish—black, purple or dark blue, in particular—interfere with accuracy. Remove these from at least one finger before using a pulse oximeter…or use the device on a toe.

•**A single low pulse oximeter reading doesn't necessarily mean a problem.** Take a few readings from both hands to rule out a bad reading before calling your doctor or visiting the emergency room—one hand might have better blood circulation than the other. If you can get one reading within normal range, there's no reason for concern—when pulse oximeters provide varied results, the highest reading is most likely to be a true reflection of your blood-oxygen levels.

How Often to Check?

I do not recommend that the general public routinely monitor their oxygen levels. Individuals with chronic health conditions that may involve low oxygen levels should discuss monitoring programs with their healthcare providers.

If an individual has been diagnosed with COVID-19 and is recovering at home, there is no perfect recipe for how often to check. Taking a reading every few hours while awake is reasonable. Make sure to check both at rest as well as during activity such as walking around. Furthermore, if new symptoms develop at any point such as chest pain or worsening cough, a quick oxygen check won't hurt.

Cannabis Use Before Surgery

Ian Holmen, MD, is an anesthesiology resident at University of Colorado School of Medicine, Aurora. His research was presented at the annual meeting of the American Society of Anesthesiologists.

If you use cannabis (including THC and/ or hemp-derived CBD products), tell your doctor and anesthesiologist before surgery. In a study of 118 patients undergoing surgery to repair leg fractures, regular cannabis users required more anesthesia, reported more pain and received 58 percent more daily opioids during their hospital stays. Regular cannabis use may affect pain tolerance.

Reduce Delirium Risk After Surgery

Background: Up to 65 percent of older adults develop postoperative delirium—sudden and severe confusion after undergoing surgery.

Recent finding: Patients who regularly exercised (walking, sports, cycling, dancing, etc.) five to six days a week before surgery were 73 percent less likely to develop postoperative delirium than those who were sedentary, according to a study of 132 men and women older than age 60 who underwent orthopedic surgery.

Even better: Those who were mentally active (for example, by knitting or doing crossword puzzles) had an 81 percent lower risk.

Susie S. Lee, MD, MS, assistant professor of anesthesiology, Albert Finstein College of Medicine, New York City.

Many Medicines Can Trigger Tinnitus

Joe Graedon, pharmacologist and cofounder of PeoplesPharmacy.com.

The condition of constant ringing in the ears can be caused by aspirin and other nonsteroidal anti-inflammatory drugs (NSAIDs), including *ibuprofen* and *naproxen*...by high doses of *acetaminophen* (Tylenol)...by some antibiotics...and by a long list of other drugs. Usually tinnitus results from long-term use, but it sometimes can occur after only a short time. It cannot be cured—treatments are designed to help people live with it. Counseling, cognitive behavioral therapy, stress reduction, sound-masking hearing aids, biofeedback therapy and other approaches may be useful.

Beware Websites Offering Online Prescriptions

Adriane Fugh-Berman, MD, professor of pharmacology and physiology at Georgetown University Medical Center, Washington, DC.

You've seen the commercials on TV, promising to fix all your intimate problems with a quick prescription—and without ever having to step foot in a doctor's office. But while skipping doctor's appointments might seem like a time- and money-saver, it also can be dangerous for your health.

These web-based companies work by promoting certain prescription drugs directly to consumers. Consumers can order those drugs without first obtaining prescriptions from their regular doctors. In some cases, the sites even push medications for uses for which they have not been approved, such as blood pressure medication to control anxiety.

These companies, which include Cove (for migraine medication), Hers (for women's health issues), Hims (for men's health issues), Kick (for anxiety drugs) and Roman (for hair loss, erectile dysfunction and other conditions), comply with health-care laws by offering an "online medical consultation," which consists of a simple online questionnaire that is reviewed by a doctor. These online doctor "visits" might be free or have a modest surcharge—often $5 to $15, but sometimes as much as $50—but their real business is selling prescription medications. And, no, they generally do not accept health insurance.

Dangers: There are many risks to the use of prescription medications without proper oversight, including serious side effects that may go unmonitored, improper dosing and dangerous interactions with other drugs or supplements that the patient is taking. Some of the conditions "fixed" by these sites actually are symptoms of more serious medical issues. If you don't see a doctor in person about your health problems, you won't learn about possible underlying causes.

It would be almost impossible for the doctors signing off on these prescriptions to uncover underlying conditions—they cannot physically examine patients…often have access only to patients' questionnaire answers, not their full medical histories… and frequently do not ask patients any follow-up questions.

What to do: Don't cut corners. See your regular doctor for diagnosis and treatment. If costs are a concern, save money not by skipping the doctor's appointment but by shopping around to find the drug for a low price at a website such as GoodRx.com or find out about patient assistance programs at NeedyMeds.org.

Managing Medication Side Effects

Ada D. Stewart, MD, president of the American Academy of Family Physicians, and a family physician with Cooperative Health in Columbia, South Carolina.

It's happened to most of us. We start taking a medication, hoping it will ease pain, wipe out an infection, or lower our blood pressure.

But soon, we have a new problem: a chronic stomach upset, headache, fatigue, or another malady.

It could be a coincidence—or it could be a medication side effect. The truth is that every medication, whether it's prescribed by a doctor or plucked off a drugstore shelf, comes with potential side effects. Even supplements can cause trouble. Some side effects, including severe allergic reactions, could be reasons for your doctor to tell you to stop taking a medication immediately. Others are so bothersome or potentially dangerous that they justify a switch to another medication or a dose adjustment. But many side effects can be managed—allowing you to keep taking a medication important to your health.

How do you sort it all out?

Start Smart

The first step should be a conversation with your doctor or pharmacist before you start taking a medication. Just taking that moment to ask what side effects are likely and what you should do if they arise could save you a lot of discomfort and worry. Your doctor should give you that information when they write a prescription, but if it doesn't happen, pipe up. Likewise, make it a habit to talk to your pharmacist. They are great sources for information on both prescription and nonprescription medications.

You can also read the literal fine print on the information sheets that come with prescription medications. But keep in mind that a long list of side effects may include some that are quite rare or not even caused by the medication. That's because drug manufacturers must report all the problems that were more common in people taking the medication than in those taking placebos in drug-approval studies. Not all of those symptoms were necessarily caused by the drug.

The information sheet will tell you which possible side effects should prompt a call to your doctor, and you should heed that advice. For example, if you are taking a statin, you should report any new muscle pain or weakness because it could be a sign of a serious condition that can lead to kidney failure. Your doctor can do lab tests to see if it's safe for you to keep taking the medication.

You should also talk to your doctor if you have side effects that makes you think about stopping your medication. You may find out that the side effect typically goes away after a while. That's true, for example, with the headaches and dizziness some people experience with blood pressure medications. Other side effects are more persistent, but often there are ways to manage them without discontinuing your medication.

Here are a few common side effects, experienced by people taking a variety of medications, and what you might do about them (keeping in mind that you should always talk with your doctor or pharmacist about your own specific symptoms).

Constipation

This is common with opioid pain killers, diuretics (water pills), antidepressants, antacids containing aluminum, and iron supplements.

Coping methods: The first thing to try is simply to drink more fluids. Most people need about eight glasses of water a day. Add fiber to your diet, especially from green leafy vegetables. If that doesn't work, try a daily fiber supplement or stool softener. It's usually best to avoid harsher laxatives, which can create new problems, including belly cramps and diarrhea.

Dry Mouth

Dry mouth is commonly experienced with antihistamines, antidepressants, and drugs known as anticholinergics, which are used to treat urinary incontinence, overactive bladder, chronic obstructive pulmonary disease (COPD), and Parkinson's disease.

Coping methods: Take frequent sips of water and stay well hydrated. Chew sugar-free gum or suck on sugar-free candies. If that's not enough, you can try over-the-counter mouth rinses, mouth moisturizers, and artificial saliva products. In some cases, your doctor may prescribe a medication to stimulate saliva flow.

Upset Stomach or Diarrhea

These side effects often occur with antibiotics, antacids containing magnesium, supplements containing magnesium, and drugs called proton pump inhibitors, which are used to treat ulcers and gastroesophageal reflux disease (GERD).

Coping methods: Be sure to follow any instructions about when and how to take your medication. Some will be gentler on your gut if you take them with food (eaten slowly and followed by a glass of water), but others must be taken on an empty stomach to be effective. If you suffer nausea after taking a medication in the morning, check with your doctor to see if you can take it at night. Don't treat yourself with an anti-diarrhea medication or probiotic supplements without checking with your doctor.

Sleepiness

Older antihistamines, some antidepressants, muscle relaxers, and narcotics can cause drowsiness.

Coping mechanisms: If you need to take the medication for just a short time, do not drive, operate heavy machinery, or perform other potentially hazardous tasks until you can stop the medication. If you need to take it for a long time, talk with your doctor about whether the sleepiness is likely to persist.

You can minimize the effects by avoiding alcohol and other substances that may add to your drowsiness. If it's a medication you can take once a day, try taking it at night. It may do double-duty as a sleep aid and affect you less during the day.

The Best General Policy

If a side effect is causing you distress, getting in the way of your normal routine or getting worse, don't stop taking it without telling your doctor. Instead, reach out and ask about coping strategies and treatment alternatives. You should also make sure that all of your health-care providers know about all the drugs and supplements you take. Your side effects may be linked to more than one medication or a different medication than the one you suspect.

Drugs That Alter Your Gut Microbiome

Anita Gupta, DO, PharmD, MPP, a pharmacist, board-certified anesthesiologist and former FDA adviser. She currently is a clinical professor at Rowan University School of Osteopathic Medicine in Stratford, New Jersey, and collaborates on design thinking in medicine at Princeton University's Keller Center. AnitaGupta.com

Antibiotics aren't the only culprit—these popular medications also can harm your overall health...

New discoveries just keep coming about the importance of the gut microbiome—that trillions-strong trove of microorganisms, including both "good" and "bad" bacteria, that live all along the gastrointestinal (GI) tract. We know that this healthy balance of bacteria not only keeps your digestion humming but also promotes overall good health.

However, certain popular medications, such as antibiotics, heartburn drugs known as proton pump inhibitors (PPIs) and oral nonsteroidal anti-inflammatory drugs (NSAIDs), have been called out for upsetting the gut microbiome's delicate balance. Now, new research is making the list even longer.

Latest development: In a study presented at a recent United European Gastroenterology Week conference, researchers from the University Medical Center Groningen in Groningen, the Netherlands, detailed additional categories of drugs that can alter the balance of good and bad bacteria.

Disrupting this balance can not only lead to troublesome side effects, such as diarrhea but also increase the risk for other health problems, such as obesity, and set the stage for serious disorders, including inflammatory bowel disease, type 2 diabetes and heart disease. Some of the same drugs have also been found to promote antibiotic resistance.

What you need to know to protect your gut microbiome...

Drugs That Change the Gut Microbiome

In addition to antibiotics, most notably, *tetracycline*...PPIs, such as *esomeprazole* (Nexium)...and oral NSAIDs, including *ibuprofen* (Motrin), the following drugs have recently been found to alter the gut microbiome...

•**Metformin.** This often is the first medication prescribed after a person is diagnosed with diabetes—or, in some cases, prediabetes.

What the recent research revealed: Use of metformin was associated with higher levels of *Escherichia coli* (E. coli) in the gut. Some strains of E. coli normally live in the gut and help with digestion, but an imbalance can be harmful, potentially leading to such problems as diarrhea and urinary tract infections.

Important: When a drug is prescribed for a specific condition—in this case, managing blood sugar—researchers noted that it's hard to tell if the gut microbiome changes are from the disease or the medication. If you're taking metformin, be sure to note any new symptoms or if the drug isn't working and contact your doctor immediately.

Alternatives to consider: A lifestyle plan focused on diet and exercise and, if medication is necessary, possibly a sulfonylurea drug, such as *glyburide* (Glynase)…or a heart-friendly diabetes drug such as the GLP-1 agonist *exenatide* (Byetta), based on a person's heart health.

• **Laxatives.** These are big gut disruptors, associated with higher, potentially harmful numbers of two types of bacteria—*Alistipes* and *Bacteroides*.

Alternatives to consider: Natural fiber products such as psyllium and, even better, eating more fiber-rich foods, such as fruit (including pears, figs, prunes and apples), beans, peas and lentils. Add them gradually to avoid bloating and gas as your GI tract adjusts to the change. Also, be sure to drink a lot of water.

• **Oral steroids.** People taking these drugs have high levels of the microbe *Methanobrevibacter smithii*, which has been associated with obesity, a known side effect of commonly used steroids such as prednisone, which is one of the steroids looked at in the study.

Alternatives to consider: There are few alternatives to oral steroids. Treatment could include IV infusions of anti-inflammatory medications, but this carries risks, such as bleeding.

• **Selective serotonin reuptake inhibitors (SSRIs).** Antidepressant medications, such as *sertraline* (Zoloft), *paroxetine* (Paxil) and *fluoxetine* (Prozac), led to increased numbers of the bacteria species *Eubacterium ramulus,* which lower the absorption of flavonoids, the powerful plant-based disease fighters.

Alternatives to consider: The SSRI *duloxetine* (Cymbalta)…a tricyclic antidepressant, such as *imipramine* (Tofranil)…or the herb St. John's wort—all of which may be less likely to increase harmful bacteria.

Worth noting: Gut microbiome changes were greater in people taking multiple medications, such as PPIs, laxatives and antibiotics. Also, people with GI conditions, including an inflammatory bowel disease or irritable bowel syndrome, which directly affect gut bacteria, may experience even greater side effects from the medications that they take.

Important: When discussing with your doctor the risk/benefit of any drug you're taking, consider whether you're using the medication temporarily or need it long-term for a serious disease such as Parkinson's disease or multiple sclerosis. Some medications are helpful, and there may not always be an effective alternative. Never stop taking a medication without consulting your doctor.

Diet: A Powerful Solution

Along with the findings on medications, the researchers reported on the effect of diet on the gut microbiome.

Using stool samples from healthy people and individuals with Crohn's disease, ulcerative colitis or irritable bowel syndrome, the researchers found that foods commonly included in a Mediterranean-style diet (such as vegetables, fruit, legumes, fish and nuts) were associated with higher levels of friendly, anti-inflammatory bacteria

Also: The findings confirmed that low-fat, fermented dairy foods, such as yogurt and kefir, increase good bacteria.

Popular Drugs That Can Lead to Eye Problems

Theresa M. Cooney, MD, associate professor of ophthalmology at University of Michigan Kellogg Eye Center in Ann Arbor and Michigan Medicine's Kellogg Eye Center in Milford. Her research has been published in *The British Journal of Ophthalmology* and other leading professional journals.

When your doctor writes you a prescription for, say, a blood pressure medication, a drug for prostate problems or even a nasal spray for your allergies, you probably don't think about your eyes. But you should.

Medications that treat a wide variety of medical conditions can lead to blurry vision, cataracts, glaucoma and even blindness.

To help protect yourself, you should get a baseline eye exam before taking one of the medications below and schedule follow-ups at the frequency recommended by your ophthalmologist (typically annually or every four to six months, depending on the drug).

Important: Be sure to report any eye-related side effects, including distorted vision or eye pain, to your ophthalmologist.

8 Widely Used Medications That Can Harm Your Eyes...

• *Hydroxychloroquine* **(Plaquenil).** This drug, which has been studied as a treatment for COVID-19, was originally used to treat malaria but now is widely prescribed for inflammatory diseases such as lupus and rheumatoid arthritis. When used for five or more years, hydroxychloroquine can cause damage to the macula, the central part of the retina where light-sensitive nerve cells are located in the back of your eye.

This side effect is insidious because symptoms usually don't occur until there's retinal damage. Even if the drug is discontinued, the impairment may be irreversible. In a recent study in *Arthritis & Rheumatology,* nearly 8 percent of lupus patients who had the highest average blood levels of hydroxychloroquine developed maculopathy, an eye disease that can result in complete loss of central vision.

Self-defense: Get a baseline eye exam by an ophthalmologist followed by annual exams...and exams as needed after five years of hydroxychloroquine use. The goal is to remain on a weight-based dosage of less than 5 mg/kg per day.

• **Steroid nasal sprays.** Like oral and topical corticosteroids, steroid nasal sprays, such as *fluticasone* (Flonase) and *triamcinolone* (Nasacort), can increase your risk for cataracts and glaucoma. Widely used for allergies, these sprays can be problematic because they are available in prescription and over-the-counter (OTC) versions—and both types carry similar risks for eye damage.

Self-defense: Do not use an OTC steroid nasal spray unless you are advised to do so by your physician. If your doctor does recommend it, try to use the medication sparingly and ask about alternative treatments that do not contain steroids. Daily nasal salt rinses can be safer and cause fewer side effects.

• *Digoxin* **(Lanoxin).** This common heart medication can cause blurry vision and halos around bright objects. These drug-induced visual changes usually mean that you have too much in your system, called digoxin toxicity.

Self-defense: If you experience eye symptoms while taking digoxin, ask your doctor to reduce the dosage. Do not make changes to your medication without consulting your physician.

• **Blood pressure medications.** When taking these drugs, blood pressure can sometimes fall too low, making you feel light-headed or dizzy. If blood pressure is consistently too low, damage to the optic nerve, called optic neuropathy, can occur due to a decreased blood supply.

Self-defense: It is often advised to take blood pressure drugs in the evening (see page 198), but if you suffer from the above symptoms, ask your physician if it is OK to avoid taking your blood pressure medication at night, when blood pressure naturally drops during sleep. Do not make any medication changes without first consulting your doctor.

• **Bisphosphonate drugs.** *Alendronate* (Fosamax) and other drugs within this class are used to help prevent osteoporosis. In rare cases, a bisphosphonate can cause inflammation of the eye called uveitis. Symptoms include eye pain, redness and blurry vision. The inflammation stops when you discontinue the drug, but always check first with your doctor.

Self-defense: If you have eye symptoms while taking a bisphosphonate, ask your physician about the osteoporosis drug *denosumab* (Prolia, Xgeva), which may be safer for your eyes.

• *Tamoxifen.* Many women with breast cancer are treated with this drug. It can be harmful to the retina, leading to distorted or blurry vision as well as cataracts. The effects are cumulative—risk for cataracts, for example, increases after using the medication for about five years.

Self-defense: If your doctor recommends this medication to reduce your risk for recurrent and/or worsening breast cancer, be sure to get yearly eye exams from an ophthalmologist.

• *Topiramate* (Topamax). Used to treat seizures and migraines, this drug can increase risk for a serious eye disease called angle-closure glaucoma. This condition results from a mainly inherited disorder, known as "narrow angle" eyes, that crowds the drainage structure of the eye, resulting in elevated eye pressure—a hallmark of glaucoma. Risk factors for narrow angle eyes include a family history of glaucoma and being farsighted. Only an eye exam, with a test called gonioscopy, can detect narrow angle eyes.

Symptoms of angle-closure glaucoma may include eye pain and headache, typically within a month of starting the drug. In severe cases, topiramate-induced angle-closure glaucoma triggers sudden blindness that is reversible if treated immediately.

Self-defense: If you develop eye symptoms while taking topiramate, see an ophthalmologist right away. If you are unable to be seen by your ophthalmologist, go to an emergency room with ophthalmologists on staff who can treat you urgently. Safer alternatives are available to treat migraines—consult your doctor for recommendations.

• *Tamsulosin* (Flomax). Commonly used by men with benign prostate enlargement, tamsulosin can weaken the iris, the colored part of the eye. When this occurs, a "floppy iris" can limit dilation during eye exams and eye surgery, which may prevent the pupil from staying open during cataract surgery. This can lead to complications, such as incomplete removal of the cataract and/or permanent damage to the iris with a permanent misshapen pupil. Women also may take tamsulosin for bladder problems and kidney stones.

Self-defense: If you have ever taken this drug, tell your eye doctor before having any eye surgery, including cataract removal. The effects of tamsulosin can linger for years. If the surgeon knows you've taken this drug, steps can be taken to greatly improve the odds of a successful eye surgery. There are alternatives to tamsulosin—discuss this with your doctor or urologist.

To Keep Your Eyes Healthy

The American Academy of Ophthalmology recommends a baseline eye exam for everyone at age 40—sooner if you have diabetes, high blood pressure or a family history of eye disease. Your ophthalmologist will tell you how often to repeat your eye exams.

Important: If you have glaucoma or narrow angle eyes (described earlier), always read drug warning labels, and don't take any prescription or OTC medication without checking with your doctor. Glaucoma warnings are found on many drugs, including those that treat urinary incontinence, acid reflux or nausea, depression and anxiety.

To find out if a drug you're taking has eye-related side effects, go to DailyMed.nlm. nih.gov, search the medication by name and click on "adverse reactions."

Problems After Gastric Bypass Surgery

Nick Calcaterra, DDS, Calcaterra Family Dentistry in Orange, Connecticut.

After undergoing gastric bypass surgery, you might begin to experience dental problems. What's going on?

Bariatric surgery causes a complex set of physiological changes to occur. As a result, patients may get more cavities, weakened tooth enamel, exposed dentin, temperature and pressure sensitivity, and a higher risk of chips and cracks.

Because bariatric surgery can change the way your body absorbs nutrients, it can lead to nutritional deficiencies that may affect your teeth. People with obesity are more likely to have gastroesophageal reflux disease (GERD), a condition that causes stomach acid to rise into the esophagus and mouth. Bariatric surgery does not always resolve this condition. Sleeve gastrectomy can even worsen it.

Eating irritating foods, eating too quickly, eating too much, or not chewing enough can trigger vomiting in people who have had a bariatric procedure. Like GERD, vomiting exposes the teeth to acid. Nearly all post-bariatric patients experience a decrease in the flow of saliva, an independent risk factor for tooth decay.

Many patients snack throughout the day and eat more sugary foods after the surgery than they did before.

To protect your teeth, first make sure your dentist knows about your surgery. He or she may recommend more frequent dental cleanings, use of a high-fluoride toothpaste such as PreviDent for daily brushing, or wearing customized trays at night. Chewing sugarless gum or candies can increase salivary flow, and acid reflux medications can reduce GERD. Follow your surgeon's guidelines to reduce the incidence of vomiting.

Key to Treating Chronic Digestive Conditions

Key to treating chronic digestive conditions such as Crohn's, celiac and irritable bowel syndrome (IBS): Testing for small intestine bacterial overgrowth (SIBO). Research shows that 50 percent to 84 percent of IBS patients have SIBO. Treating the bacterial overgrowth can eliminate symptoms. Diagnosis is via a 10-minute breath test (cheaper and more accurate than endoscopy), where the patient takes the carbohydrate lactulose. Those with SIBO show premature metabolism in the small intestine.

Typical treatment: Antibiotics and repopulating the gut with probiotics.

Niket Sonpal, MD, board-certified gastroenterologist and an assistant professor at Touro College of Osteopathic Medicine, New York City.

Are PPIs OK?

Jesse P. Houghton, MD, FACG, adjunct clinical assistant professor of internal medicine, The Ohio University Heritage College of Osteopathic Medicine, Athens, Ohio.

If you take *omeprazole* (Prilosec) for gastroesophageal reflux disease (GERD), you might be wondering...Is long-term use safe? *Here's one physician's view...*

Omeprazole is a proton pump inhibitor (PPI), a medication prescribed for heartburn, GERD, peptic ulcer disease, and Barrett's esophagus.

There has been a lot of bad press regarding these medications. Reported side effects include bone fracture, dementia, kidney problems, increased risk of Clostridium difficile infection, increased risk of gastroenteritis, pneumonia, and low levels of magnesium, calcium, and iron.

However, clinical trials have not proven that PPIs cause any of these conditions, only that they are associated with them. When other researchers looked more closely at these studies, they often found flaws with them and what we call confounding factors. For example, patients at increased risk for dementia may also be more likely to have conditions that required a PPI. Therefore, I consider these drugs to be safe, and if my patients find relief with them, I advise them to continue taking them.

Some patients may prefer a histamine-2 blocker medication, such as *famotidine* (Pepcid). The U.S. Food and Drug Administration requested that manufacturers withdraw another H2 blocker, *ranitidine* (Zantac), from the market because of contamination with a potential carcinogen called *N-Nitrosodimethylamine,* but the agency did not find the same contaminant in famotidine.

NSAIDs Do Not Make COVID-19 Worse

Anton Pottegård, PhD, is professor of pharmaco-epidemiology at University of Southern Denmark, Odense, and leader of a study published in *PLOS Medicine*.

Early in the pandemic, the health-care community was concerned that non-steroidal anti-inflammatory drugs such as *ibuprofen, naproxen* and *diclofenac* might cause worse outcomes for people infected with COVID-19. A new study of 9,000 patients shows no correlation between NSAID use in the period up to a positive COVID-19 test and increased hospitalization, ICU treatment or deaths.

A Natural Medicine Advocate at the Hospital Emergency Department

Andrew Rubman, ND, medical director of Southbury Clinic for Traditional Medicines in Southbury, Connecticut. SouthburyClinic.com

The patient: "James" is a retired architect who has been a patient of mine for years. When he called in complaining of chest pain and shortness of breath, I immediately sent him to a local hospital. He asked me to come and "run point" for him there—to be his advocate—a request I could not refuse.

What I did for him in hospital: James needed critical care evaluation and had me listed as "one of his PCP's" (primary care physician). In Connecticut, hospital privileges are not afforded to naturopathic doctors (my degree), nor does Medicare, a federal program, cover my services, so James retains a local MD as his "backup Medicare doc" to cover hospitalizations. I did meet James when he arrived at the hospital by ambulance and coordinated his intake in the emergency department. I told James that I would help him understand the intended procedures and emphasized that he needed to agree to everything that the doctors wanted to do for him.

How his care proceeded: As procedures progressed and findings were acquired, I discussed with James the good news that he showed no signs of a heart attack but that his heart showed a sensitivity to stress, which was the probable cause of what the hospitalist, cardiologist and I concurred was a "transient atrial fibrillation"—a temporary rapid heartbeat that is often associated with passing chest pain.

How we addressed his problem: James agreed with everyone that he should be on a single medication, a beta blocker, with a very light dose to quiet down the irritability of his heart. He also agreed to wear a 24-hour heart monitor and report back to cardiology for analysis. He was able to be discharged after only five hours in the hospital, a very short stay by today's standards.

The patient's progress: James has been "out of the shop" now for a few weeks and has started on a supportive regime with me including...

- **Co-enzyme Q10** to improve heart contraction and blood flow.

- **L-carnitine** to enhance the heart's ability to deal with times of lowered oxygen as occurs with fibrillation.

- **A special calcium, magnesium and potassium supplement** designed to target heart stability.

His cardiologist likes what he is seeing... the 24-hour heart monitor was clear...and he is even thinking of having James discontinue the beta blocker—albeit "not so fast." Ah, conventional medicine!

The Pros and Cons of Chiropractic Care

Laurie Steelsmith, ND, LAc, medical director of Steelsmith Natural Health Center in Honolulu, where she has a busy private practice, and is an associate clinical professor at Bastyr University. She is coauthor of three books—*Natural Choices for Women's Health, Great Sex, Naturally* and *Growing Younger Every Day.* DrSteelsmith.com

While I've long lived by the philosophy that our bodies are more than capable of healing themselves, I recently experienced a subluxation in my lower spine that left me pursuing outside measures. I wanted my life back—and fast— and so I booked a chiropractic session for the lumbar (L4) adjustment I knew I needed. (*To note*: The L4 is the second lowest vertebrae on your spine.) I went with a veteran chiropractor in the area who had not only 20 years of professional experience under his belt but also came highly recommended. His manipulations seemed sound; his bedside manner was great. But after dropping his entire body weight on the right side of my body in what's known as a high-velocity manipulation, I was left with a dislocated rib that, a month later, had yet to fully heal.

Which got me thinking about chiropractic care in general. How many of us walk blindly into an office and end up with zero results, or, worse (way worse), an injury? How many of us still believe that chiropractic care is the only way to approach musculoskeletal pain? And how many of us know what to do when an injury, such as the one I endured, happens?

My recent experience notwithstanding, I believe chiropractors can work wonders, offering incredible relief and lasting healing. But, as *U.S. News and World Report* asserts, chiropractic care is "not without risk." As with anything associated with your health, it's imperative for you to be proactive. With this in mind, here are the pros and cons of chiropractic care, the two primary techniques offered, how to choose a chiropractor—and the alternative forms of treatment you may want to seek out.

But first: What is chiropractic care, anyway?

Chiropractic care may seem like a modern invention but it dates back hundreds of years. The healing technique—which is derived from the Greek words "cheir" (or hand) and "praktos" (or done), and is translated as "done by hand"—is often attributed to Daniel David Palmer, an advocate of alternative medicine who maintained that he enabled a deaf man to hear again after conducting a spinal manipulation.

The lure of this persisted—and escalated. Today, the American Chiropractic Association reveals that there are more than 70,000 active chiropractors in the US. It's the third most popular form of health care, right below primary care and dentistry. Canada, Australia, Great Britain and Japan are just a few of the other countries who "recognize and regulate" chiropractic care as a means of health care, the ACA reports.

To the 62 percent of Americans who have had neck and back pain significant enough to obtain help from a health-care professional, the prevalence of chiropractic care may seem like a boon. And, indeed, it can be, in that a skilled chiropractor may be able to assist with everything from sciatica (a condition in which a pinched nerve in the lower spine results in leg pain and numbness) to headaches. Chiropractors live by the tenet that a host of health conditions—from back pain to achy wrists— result from misalignments in the body's underlying structure, including the skeleton and joints. To this end, they use different adjustments to properly align your frame.

The Two Main Types of Chiropractic Adjustments— and Their Risks and Rewards

While there are well over 100 types of adjustment techniques used by chiropractors, most rely on roughly 10, *Arizona Pain* reports. *Of these, the two most popular are the following...*

• **Spinal Manipulation (High-Velocity Low-Amplitude Thrust).** As *Spine Health/ Veritas* reports, "The most frequently used chiropractic technique, spinal manipulation, is the traditional high-velocity low-amplitude (HVLA) thrust." This manipulation, they also report, "often results in an audible 'pop,' as chiropractors use their hands to apply a controlled sudden force to a joint while the body is positioned in a specific way."

While the "pop" you may hear in this sort of adjustment shouldn't be cause for concern— it's gas being released by joints—a study in the *American Journal of Medicine* indicates that these manipulations are not risk-free. "Data from prospective studies suggest that minor, transient adverse events occur in approximately half of all patients receiving spinal manipulation," they report—which, while "minor," is a lot. Meanwhile, more serious injuries can occur, such as disk herniation, dislocated ribs (as in my case), blood flow issues and cauda equina syndrome—a rare condition, affecting the nerves in the lower spine, that requires urgent surgery. Notably, in 2016, the model Katie May died from a stroke believed to be induced by a chiropractor's neck manipulation—two years after the American Heart Association released a statement stating that getting your neck adjusted by a chiropractor or osteopathic doctor may be linked to an elevated risk for stroke.

On another note, while the use of HVLA has declined in recent years, the *Journal of Bodywork and Movement Therapies* contends that the risks of this technique—the same I recently received—"are low, provided patients are thoroughly assessed and treated by appropriately trained professionals." When it works, this manipulation can produce positive, though short-term, outcomes for people with low back pain, *The British Medical Journal* reports, but WebMD warns that people who have "osteoporosis, spinal cord compression, or inflammatory arthritis, or who take blood-thinning medications, should not undergo spinal manipulation."

• **Spinal Mobilization (Low-Force or Gentle Chiropractic Techniques).** The aim of spinal mobilization mirrors HVLA—to restore and improve function—but it utilizes a slower, gentler approach. Chiropractors, or patients themselves, may choose to use this milder method for a number of reasons, including osteoporosis, bone pathology, obesity, and sensitive nervous systems.

Several techniques are called upon under this version of chiropractic therapy, but one of the most popular is what's known as the activator method. Using a hand-held, spring-loaded, manual tool, which offers a low-force impulse, a chiropractor uses this technique to evaluate "leg length, perform muscle testing, and adjust the spine or extremity joints using the Activator tool," says Steven Yeomans, DC, FACO. Several studies have shown enhanced range of motion after spinal mobilization, as well as improved sciatica, low back pain, and shoulder movement. What's more, while this more moderate approach to treatment may result in tenderness and even some pain, it is overall safe, the National Institutes of Health reports.

What to Look for in a Chiropractor—and What to Do When You Enter Their Office

Don't go with the first chiropractor in your area that pops up on a Google search. Rather, ask your primary care physician or naturopathic doctor for a referral, or ask a trusted loved one to recommend someone—the caveat being, of course, that every personality and body is different and you shouldn't work with someone who feels intuitively wrong to you. Ensure they're licensed, and have obtained a Doctor of Chiropractic degree from a Council on Chiropractic Education (CCE)–accredited college. Find out how long they've been practicing, and learn whether they specialize in a certain field, such as sports medicine.

Once you've found someone you believe you can trust, be sure to tell them about the nuances of your condition and your physical form. For example, years of yoga, as well as completion of my yoga teacher training, has rendered me flexible, which makes me harder to adjust, and when not adjusted correctly could put me at an increased risk for spinal manipulation injuries. Other yogis—as well as dancers, springboard divers, gymnasts and athletes that require a great deal of flexibility to excel in their sport—may also have a difficult time with HVLA adjustments. People who have an inherited condition called Ehlers-Danlos Syndrome, which results in a defect in the production of collagen and hyperelastic joints, should also not receive HVLA manipulations. And those with osteoarthritis need to make their severity of pain clear to their chiropractor. If I had it to do over, I would have asked for the low-force adjustment with an activator instead of the high-velocity adjustment.

Further, be sure the chiropractor explores your different treatment options with you. Refrain from going with chiropractors who insist on "packages," or who don't take a holistic perspective of your health. Ask your chiropractor to tell you what they plan on doing during your session, and empower yourself to say no when something doesn't seem right. Acknowledge that soft tissues—your ligaments and tendons—are what pull bones out of place, and take a good amount of time to heal. (In other words, don't rush it.)

Should you suffer an injury at a chiropractor's hands, be aware—and persistent—about what you, as a patient, deserve. Seldom is legal action the solution (although this is case by case) but care and compassion are an enormous part of the overall healing process—and this should manifest in their foll0w-up treatment, communication and compensatory efforts.

Here's what happened in my follow-up after my injury…

I called the practitioner and told him that I thought my rib could be broken. He told me to follow up with a physician and let him know if it was. The MD thought it was dislocated. The chiropractic doctor that I had seen in the past—who he was subbing for—called me and had me in for a free follow-up visit. She did some deep tissue work and acupuncture and she called numerous times to check in afterwards. Meanwhile, the chiropractor who injured me didn't follow up until weeks later. I told his office manager he gets an F in follow-up. Of course, I know that I will never get the HVLA kind of adjustment again.

Alternative Forms of Treatment

If you're one of the 85 percent to 90 percent of people who suffer from back pain (or other musculoskeletal issues), do know that chiropractic care isn't the only form of treatment available.

• **Massage** may offer effective, albeit modest relief.

• **Acupuncture** can provide respite for those who have chronic back pain, osteoarthritis, and headaches, with minimal side effects (although keep in mind that the results of several studies on acupuncture have had limitations).

• **Osteopathic Manipulative Medicine** has demonstrated efficacy as well, with data showing that it can be not only valuable for treating chronic low back pain but also have results lasting up to a year.

• **Dozens of targeted exercises can alleviate pain,** while researchers show that exercising in general can increase blood flow to the lower back area, which can decrease stiffness and accelerate the healing process. Strengthening your body, and making it more resilient, can improve musculoskeletal complications as a whole.

• **Yoga** is as effective as standard physical therapy for treating moderate to severe chronic low back pain, reports the National Institutes of Health.

Chapter 8

HEART AND STROKE HEALTH FOR WOMEN

Heart Disease in Women: A New Paradigm for Prevention & Treatment

As women actresses walked the red carpet at the 2018 Golden Globe awards dressed in black in order to lend their support to the #metoo movement, I was touched by the notion that women are increasingly standing up for each other and coming together for the betterment of all women's lives. As this consolidation of purpose is occurring, I can't help thinking that we can do even more.

Shouldn't there be a movement as powerful and significant as #metoo that could shed light on the fact that more women continue to die from heart disease than from any other cause? And—that this is largely preventable?

I have been involved with the Go Red for Women movement, an initiative created by the American Heart Association, that has been educating and empowering women to take care of their hearts and their heart health for over a decade. Yet, after all this time, I still become infuriated every time I see the statistics that women are still under-diagnosed, still provided with less life-saving treatment, still referred less often for procedures that might actually result in more successful outcomes for them.

The bias—to treat women heart patients like men heart patients—still exists and has resulted in the deeply disturbing reality that when women get heart disease, they are more likely to die or to do much more poorly afterwards, including being more likely to suffer a subsequent heart attack.

#Metoo has sparked a lot of important, if difficult, feelings for all of us, both women and men. Many are finally coming to more fully understand the collective reality of women's lives. This is a very good thing, because if we viscerally understand #metoo, then maybe we have a chance to understand #GoRed in a similarly urgent way.

The bottom line across the board is that women are paying a deep price just for being women, whether that involves being the victim of sexual assault or misconduct...or being the victim of an antiquated health-care system that does not see and understand how heart disease manifests in and kills women.

Dr. Suzanne Steinbaum is a cardiologist who has devoted her career to the treatment of heart disease through early detection, education and prevention. She is author of *Dr. Suzanne Steinbaum's Heart Book: Every Woman's Guide to a Heart Healthy Life.* DrSuzanneSteinbaum.com

Just to give you an example, which sheds light of how pressing this issue is for all women, a study was done simulating male and female patients going into the emergency room. The actors recited the same script about their symptoms to the ER doctors. What happened? The male actors were admitted to the hospital with the diagnosis of possible heart attack; the women actors were sent home with the diagnosis of "anxiety." Really? With the same script and the identical symptoms, this is still happening? We are victims of stereotypes, misconceptions, callousness or, worse, disregard.

The good news is that the research is finally catching up to the reality. In the last decade, we have made significant progress in the study of women and heart disease. *The Guidelines for the Prevention of Cardiovascular Disease in Women*, last updated in 2011 by the American Heart Association, showed the profound impact of hypertension, diabetes and depression on women's hearts and explained that pregnancy can be a sort of "metabolic stress test" because there are many warning signs of future heart disease in pregnant women. That is progress.

There are also the *Guidelines for the Prevention of Stroke in Women*, issued jointly by the American Heart Association and the American Stroke Association in 2014, showing that pregnancy, hormones and migraines all contribute to the risk of stroke. Furthermore, the American Heart Association's Scientific Statement from 2016 about Acute Myocardial Infarction in Women sheds light on how women who have had a heart attack are less frequently referred to life-saving treatment and are less likely to be prescribed medication to prevent complications, improve quality of life and to prevent a second heart attack. (Note that "myocardial infarction" is the medical term for heart attack.)

This is all significant—then again, the change isn't happening fast enough. We are still seeing more women dying of heart disease, and heart disease still causes more deaths in women than all cancers combined.

I propose a new paradigm, not just in cardiology but across the board at all levels of women's health care, from OB-GYN to general practitioners. I propose that we focus on the preventive aspects of heart health and provide active and effective strategies for early detection of disease in every at-risk woman before there are clinical manifestations. And every at-risk woman is every woman.

I believe that in order to change these statistics, we have to change the culture, which, as we all know, is a slow process. In the meantime, women (and I include myself of course) need to take charge of their hearts and implement the preventive strategies that we already know. *These include…*

- **Understanding the huge impact of psychosocial risk factors on women's hearts,** and addressing problems like depression and social isolation.

- **More aggressive screening in women with any family history of heart disease,** but especially for those with multiple risk factors.

- **Taking seriously any hypertension or diabetes during pregnancy,** since heart disease in women typically begins with endothelial dysfunction, which can be detected in pregnancy. (Endothelial cells line the heart and blood vessels.)

- **Regularly ordering screening tests that look for plaque in the arteries,** such as coronary artery calcium scores or carotid dopplers, as part of annual health exams in women over 40. The goal must be to find disease before it starts.

I believe we can beat the number-one killer of all women if doctors decide to make a real commitment to diagnosing earlier in the disease process, and if women decide to implement lifestyle changes and, if necessary, medications to prevent progression. This goal is multi-fold and necessitates the participation of women patients, doctors, and the medical system in general. But that is the nature of real change. We all need to collaborate on this significant venture.

As women's needs are increasingly coming to the forefront of the cultural mindset, let's take advantage of this momentum to use the tools we have to become less reactive within the framework of the current paradigm of women's health care, and more proactive in caring for women's hearts in ways that are effective. It's time to set aside opinions, old ways, and traditional methods in favor of the current data, because so far, our opinions have been selling women short.

It is (literally!) heartbreaking that this is the current state of medicine. so let's change that. I think it has become clear that the time is now.

Heart Failure Is Deadlier for Women

Study by researchers at University of Bergen, Norway, published in *Nature Medicine*.

This is because only half the heart-failure cases in women are caused by a heart attack—which can be treated. The other half of female patients usually have heart failure because of long-term untreated high blood pressure, which leads to progressive stiffening of the heart muscle—a condition that cannot be effectively treated. Doctors need to be sure that high blood pressure in women is treated more aggressively and that other risk factors for heart failure, including obesity and type 2 diabetes, are identified and treated.

Heart Attack or Passing Panic?

Sam S. Torbati, MD, emergency medicine physician and medical director of the Ruth and Harry Roman Emergency Department at Cedars Sinai Hospital in Los Angeles.

You have a sudden onset of chest pain, trouble breathing, sweating, nausea, dizziness, and a terrifying sense of impending doom-the classic symptoms of a life-threatening heart attack. But they are also classic symptoms of a passing panic attack.

If you are having a heart attack, time is not on your side. The sooner you get to the emergency room (ER), the sooner they can get a stent in your heart and restore blood flow. Any delay means more damage to your heart muscle.

On the other hand, if it is just a panic attack, it will pass in about 20 minutes. You really don't want to have an ambulance show up at your house or drop you at the ER with all your symptoms gone as quickly as they came. What should you do?

When to Call 911

Unfortunately, there is not enough difference between symptoms of a heart attack and a panic attack for you to know what to do at home. Classic heart attack symptoms are new chest pain, shortness of breath, dizziness, and sweating. Classic heart attack chest pain is a sensation of tightness, squeezing, and heaviness, with pain radiating to your jaw or arm.

In a panic attack, chest pain may be less severe and limited to the front of your chest. However, many people with a heart attack have that type of chest pain, so the type of pain is not a reliable indicator.

Heart attack may be more likely if you are over age 40 and you have risk factors for a heart attack or you already know you have heart disease. Risk factors include a family history of heart attack, high blood pressure, diabetes, obesity, high cholesterol and smoking.

The worst mistake you can make is to assume you are having a panic attack and show up at the ER hours later or the next day still having chest pain. By this time the damage is done. You may still get a stent placed, but the consequences of your heart attack may affect the rest of your life. It would have been much wiser to show up at the ER without any symptoms. You might feel a bit embarrassed, but your ER doctor would rather see you embarrassed than debilitated.

Don't Drive Yourself

Don't ever take a chance on driving to the ER. Calling 911 gets you there safely and quickly. Traffic will move out of the way. Paramedics can start treatment in the ambulance, and they can call ahead to get the ER and the stent room ready for you. This is the only way to go when you might be having a heart attack.

When to Wait

A panic attack usually peaks and passes quickly. If you are under age 40 with no history of heart disease or risk factors, and you have a history of panic attacks in the past, you can try some relaxation techniques and deep breathing to see if your symptoms will pass. If they last longer than 20 to 30 minutes, call 911.

A panic attack is a sudden episode of intense fear when there is no apparent danger. Panic attacks are not life-threatening, even though they may feel that way. Symptoms peak within minutes. After the attack you may feel tired and drained. Even though you did not need to call 911, you should still call your doctor. Panic attacks tend to get worse and more frequent without treatment.

Beware of This Myth

You may have heard that panic attacks come out of the blue when you are resting, but a heart attack usually occurs during exercise. That is true for chest pain called angina, but not for a heart attack. Most heart attacks occur without exertion or warning.

Finally, remember that the difference between a heart attack and a panic attack is not like the difference between a sprained ankle and a broken ankle. As they say in the ER, time is muscle. If in doubt, call 911.

Mediterranean Diet Beats Low-Fat Diet for Heart Attack Patients

Study titled "Mediterranean Diet and Endothelial Function in Patients with Coronary Heart Disease: An Analysis of the CORDIOPREV Randomized Controlled Trial," by researchers at Maimonides Biomedical Research Institute of Cordoba, Spain, published in *PLOS Medicine*.

Diet is an important part of a heart-healthy lifestyle. Numerous studies show that both a low-fat diet and a Mediterranean diet can help people with high cholesterol or obesity reduce their risk of coronary heart disease (CHD) that leads to heart attacks. But which diet works better?

Recent development: A new study from researchers at Maimonides Biomedical Research Institute of Cordoba, Spain, is the first study to show that diet can reduce the risk of a second heart attack in people who have already had a CHD event. They compared a Mediterranean diet with a low-fat diet and found that both diets helped, but the Mediterranean diet worked significantly better.

When someone has CHD, the inner lining of the arteries that supply heart muscle is damaged. This lining is called the endothelium. Repair of the endothelium and endothelial function are the keys to recovery and prevention of another heart attack. The research team wanted to find out which type of diet worked better for reversing endothelial damage in heart attack patients.

Study details: Just over 800 patients with a heart attack history obtained endothelial testing that included measuring endothelium flexibility, called flow-mediated dilation (FMD). Better FMD means that there is better blood flow during stressful events or exercise. The researchers also measured the ability of the endothelium to produce cells that repair damage. These cells are called endothelial progenitor cells (EPCs).

The patients were then equally divided into two diet groups for one year. *One group was put on a low-fat diet and the other on a Mediterranean diet...*

•**The low-fat diet consisted of 12 percent monounsaturated fatty acids (MUFAs),** 28 percent fats and more than 55 percent carbohydrates. This diet featured a reduction in all fats, increased complex carbohydrates (like whole grains), low-fat dairy and avoidance of nuts, red meat, sweets and pastries.

•**The Mediterranean diet consisted of 22 percent MUFAs,** 35 percent fats and less than 50 percent carbohydrates. It featured virgin olive oil, fruits and vegetables, and three weekly servings of fish, legumes and nuts. Patients were asked to cut back on meats—especially red meat—and to avoid margarine, butter and added sugar.

Results: At the end of one year, endothelial testing was repeated. Patients on the Mediterranean diet had doubled their FMD and improved their EPCs by over 60 percent compared with the low-fat patients. The research team concluded that the Mediterranean diet led to better endothelial function and repair and that the Mediterranean diet can be recommended as the best diet for reducing risk in patients with CHD.

Omega-3 Supplements Really Do Help Prevent Heart Disease

Study titled "Effect of Omega-3 Dosage on Cardiovascular Outcomes: An Updated Meta-Analysis and Meta-Regression of Interventional Trials," by researchers at Global Organization for EPA and DHA Omega-3s, Salt Lake City, et al., published in *Mayo Clinic Proceedings.*

Cardiovascular disease (CVD) is the leading cause of death in the US. One prevention strategy has been the use of omega-3 supplements, which contain eicosapentaenoic acid (EPA) and docosahexaenoic acid (DHA), the two main fatty acids that have been shown to protect against CVD.

Studies of omega-3 supplements have not consistently shown positive results, but a new review of 40 clinical studies, published in *Mayo Clinic Proceedings*, gives strong evidence that there are substantial benefits. The 40 studies included more than 135,000 participants. This evidence includes and builds on a review from the Harvard School of Public Health that found similar benefits when reviewing the 13 largest omega-3 clinical trials in 2019.

The researchers examined randomized control trials, which means the studies compared benefits in people taking omega-3 supplements with people not taking supplements. The trials indicated that the percentage at which omega-3 reduced the risk of heart attack and deaths from heart attack and coronary events such as angina, stroke, heart failure and peripheral artery disease.

The review of these studies, when taken all together, found these key benefits for people taking omega-3 supplements versus people not taking the supplements...

•**A 35 percent reduced risk of death from heart attack.**

•**A 13 percent reduced risk of heart attack.**

•**A 10 percent reduced risk of coronary events.**

•**An overall decreased risk of death from coronary disease of 9 percent.**

The studies included omega-3 doses from 400 mg to 5,500 mg per day. As the amount of omega-3 used in the research increased, so did the benefits. Adding 1,000 mg per day decreased the risk of heart disease and heart attack. Heart attack risk went down by about 9 percent for each 1,000 mg added up to 5,500 mg.

Takeaway: Although omega-3 fatty acids can be obtained from eating fatty fish such as salmon, anchovies and sardines, very few people eat enough of this kind of seafood to get substantial benefits. The researchers recommend taking 1,000 mg to 2,000 mg of omega-3 supplements every day as an inexpensive and safe way to improve heart health and reduce heart disease risk.

Note: Because omega-3 supplements may increase bleeding risk, speak to your doctor before starting to use these supplements if you take a blood thinner.

New Way to Help Treat Heart Failure

Martin Gerdes, PhD, professor and chair of biomedical sciences at New York Institute of Technology College of Osteopathic Medicine, Old Westbury, New York, and leader of a study published in *Frontiers in Physiology.*

Low levels of thyroid hormone T3 in cardiac tissue are associated with heart failure, but doctors have hesitated to treat with T3 for fear of potential overdosing and causing harm. Research now shows the serum biomarker BNP, determined with a blood test, tracks with cardiac tissue T3 levels and can be used to guide T3 dosing to improve safety.

Hot Flashes and Night Sweats Are Linked to Heart Attack

Study by researchers at University of Queensland, Brisbane, Australia, published in *American Journal of Obstetrics and Gynecology.*

Data from 25 studies covering more than 500,000 women show that those who experience hot flashes and night sweats are at increased risk for nonfatal angina, heart attacks and stroke. For premenopausal women, the increased risk averages 40 percent, and for postmenopausal women, 70 percent—and the more severe the symptoms, the higher the risk. If you have either symptom, be sure you're closely monitoring your heart health.

How Hard Are You Exercising?

Barry A. Franklin, PhD, director of Preventive Cardiology/Cardiac Rehabilitation at Beaumont Health in Royal Oak, Michigan. He is past president of the American Association of Cardiovascular and Pulmonary Rehabilitation and a member of the *Bottom Line Health* advisory board.

When using cardiovascular equipment at the gym or at home, you may have seen a measurement called METs on the dashboard. The term metabolic equivalents, or METs, is a representation of the oxygen requirements of an activity.

One MET equals the amount of oxygen the body uses at sitting rest, so if you exercise at three times your resting energy expenditure, you are working at 3 METs.

Not only do METs measure the work needed for an activity, but they are also used to measure a person's exercise capacity—a predictor of survival and longevity. Exercise professionals and physicians use METs data to classify fitness as poor, average, or good, and to prescribe activities that are safe and effective.

Measuring METs Capacity

The most accurate way to measure exercise capacity is to have a progressive treadmill test. As you walk or run on a treadmill, the medical professional who is administering the test will increase the speed until you reach your highest possible workload while measuring your oxygen consumpton. The longer you exercise on the treadmill, the higher your MET capacity.

The average healthy young to middle-aged adult has an aerobic fitness level of 8 to 12 METs, while an elite endurance athlete's may be as high as 25 METs. Heart failure patients and those who are elderly or morbidly obese could have fitness levels as low as 2 to 4 METs.

A good fitness capacity is based on your sex and age (table 1).

Table 1. Good Exercise Capacity		
Age	Sex	Net Capacity
45 years	Men	12
	Women	8
55 years	Men	10
	Women	7
65 years	Men	9
	Women	6
75 years	Men	8
	Women	5

Boost METs to Reduce Risk

There's good reason to work to increase your MET capacity: New studies indicate that for each MET increase, patients reduce their likelihood of dying from a heart attack by about 15 percent. Thus, an inactive person who gradually increases his/her MET capacity from 5 to 8 could reduce the risk of dying from heart disease by approximately 45 percent.

To attain a good METs exercise capacity, you should exercise at an appropriate METs intensity (table 2).

Table 2. Goal Exercise Intensity		
Age	Sex	Goal Exercise METs
40–49 years	Men	7–9
	Women	5–7
50–59 years	Men	6–8
	Women	5–6
60–69 years	Men	5–7
	Women	4–5
70–79 years	Men	5–6
	Women	3.5–4.5

If you are exercising below these intensities, you should strive over the next three to 12 months to gradually increase your MET exercise training intensities. If you develop symptoms such as chest pain/pressure, lightheadedness, fast or irregular heart rate, or unusual shortness of breath as you increase your exercise intensity, stop exercising and seek medical evaluation.

Estimating METs

If you are walking on a treadmill without a METs counter, you can estimate your energy expenditure with a simple calculation. Walking on a flat surface at 2 mph uses about 2 METs. Each 3.5 percent grade increase adds another MET to the energy expenditure. Walking at 3 mph uses about 3 METs. At that speed, each 2.5 percent increase in treadmill grade adds another MET. So walking at a pace of 3 mph on a 7.5 percent grade would be about 6 METs.

You can also estimate METs by measuring your heart rate. In general, each 10 beat-per-minute (bpm) increase in heart rate corresponds to an additional MET in energy expenditure.

Conclusions

For previously inactive adults, moderate-to-vigorous physical activity, which corresponds to 3 or more METs, may increase your MET capacity and decrease your risk of future cardiac events. By gradually achieving your goal training intensity, you'll attain a good level of aerobic fitness and likely experience the maximal survival benefit of exercise.

Silent Heart Attacks

Rekha Mankad, MD, a noninvasive cardiologist. She is the director of the women's heart clinic and the director of the cardio-rheumatology clinic at Mayo Clinic in Rochester, Minnesota.

When we think of heart attacks, a common image comes to mind: a person clutching his or her chest, doubled over in pain. But it's quite possible to have a heart attack without chest pain, especially if you're a woman. In fact, it's possible to have no symptoms at all.

The lack of symptoms doesn't mean these events are insignificant, though. They can cause long-lasting damage that goes untreated and increases the risk for a second—and potentially fatal—cardiovascular event.

How Can It Be Silent?

Often, people learn they experienced a silent heart attack only when imaging shows evidence of previous heart damage. While some people recall no symptoms at all, others look back and recognize that they felt something—just not a classic heart attack symptom.

They may have felt indigestion, a pulled chest muscle, or flu symptoms. They may have had sweating, lightheadedness, nausea, or shortness of breath. Or they may have had very mild classic symptoms—chest pain and pressure, or pain in the arm, neck or jaw—that didn't feel severe enough to cause alarm.

Gender Differences in Silent Heart Attacks

Women more commonly experience these kinds of nontraditional symptoms, possibly because they are more likely to have blockages in the smaller arteries that supply blood to the heart, in addition to the main arteries.

But while the symptoms of a silent heart attack may be different, the underlying process is the same: Blood flow to the heart is blocked, potentially damaging the heart muscle.

Risk Factors

The risk factors for a silent heart attack are no different from a traditional one...

- **Advanced age.** Men ages 45 or older and women ages 55 or older are more likely to have a heart attack.

- **Excess weight.** Even being somewhat overweight is a risk factor, and the risk rises along with body mass index.

- **High blood pressure.** The excess strain from high blood pressure causes the coronary arteries to stiffen and narrow.

- **High cholesterol.** Strive to keep your total cholesterol under 200 milligrams per deciliter (mg/dL) and your LDL ("bad") cholesterol under 100 mg/dL. If you have coronary artery disease, aim for less than 70 mg/dL.

- **Lack of exercise.** You need 150 minutes per week of moderate-intensity aerobic activity or 75 minutes per week of vigorous aerobic activity, or a combination of both.

- **Tobacco use**

- **Family history of heart disease.** This is a significant risk factor, but it does not increase the likelihood of symptoms being vague or silent.

- **People with diabetes** may have a higher likelihood of silent events, particularly if they also have neuropathy.

Future Risk

A person who has experienced a silent heart attack has an elevated risk of having another attack. Because they didn't know they had an event, they had no medical intervention to limit damage to the heart. Further, there are no clues to guide ongoing monitoring. If you are concerned that you may have had a silent heart attack, talk to your doctor about your symptoms to see if you should undergo testing.

Whether that testing reveals a prior heart attack or not, you can immediately begin to lower your risk of a first or subsequent event by following a heart-healthy diet, reducing stress, exercising, losing weight, and managing other conditions like diabetes and high blood pressure.

If you are concerned that you may have had a silent heart attack, talk to your doctor. A medical professional can review your symptoms and health history, and a physical exam can help determine if you need more tests.

A Novel Way to Predict Heart Failure Prognosis

The study titled "Prognostic Value of Pupil Area for All-Cause Mortality in Patients with Heart Failure," by researchers at Kitasato University Hospital, Kanagawa, Japan. The research was published in *ESC Heart Failure*, a journal of the European Society of Cardiology.

For many people with heart failure, the condition can be devastating. Almost half of all those admitted to a hospital for this health problem die within one year.

In the face of such a dire prognosis, people with heart failure—especially those who are at high risk for hospital admission or death from the condition—could benefit from starting cardiac rehabilitation or trying other therapies sooner. The challenge comes in identifying those high risk cases.

It's been shown that when heart failure worsens, it typically disrupts the body's autonomic nervous system, which regulates such functions as heart rate, digestion and respiration. This is usually identified by changes in heart rate, but this method is not reliable in patients with atrial fibrillation, a heart rhythm disorder that occurs in 20 percent to 50 percent of people with heart failure.

In an effort to find another way of detecting worsening heart failure, researchers at Kitasato University Hospital in Kanagawa, Japan, decided to investigate whether pupil size—a method that has been used to evaluate autonomic function in people with Parkinson's disease and diabetes. Because the autonomic nervous system also controls how the pupils of the eyes open and close, the researchers theorized that pupil size could be a predictor of heart failure severity.

Study details: To test this approach, researchers measured the pupil size of 870 patients (average age 67) who were hospitalized for heart failure. To prevent any changes that could occur if the patients' pupils reacted to light or movement, the study participants wore goggles that blocked such effects.

After five minutes, the patients' pupils were photographed inside the goggles, and the pupils were rated as above or below average size. With this data, the researchers set out to analyze whether pupil size would predict readmission to the hospital and/or death from heart failure.

Research findings: After about two years, 131 of the study participants had died and 328 had to be readmitted to the hospital for heart failure. After comparing the patients' pupil sizes to their outcomes, the researchers discovered that those with larger pupils had an 18 percent lower risk of being readmitted to the hospital for heart failure and a 28 percent lower risk of dying from any cause. These results were adjusted for factors that could affect the progression of heart failure, such as body mass index (BMI) and kidney function.

Takeaway: Based on these findings, which were published in the European Society of Cardiology journal *ESC Heart Failure,* the investigators concluded that pupil size is a convenient and effective way to predict heart failure risk.

"Pupil area can be obtained rapidly, easily and non-invasively," explained study author Kohei Nozaki, PT, MSc, of Kitasato University Hospital's department of rehabilitation. "Our study indicates that it could be used in daily clinical practice to predict prognosis in patients with heart failure, including those who also have atrial fibrillation."

With this information, doctors could then be sure to urge heart failure patients with small pupils to get more physical activity and possibly undergo cardiac rehabilitation to help improve their heart condition, according to the researchers.

Note: Pupil size measurement for heart failure should not be used in individuals with severe retinopathy or other eye diseases.

Carpal Tunnel Syndrome: A Harbinger of Heart Failure?

Brett W. Sperry, MD, a cardiologist and director of the Cardiac Amyloidosis Program at Saint Luke's Mid America Heart Institute and an assistant professor of medicine at the University of Missouri-Kansas City.

When wrist pain and numbness strike both hands, a process that also affects the heart may be to blame.

What do concert pianists and construction workers have in common? The same thing that typists, surgeons and cake decorators do: a high incidence of carpal tunnel syndrome (CTS).

The carpal tunnel is a channel formed by eight small bones on three sides and a ligament on the fourth. The median nerve runs through the tunnel, along with nine tendons that help move the fingers. When the tunnel is narrowed or the tissues around the tendons (called the synovium) swell, pressure on the nerve can result in pain, tingling and numbness. That swelling is most often caused by repetitive hand motions or illnesses such as diabetes and hypertension.

For about 10 percent of patients, however, CTS has a different cause, one that makes it a harbinger of heart failure. That's because the CTS symptoms in these patients, which always appear in both wrists, come from a condition called amyloidosis.

Understanding Amyloidosis

Proteins are made of amino acids that are strung together like a strand of pearls. To function properly, that strand must form into a 3D structure. About 30 different proteins can fold incorrectly, creating insoluble clusters (amyloid fibrils) that can build up in different parts of the body. Amyloidosis can be localized to a single area or widespread, and it can affect any major organ.

When a protein called transthyretin misfolds and builds up in the heart, it leads to a condition that can stiffen the heart and ultimately lead to heart failure (transthyretin amyloid cardiomyopathy). This same misfolded protein has been found in biopsies of people undergoing surgery for bilateral CTS—typically five to 10 years before the appearance of heart failure symptoms.

Early Warning System

Early warning of amyloidosis can be life-changing. Once amyloid deposits are in the heart, it's extremely difficult to get rid of them, but there are several effective ways to prevent them from forming. When patients undergo surgical treatment for bilateral CTS, they can start this process by asking the surgeon to take a biopsy and send it to a pathologist to look for amyloid deposits. If there's evidence of misfolded proteins, an amyloidosis specialist can begin preventive care and monitor the heart. The sooner this process begins, the better the results.

In the early stages of prevention, simple, low-cost, over-the-counter products can be quite valuable.

• **Green-tea extract.** Epigallocatechin-3-gallate (EGCG), a catechin in green tea, helps prevent the formation of amyloid fibrils. The recommended dosage is 600 to 800 milligrams (mg) per day. Don't take any more than that, though. High doses can lead to liver issues.

• **Curcumin** can also disrupt fibril development, at least in test-tube and animal studies. Curcumin is one exception to the advice to get your nutrients from foods before supplements. Although the spice turmeric contains curcumin, the concentration isn't high enough to provide therapeutic benefits.

Curcumin is poorly absorbed in the gastrointestinal tract, but products that use nanoparticle formulations or contain fat or black pepper may increase absorption. Ask your physician for a product recommendation.

• ***Diflunisal*** is a prescription nonsteroidal anti-inflammatory drug that may prevent misfolding proteins from forming amyloid deposits in the heart.

• *Tafamidis* (Vyndaqel, Vyndamax) is a newly approved drug that is indicated for people who already have heart disease. While the aforementioned medications have some evidence of benefit in small studies, tafamidis has shown strong improvements in duration and quality of life and has no side effects, but it's expensive.

Other Signals

Two other orthopedic conditions can be associated with amyloidosis too. About 20 percent of patients undergoing surgery for spinal stenosis have amyloid deposits in the spinal canal, so a biopsy specimen at the time of spinal stenosis surgery could be a good idea.

Another condition that raises a red flag is a bicep tendon rupture. In this condition, when a person flexes the bicep muscle, there may be a small bulge near the elbow. That bulge is caused by the muscle curling back. This is very rare, so if I see it, especially in a person over age 60, I suspect amyloidosis.

The Takeaway

There are three types of cardiac amyloidosis: One comes from aging and is much more common in men over age 70. A second, hereditary form strikes younger, black men and women, usually in their 60s and 70s. A third type is related to a bone marrow problem and can be more rapidly progressive, though it is rarer.

If you are under 50 and have CTS in only one hand, it does not suggest amyloidosis. Bilateral CTS doesn't mean you have amyloidosis, but if you have a scheduled surgery for bilateral symptoms (or spinal stenosis), request a biopsy. It costs about $30 and can provide valuable information.

If you do test positive for amyloidosis, look for an amyloidosis specialty center for care. Because this condition can affect nearly every major organ, a dedicated center staffed by a variety of specialists can offer the most comprehensive care. If you do not live near a center or are unable to travel to one, then work with a cardiologist and your physician.

Busting the Cholesterol Myth

Stephen Sinatra, MD, an integrative cardiologist and the founder of the New England Heart Center in Manchester, Connecticut. Dr. Sinatra is the author of *The Great Cholesterol Myth* and *Reversing Heart Disease.* HealthyDirections.com/dr-stephen-sinatra

Every year, doctors in America write 240 million prescriptions for statins, such as *simvastatin* (Zocor) or *atorvastatin* (Lipitor), to lower "bad" LDL cholesterol and reduce the risk of heart disease.

But here's a little-known fact: Although statins lower LDL, as advertised, for most people, that reduction doesn't translate to a lower risk of heart disease.

Looking at the Data

In new research published in the *British Medical Journal* (BMJ Evidence-Based Medicine), three cardiologists analyzed the results of 35 studies on lowering LDL cholesterol with statins or other cholesterol medications. Nearly half of the studies failed to show that taking statins or other LDL-lowering medications reduced the risk of developing cardiovascular disease (CVD), and 75 percent showed no reduction in rates of death from heart disease.

What's more, there was no consistent correlation between lowering LDL and cardiovascular protection. In many of the studies, large drops in LDL levels produced no reduction in heart attacks, strokes, or deaths from CVD. In others, failure to significantly decrease LDL did not lead to more heart attacks, strokes, and deaths from CVD. In fact, in 14 of the 35 studies, a failure to decrease LDL reduced the risk for heart attacks and strokes. The researchers noted that, in the United States, cardiovascular deaths are increasing despite the rising use of statins and lower levels of cholesterol overall.

The only proven and reliable benefit of statins for CVD is for men under 75 with heart disease or a previous heart attack or stroke. Statins work in this case by thinning the blood and reducing inflammation, not by lowering LDL.

Questioning the Prevailing Theory

The study authors concluded that using statins and other drugs to reduce the risk of CVD is a failed strategy.

They wrote: "Considering that dozens of randomly controlled trials of LDL-cholesterol reduction have failed to demonstrate a consistent benefit, we should question the validity of this theory. In most fields of science, the existence of contradictory evidence usually leads to a paradigm shift or modification of the theory in question, but in this case, the contradictory evidence has been largely ignored, simply because it doesn't fit the prevailing paradigm."

How Did the Experts Get It So Wrong?

The main factor behind the persistence of the prevailing paradigm is profit—for the food industry and for drug companies. In the 1960s, the dietary causes of heart disease were still a matter of debate—with many scientists asserting that cholesterol-raising saturated fat found in meat, dairy, and eggs was the culprit, and others pointing to artery-damaging sugar. The debate was largely decided by a seemingly definitive 1967 study conducted by Harvard scientists and published in the prestigious *New England Journal of Medicine*. It reviewed the link between sugar and heart disease and concluded sugar did not play a role in heart disease, and that the only dietary factors of importance were fat and cholesterol.

But recent investigative research revealed that the study was secretly funded, designed, and directed by the Sugar Research Foundation—a trade group dedicated to the profitability of sugar.

LDL-lowering statins came on the market in the 1990s and were heavily promoted by drug companies as the answer to heart disease. However, the results of statin-supported research were consistently exaggerated by those same drug companies and the scientists they funded—as demonstrated by the new *BMJ* study.

The Real Risk

What is significantly more worrisome than high cholesterol is insulin resistance. This condition doesn't account for 100 percent of heart disease, but it predicts CVD better than any other variable studied. Research by the late Gerald Reaven, MD, of Stanford University, showed that insulin resistance dramatically increases the risk of heart disease. Other researchers found that insulin resistance was the only significant predictor of a second heart attack, while LDL cholesterol had no predictive value.

A hormone manufactured by the pancreas, insulin ushers blood sugar (glucose) out of the bloodstream and into muscle cells, where it is used for energy. But in an estimated 50 percent of Americans, insulin doesn't work that way. That's because excessive stress and a daily diet rich in refined carbohydrates trigger the pancreas to pump out unnatural amounts of insulin—so much that the muscle cells begin to resist the hormone. Instead, the glucose is stored in fat cells. Those cells release a flood of inflammatory chemicals—and inflammation is one of the major causes of CVD. It makes arteries vulnerable to artery-clogging plaque. Insulin resistance also causes high blood pressure; increases triglycerides; lowers heart-protective HDL cholesterol; and increases small, dense LDL particles. This subtype of LDL is dangerous because—in contrast to large, fluffy LDL particles—it can burrow into arteries.

Are You Insulin Resistant?

Fortunately, there is a simple way to figure out if you're insulin resistant: Measure your waist. Men with waist sizes of 40 inches or more are almost certainly insulin resistant, as are women with waist sizes of 35 inches or more. However, about one in 10 people with insulin resistance are slim—their sugar-generated fat isn't right under their skin, but invisibly wrapped around their abdominal organs, a form of fat scientists call visceral.

Another giveaway is the ratio of your triglycerides divided by your HDL. An ideal ratio is 2 or under.

Addressing Insulin Resistance

The best way to eliminate insulin resistance is by changing your diet.

- **Sugar is the biggest threat** to your heart. Cut out soda, processed cereals, pasta, bread, cakes, candies, pastries, and doughnuts.

- **Avoid trans fats,** a highly inflammatory form of fat that has been removed from much of the food supply, but may still be found in non-dairy creamers, margarine, ramen noodles, energy bars, and fast food

- **Don't eat processed meats,** such as salami, sausages, hot dogs, luncheon meats, and bacon. They contribute to inflammation and heart disease.

- **Cut back on omega-6 fats,** which are found in vegetable oils such as corn, canola, and soybean. They're also pro-inflammatory.

Eat This Instead

Research shows the higher the average daily consumption of vegetables and fruits, the lower the chances of developing CVD.

- **Eat five to nine half-cup servings of vegetables and fruits each day.** The most protective are green, leafy veggies, such as spinach and kale, and cruciferous veggies, such as cauliflower and broccoli. Berries and cherries are also loaded with anti-inflammatory compounds.

- **Wild Alaskan salmon, sardines, and anchovies** are loaded with anti-inflammatory omega-3 fatty acids and are low in mercury. Eat these at least twice a week.

- **Eat more nuts.** Five large studies have found a consistent 30 to 50 percent lower risk of heart disease or heart attacks linked to eating nuts several times a week.

- **Eat more beans.** One study found that one serving of beans daily lowered the risk of a heart attack by 38 percent. Eat a serving of beans or lentils at least four times a week.

- **Favor dark chocolate for dessert.** It's rich in flavanols, a heart-protecting antioxidant. Research has found that regular chocolate consumption reduces CVD by 37 percent. Look for a product with no less than 60 percent cocoa. Eat one or two squares four to six days a week.

- **Use only olive oil.** Dozens of studies show it's one of the healthiest fats for the heart.

- **Use more garlic.** It lowers blood pressure and thins the blood. In one study, people who used garlic powder regularly for four years had a 2.6 percent regression in arterial plaque—while people who used a placebo powder had a 15.6 percent increase.

Supplement Superstars

I've used these two science-backed nutritional supplements (and many others) in my practice for decades—and they're superb for protecting and restoring the health of the heart.

- **Coenzyme Q10 (CoQ10) helps create cellular energy from nutritional fuel.** And the heart—which beats more than 100,000 times a day—is dependent on the energy-generating power of CoQ10. It also helps protect against the side effects of energy-depleting statins.

Recommended dose: At least 100 milligrams (mg), twice a day.

- **The mineral magnesium can help prevent and manage both insulin resistance and high blood pressure.** It also helps stop the calcification that underlies clogged arteries.

Recommended dose: 400 mg daily. (Magnesium supplementation is not recommended for anyone with kidney disease.)

Stress Is Hard on Your Heart

Chronic stress is a major instigator of inflammation and high blood pressure and weakens your heart. Use the relaxation response exercise every day for 10 to 20 minutes to decrease heart rate, lower blood pressure, slow breath, and relax the muscles. Sit quietly in a comfortable position with your eyes closed. Deeply relax all your muscles, beginning at your feet and progressing up to your face. Breathe through your nose. Become aware of your breathing. As you breathe out, say one word silently to yourself.

3 Questions to Ask Before You Start Statins: Personalizing Your Risk Profile

Jamal S. Rana, MD, PhD, award-winning heart researcher, preventive cardiologist and chief of cardiology at Kaiser Permanente's Oakland Medical Center and president-elect of American College of Cardiology, California Chapter. He has published more than 125 peer-reviewed studies in scientific journals and made numerous national and international presentations.

Cardiovascular disease remains the leading cause of death in the US. To help combat unnecessary deaths, national guidelines by the American College of Cardiology/American Heart Association (ACC/AHA) suggest that in addition to a healthy lifestyle, people at risk should talk with their doctors about taking cholesterol-lowering statin drugs. Research shows that these drugs help stop buildup of plaque in arteries, a main risk factor for heart attack and stroke, and may stabilize already built-up plaque.

Although statins were initially approved to reduce high cholesterol levels, the definition of "high cholesterol" has changed through the years, as has the consideration of statins for other related health concerns. In addition to those with established heart disease, statins now are recommended for people

ages 20 to 75 with an LDL-cholesterol level of 190 mg/dL or higher...patients with diabetes ages 40 to 75 (have a risk-benefit discussion with your doctor if you're younger or older)...or with a 10-year calculated risk for heart disease of 7.5 percent or higher (more on this factor below). Some of these criteria are clear-cut, but others are more of a gray area. Here's what you need to know before you say "yes" to a statin prescription.

Two Types of Prevention

When considering statins to prevent heart attack and stroke, there really are two types of prevention. Primary prevention relates to people who have never had either of these events and are trying to prevent one from happening in the first place. Secondary prevention relates to people who already have had a stroke or heart attack, which puts them at high risk for a second one in the future.

There's no controversy regarding the benefits of statins for secondary prevention. All people who have had a heart attack or stroke, in addition to striving for a healthy lifestyle with exercise and a healthy diet, should be taking statins. For these patients, it is a lifelong commitment as they remain at high risk for a future event.

The statin decision is more nuanced when it comes to primary prevention. The guidelines recommend them for a broader range of people than ever before due to our better understanding of risk enhancers. But the value of statins has to be evaluated in the context of your personal health history and weighed against the concern surrounding side effects, such as muscle pain or weakness, headaches and dizziness. A careful evaluation of the combined answers to three key questions can help clarify whether these statins are right for you.

The 3 Questions

1. What is my ASCVD Risk Score? At the heart of the widening scope of who should take statins is the Atherosclerotic Cardiovascular Disease (ASCVD) Risk Estimator, created by the ACC/AHA and used by doctors to evaluate their patients. You can take it online at https://bit.ly/2TBlmpC.

After plugging in information—such as cholesterol (total, HDL and LDL), blood pressure, age, race, gender and whether you have diabetes or are or were a smoker—the tool rates your 10-year risk of having a heart attack or stroke. You'll note that there are no questions about diet or exercise in this questionnaire. If you are exercising regularly and eating well, your blood pressure and cholesterol levels would reflect the impact of those healthful behaviors.

Results fall into four categories…

Low: Below 5 percent

Borderline: 5 percent to 7.4 percent

Intermediate: 7.5 percent to 19.9 percent

High: 20 percent or greater.

Interpreting the low and high scores is very easy. If you have a low score, statins generally are not recommended—you can feel reassured that you're in good shape. If you're at high risk, many doctors recommend starting a statin—its preventive benefits have been proven. You may be able to lower the dose over time by making healthy lifestyle changes.

If your score is borderline or intermediate, the statin decision is more nuanced. Also, no risk calculators are perfect. In research conducted at Kaiser Permanente, we found that there was risk overestimation among adults without diabetes between ages 40 and 75, which could lead to unnecessary statin therapy. In fact, at Kaiser Permanente, we are in the process of implementing our own calculator that will address this problem. But for now, the ACC/AHA ASCVD Risk Estimator is a useful tool.

Benefits to knowing your ASCVD Risk Estimator score: Your result can trigger a useful discussion with your doctor and encourage you to look at lifestyle habits that could help reduce your risk for heart disease. A healthy lifestyle remains the cornerstone of prevention of heart disease and stroke. Rather than starting statins, you might try to lower your risk through improved diet, exercise and, if you smoke, quitting.

2. Do I have any "risk enhancers"? *These factors increase your heart attack and stroke risk but currently are not part of the ASCVD Risk Estimator questionnaire…*

• **Having a family history of premature heart disease**—before age 55 in men…age 65 in women

• **Having LDL cholesterol of more than 160 mg/dL**

• **Having metabolic syndrome,** a group of risk factors that include high triglyceride levels, high blood sugar, high blood pressure and excessive body fat around the waist

• **Having chronic kidney disease**

• **Having an inflammatory condition** such as rheumatoid arthritis, psoriasis or HIV/AIDS

• **Menopause before age 40**

• **Having had a pregnancy-related circulatory condition such as preeclampsia**

• **Being part of a high-risk ethnic group,** such as South Asian

• **Having a biomarker such as Lp(a)** (a type of low-density lipoprotein—LDL—cholesterol) levels of 50 mg/dL or higher.

3. What is my CAC score? A low-radiation imaging test detects the level of coronary artery calcium (CAC) buildup in your arteries. The presence of such plaque buildup is associated with risk for future heart attacks. If there is a question about the merits of taking a statin, having this test may help indicate whether you will benefit. Results are given as a number, from zero to, in some cases, more than 1,000.

0: This shows no calcium or calcified plaque buildup so no statin would be recommended in the absence of diabetes, family history of premature heart disease and smoking.

1 to 99: You have some degree of calcium buildup that can help guide the statin decision-making process. Having a lower number might allow you to put off statins and adopt a lifestyle of good habits. However, if you're over age 55 and have plaque development and are at the higher end of this range despite a healthy diet and regular exercise, taking a statin merits consideration.

100 and over: This score suggests that statin therapy should be considered.

A recent study published in *Circulation: Cardiovascular Imaging* added to our understanding of the CAC score and differences in how it predicts heart attack and stroke. *It found that…*

• **The 10-year risk level for both heart attacks and strokes for those with scores of 1 to 99 is below 6 percent.**

• **At scores of 1 to 99, stroke risk is higher than heart attack risk for women…and the reverse for men.**

• **With a CAC score of 100 or higher, the 10-year heart attack risk jumped above 12 percent for men and 8 percent for women.** Stroke risk averaged 8 percent, with a woman's risk again higher than a man's.

Benefits to knowing your CAC score: As a real-time snapshot, the CAC is a visual reinforcement of your risks and can help encourage lifestyle changes even if you've been resistant.

If Your Doctor Suggests Statins…

If statins seem wise for you, ask your doctor if you can take a low dose to minimize any side effects.

While natural practitioners may recommend supplements of CoQ10 and/or vitamin D to help prevent statin side effects, their effectiveness has not been demonstrated in randomized control trials. However, both have good safety profiles, so there is no harm in trying them to see if they help.

When There's Time to Put Off Statin Therapy

The first and foremost step in preventive cardiology is lifestyle changes—following a plant-based diet focused on vegetables, fruits, whole grains, nuts and seeds, and unsaturated fats (such as olive oil)…eating less

animal protein and minimal added sugars… getting more exercise…and losing weight if needed. Losing just 5 percent to 10 percent of excess body weight can lead to significant improvement in cholesterol as well as blood pressure.

We know these changes are more difficult than taking a pill, but remember that statin therapy is not an alternative to healthy eating and exercise—it's an added preventive measure to consider when those steps aren't enough.

Most People Don't Benefit from Low-Dose Aspirin

Thomas M. Maddox, MD, MSc, professor of medicine (cardiology) and executive director of the Healthcare Innovation Lab at BJC HealthCare/Washington University School of Medicine in St. Louis. Healthcare InnovationLab.org

---

As effective as taking a daily low-dose aspirin can be for some heart issues, it's definitely not for every heart condition. And, according to a new almost-five-year study published in *Neurology*, low-dose daily aspirin does nothing to prevent dementia or slow cognitive decline either.

For most people, studies reaffirm that the increased risk for internal bleeding outweighs the benefits of low-dose daily aspirin. Yet many who shouldn't take it still do.

Daily aspirin is recommended only for preventing a second heart attack or second stroke, and it is therefore prescribed only following a heart attack, stroke or diagnosis of peripheral arterial disease, which increases heart attack and stroke risk.

While a family history of heart disease or high calcium scores on a coronary CT scan also appear to increase cardiovascular risk and may prompt more aggressive prevention measures, statins, blood pressure control, smoking cessation and lifestyle changes such as improved diet and exercise are the best strategies to prevent a first heart attack or stroke. Aspirin may be useful in select individuals but generally is not part of a primary prevention strategy.

A review of observational studies published in *Annals of Oncology* found continued evidence that regular aspirin use plays a role in reducing risk for colon and other digestive tract cancers, and prior studies have found that it helps prevent recurrence of some cancers, especially breast cancer. These associations are intriguing, but the effect of aspirin on cancer prevention has not been evaluated in a rigorous, randomized controlled trial—medical research's gold standard. Until then, aspirin shouldn't be taken solely to reduce cancer risk.

If you are currently taking aspirin daily, ask your doctor about removing it from your regimen. If he/she recommends that you continue, be sure to be monitored for signs of bleeding.

"Broken-Heart Syndrome" and COVID-19

Study by researchers at Cleveland Clinic, Ohio, published in *JAMA Network Open.*

Stress-induced cardiomyopathy, known informally as broken-heart syndrome, happens when heart muscles weaken, causing chest pain and shortness of breath. Symptoms resemble those of a heart attack—but are triggered by stress, not arterial blockage. A new study suggests that the syndrome is increasing in people who are being seriously affected by the physical, emotional and social stresses associated with the pandemic. Patients with broken-heart syndrome usually recover within weeks, but in rare cases, the condition can be fatal.

Nocebo-Effect May Explain Many Side Effects of Statins

Study by researchers at Imperial College London, published in *New England Journal of Medicine.*

"Nocebo" is the opposite of placebo—it means that expectation of negative symptoms leads to experiencing those symptoms. Up to one-fifth of people taking statins report fatigue, muscle aches, joint pain or nausea—but clinical studies consistently show a lower percentage of these side effects. In new research, study participants were given four bottles of statins, four bottles of identical-looking placebos and four empty bottles. Participants took the pills—or abstained from them—in a randomly prescribed order for a month at a time. The researchers found that 90 percent of the negative effects experienced by the patients occurred even when they took placebo pills.

Sudden Cardiac Arrest May Not Be So Sudden

Study of 28,955 people who had cardiac arrest outside a hospital between 2001 and 2014 by researchers at Copenhagen University Hospital Herlev and Gentofte, Hellerup, Denmark, presented at the European Society of Cardiology Congress 2020 in Sophia Antipolis, France.

More than half the people who suffered cardiac arrest contacted doctors with symptoms such as shortness of breath, chest discomfort and heart palpitations during the two weeks before the event. A statistical analysis found that, on average, 26 percent of patients who eventually had cardiac arrest were in contact with their primary physician each week—and at two weeks before cardiac arrest, the percentage rose to 54 percent. Cardiac arrest, an electrical malfunction that causes a sudden loss of heart function, is fatal within minutes if left untreated—less than 10 percent of victims survive.

Blood Pressure Mistakes

Raymond R. Townsend, MD, professor of medicine and director of the Hypertension Program at the Hospital of the University of Pennsylvania in Philadelphia. His research has been published in leading medical journals, including *The New England Journal of Medicine, Annals of Internal Medicine, The Lancet* and *JAMA* (*Journal of the American Medical Association*). He has worked as part of the US and Canadian groups that generate the guidelines for blood pressure evaluation and management.

O ver the course of your lifetime, you're likely to get your blood pressure measured dozens—if not hundreds—of times by your doctors. After all, blood pressure is the most important indicator of a person's risk for heart disease, stroke and other chronic diseases.

But what if a good number of those blood pressure readings are inaccurate?

Depending on the type of error that occurs during testing, you could be misdiagnosed with high blood pressure (hypertension)...or you could have hypertension that goes undetected and untreated, increasing your risk for a heart attack or stroke.

Most of these errors raise the systolic (top number) reading—the one that doctors watch most closely as you age. That's because diastolic (bottom number) readings peak around age 50 to 55 and may decline thereafter. Systolic numbers, on the other hand, may keep going higher.

There are guidelines for getting accurate blood pressure readings, but most people don't know them and they're often overlooked by health-care providers. In research published in *The Journal of Clinical Hypertension*, my colleagues and I studied how well medical students followed the guidelines. Only one of the 159 participants followed all 11 steps looked at in our research.

Other research found that even seasoned medical providers make the same mistakes, especially those using a sphygmomanometer, a blood pressure monitor with an inflatable cuff, a manually operated bulb and an aneroid (nonmercury) gauge that the doctor uses with a stethoscope. (Mercury sphygmomanometers have traditionally been the "gold standard.") Human errors still are being made even with meters using the oscillometric method that relies on an automated electronic pressure sensor that is interpreted by the person conducting the test.

Among oscillometric monitors, fully automated electronic devices are the most reliable. They record multiple readings as you sit undisturbed without any medical staff in the room. Yet even if your doctor's practice has this state-of-the-art device, testing guidelines need to be followed to get the most accurate measurement.

Steps for BP Accuracy

To ensure your blood pressure is being measured accurately, follow these steps from the American Heart Association (AHA) and the American Medical Association (AMA)...

1. On the day of your test, avoid caffeine, exercise and smoking (there's never a good time to smoke!) for at least 30 minutes beforehand.

2. Empty your bladder. Waiting in an exam room with a full bladder can increase your blood pressure.

Helpful: When you arrive at the doctor's office, ask if a urine sample is needed. If not, heed nature's call before going into the exam room. If a sample is necessary, request a cup so that you can empty your bladder before seeing the doctor.

3. Sit in an armchair with your back supported...uncross your legs...and place both feet flat on the floor or on a low stool.

4. Support your forearm on the arm of the chair. Blood pressure is lower when the measurement site is above heart level...and higher when the measurement site is below heart level.

5. Rest for five minutes before the test. This is essential to get blood pressure to its baseline (the treatment target).

6. Make sure the correct cuff size for your weight is used. Many practices have only the one size cuff that came with the equipment. But a small, medium, large and extra-large cuff should be available to account for differences in body weight. Though less common than getting a too high blood pressure reading, an inaccurate low reading can result if a medium or large cuff is used on a petite woman, for instance, and high blood pressure could be missed.

7. Make sure the cuff is placed over a bare arm or nothing more than very thin fabric—slip your arm out of your clothes if necessary. Thick shirts and sweaters reduce the oscillations detected by the blood pressure device. The cuff should be placed on the upper arm, level with your heart.

8. No chitchat. Talking can raise blood pressure by up to 15 mmHg—likely due to activation of the brainstem centers that govern our focusing of attention.

9. Don't use or even look at your cell phone. And skip the magazines. Such activities activate the brain centers that govern blood pressure and heart rate.

Important: Have your blood pressure taken in both arms if you've never had that done before—there can be a 10 mmHg to 15 mmHg difference between the right and left arms. The arm that gives the higher reading is the one to use for future readings.

Correcting Mistakes

Once you know how your blood pressure should be measured, you (as the patient) should speak up if missteps are being made. It's your health at risk.

What's more, that blood pressure reading is going into your medical record. If the numbers are incorrect, it can result in a misdiagnosis of hypertension when it is not present, for example, or overtreatment, which can result in dizziness and lightheadedness.

Talk to the doctor if the guidelines weren't followed when he/she, a nurse or medical assistant tested your blood pressure. If your doctor doesn't listen, get a new one. That may sound harsh, but controlling blood pressure is among the most effective strategies to

help people live longer and without chronic disease, so it needs to be done correctly.

Best At-Home BP Testing

We all benefit from keeping an eye on our blood pressure, but it's especially important to monitor it if you've been diagnosed with hypertension.

There are good oscillometric devices for home use. You can buy a high-quality device online for less than $100. Manufacturers such as Omron and Welch Allyn have developed monitors that have been scientifically validated. For a list of validated blood pressure devices, go to the AMA site ValidateBP.org.

If you don't yet know which arm has the higher reading, take your blood pressure in both arms and use the higher one for future measurements.

Keep a log, and bring it with you to doctor appointments. Once a year, bring along your home monitor and have it checked for accuracy against a mercury sphygmomanometer or comparable device. Readings from a device that is not properly calibrated may be consistently 5 mmHg or more higher or lower. Aneroid devices can be sent back to the manufacturer for recalibration, while oscillometric devices will need to be returned or replaced.

Be sure to ask your doctor how often you should check your blood pressure at home. He may advise you to take it daily, for example, starting two weeks after you have changed blood pressure medications.

What to do: Before taking any blood pressure medication, take two measurements one minute apart in the morning...and two readings, also a minute apart, in the evening, and average the two sets.

If the readings aren't in line with your doctor's office reading—especially if they are higher at home—it could be a sign that you need more medication or coaching to better stick with your regimen. Not taking medications as directed is the biggest problem among people with hypertension.

Long Work Hours Are Linked to High Blood Pressure

Xavier Trudel, PhD, assistant professor, social and preventive medicine department, Laval University, Quebec, Canada, and leader of a study of more than 3,500 people, published in *Hypertension*.

People who worked 49 or more hours per week had a 70 percent greater chance of having masked hypertension—a type that may go undetected during routine medical exams. And they had a 66 percent greater likelihood of having sustained hypertension—elevated readings both in and out of a clinical setting. Working 41 to 48 hours a week was linked to a 54 percent greater chance of masked hypertension and 42 percent higher likelihood of sustained hypertension. The five-year study did not look into possible nonwork sources of stress-related hypertension, such as family matters, and it included only white-collar workers.

Low Blood Pressure: No Symptoms? No Problem

Nieca Goldberg, MD, medical director of NYU Women's Heart Program; senior advisor, women's health strategy, NYU Langone Health; clinical associate professor, NYU Grossman School of Medicine. She hosts the radio show "Beyond the Heart" and is the author of *The Women's Healthy Heart Program: Lifesaving Strategies for Preventing and Healing Heart Disease* and *Dr. Nieca Goldberg's Complete Guide to Women's Health*. DrNieca.com

Blood pressure that rises over the standard goal of 120/80 millimeters of mercury (mmHg) gets plenty of attention, but it can dip well below those numbers, too. Let's take a look at what that means.

Your blood pressure reading measures the force of blood pushing against the walls of your blood vessels. The systolic (top) number

Blood Pressure Meds at Night

Take blood pressure meds at night rather than in the morning. It cuts the risk for death from heart or blood vessel problems by 66 percent. Sleeping—not waking—systolic blood pressure is the most significant measure of heart disease risk. Talk to your doctor about the best way to make the switch to nighttime treatment.

John A. Osborne, MD, PhD, is medical director of State of the Heart Cardiology in Southlake, Texas, commenting on a study published in *European Heart Journal*.

is the amount of pressure when the heart pushes blood out to the body, and the diastolic (bottom) number represents the pressure on the blood vessels between beats.

Blood pressure changes throughout the day. It's lowest at night and highest when you wake up. It's affected by your position, your breathing, your stress level, and your diet—salt and caffeine can cause it to spike.

If your systolic pressure is consistently under 90 mmHg or your diastolic pressure stays under 60 mmHg, your blood pressure is considered low. If you don't have any symptoms, this is nothing to worry about, but some people experience dizziness, lightheadedness, nausea, and fainting.

Causes of Low Blood Pressure

The healthiest cause of low blood pressure is simply being fit, which makes the arteries more flexible. The heart doesn't have to pump as hard to push blood through them, so pressure drops.

A less benign cause is dehydration. Reduced fluid in the body means less pressure against the blood vessels. Exercise, heat, not drinking enough fluids, vomiting, and diarrhea can increase the risk.

More serious causes of low pressure include severe bleeding, severe anemia, and infection. Medical conditions such as low heart rate (bradycardia), heart valve problems, heart attack, and heart failure can lower blood pressure, as can low blood sugar, parathyroid disease, adrenal insufficiency, and, sometimes, diabetes.

Medications such as diuretics, beta blockers, calcium-channel blockers, angiotensin-converting enzyme (ACE) inhibitors, antidepressants, and drugs used to treat erectile dysfunction can also be culprits. If you take medication for high blood pressure and lose weight, you may experience low blood pressure symptoms, too.

Orthostatic Hypotension

Some people experience a sudden and transient drop in blood pressure when they change position from lying down to sitting or from sitting to standing. Called orthostatic hypotension, this drop can cause dizziness, lightheadedness, blurred or tunnel vision, and fainting. Like any low blood pressure, it can be caused by dehydration, diabetes, heart problems, excessive heat, and some neurological disorders.

Managing Symptoms

If you're experiencing bothersome symptoms from low blood pressure, start with drinking more water. Eating more salt can help, too. In severe cases, doctors may recommend drinking an electrolyte solution, such as Pedialyte, to increase volume in the blood vessels.

Why the Sight of Blood Makes Some People Faint

Another harmless but unpleasant cause of a sudden drop in blood pressure is the vasovagal response, which occurs when part of the nervous system responds to a trigger, such as the sight of blood, with a sudden decrease in heart rate and blood pressure. It reduces blood flow to your brain, which can cause fainting. Other common triggers include standing for a long time, heat exposure, and fear of bodily injury or a medical procedure. If you feel it coming on, try contracting the muscles in your arms, hands, feet, and legs to interrupt the reflex.

All About Resting Heart Rate

Jessica DeLuise, MHS, PA-C, CCMS, a physician assistant at American Family Care in Conshohocken, Pennsylvania. She is a wellness expert, TV personality, and certified culinary medicine specialist. Her TV show, *Eat Your Way to Wellness*, is now streaming on Amazon Prime.

Resting heart rate (RHR), the number of times your heart beats per minute (bpm) while you're at complete rest, serves as an indicator of overall physical fitness and can help predict your future risk of cardiovascular disease.

You can easily measure your RHR at home. According to the American Heart Association, the best time to test your RHR is first thing in the morning, before you've gotten out of bed, ideally after a good night's sleep. Use your index finger and middle finger to find the pulse in your wrist, just below your thumb (in the radial artery). When checking your pulse, do not use your thumb. It carries its own pulse, which can be confusing and provide an inaccurate RHR.

Count the number of beats you feel in one minute to determine heart rate. Or count for 15 seconds and multiply by four.

You can also use a heart rate monitor device, such as a Fitbit or Apple Watch, to measure heart rate. Once per week, check your pulse manually and match it up to the reading on the device to ensure accuracy. For healthy adults, 60 to 100 bpm is considered a normal heart rate range.

When RHR Is Too High

Stress levels, caffeine consumption, and over-the-counter or prescription drugs may cause RHR to go up temporarily, but if your rate is consistently or frequently over 100 bpm, alert your physician. This may be an indication that you have a fast sinus rhythm known as tachycardia or an irregular rhythm.

If you do not have an underlying health issue, here are some simple ways to lower your RHR...

• **If your physician approves,** exercise at a moderate level for about 30 minutes on most days of the week. Exercise can increase cardiovascular health and, in turn, may lower heart rate.

• **Lose weight if necessary.** If you need any resources and referrals, talk to your health-care practitioner or visit TheWellness Kitchenista.com.

• **Reduce stress through relaxation exercises, journaling, or lifestyle changes.** People have found success through daily meditation, tai chi, and other stress-busting techniques.

• **Avoid tobacco products,** and limit alcohol, processed and refined foods, and caffeinated beverages.

When RHR Is Too Low

Some professional or seasoned athletes may have RHRs that safely dip as low as 40 to 50 bpm, but if you're not an athlete and have an RHR under 60 bpm, I recommend being evaluated by your health-care provider. Slow heart rate, or bradycardia, may cause insufficient blood flow and result in fatigue, dizziness, or shortness of breath.

Using RHR for Exercise

Once you know your RHR, you can use it to determine your maximum heart rate (MHR) and to set a goal range to attain during exercise. MHR varies by age, exercise tolerance, cardiovascular status, and heart arrhythmia.

Ideally, you should talk to your health-care provider to determine your safe ranges and goals, but you can also estimate your target zone with a series of calculations called the Karvonen method (see table).

TABLE: THE KARVONEN METHOD	
Calculate MHR by subtracting your age from 220.	**Example: Age 50, RHR 70** 220-50 years old = 170
Subtract your RHR from your MHR.	170-70 = 100
Multiply the number from step 2 by 50 percent, and then add your RHR back in. That number is the lowest heart rate that would be considered moderate activity.	100 x 50 percent = 50 50 + 70 (RHR) = 120 bpm
Redo the calculation from step three but use 70 percent to calculate the upper level of moderate exercise.	100 x 70 percent = 70 70 + 70 = 140 bpm
Do it one more time but use 85 percent to determine the top end of the vigorous exercise goal.	100 x 85 percent = 85 85 + 70 = 155 bpm
Monitor your heart rate during exercise to gauge intensity.	Moderate: 120 to 140 bpm Vigorous: 141 to 155 bpm

Training for a First-Time Marathon

Charlotte H. Manisty, MD, consultant cardiologist, Barts Heart Centre and University College Hospitals, both in London, and senior author of a study published in *Journal of the American College of Cardiology.*

Training for a first-time marathon reverses aortic stiffening—the "hardening of the arteries" that raises cardiovascular disease risk. Researchers measured aortic stiffening in 138 untrained healthy people before and after they trained for and ran the London Marathon. Their training plan—17 weeks of scheduled walking, running, core exercises and stretching—reversed stiffening by 9 percent, equivalent to a four-year reduction in "aortic age."

Mealtime Linked to Heart Health

Nour Makarem, PhD, associate research scientist, Columbia University's Vagelos College of Physicians and Surgeons, New York City.

*R*ecent study: Researchers evaluated the heart health of 112 women at the beginning and end of a 12-month study. The women kept food diaries for one week at the time of the heart assessments.

Finding: Every 1 percent increase in calories consumed after 6 pm increased the risk for high blood pressure and body mass index as well as poorer long-term control of blood sugar. Although the study was done on women, previous research found a similar association in men.

When It Seems Like You're Wearing a Heart Monitor Too Long...

Erin D. Michos, MD, MHS, associate professor of medicine, division of cardiology, The Johns Hopkins School of Medicine, Baltimore.

A heart-rhythm monitor is something that is worn continuously to give your doctor a better picture of your heart's activity. There are different types of heart monitors. Examples include Holter monitors, cardiac event recorders, mobile cardiac telemetry and Zio patches.

Heart monitoring can be ordered for many reasons.

Examples: It may be prescribed when symptoms such as syncope (passing out), near syncope (nearly fainting) or significant, bothersome palpitations (heart racing) indicate the possibility of an abnormal heart rhythm (arrhythmia).

The Holter monitor is usually used for 24- or 48-hour periods, but if symptoms don't

A Flavanol-Rich Diet Lowers Blood Pressure

Researchers objectively measured indicators of dietary intake among more than 25,000 adults and found that those who consumed the most flavanols—compounds that promote circulatory health—had lower blood pressure. Flavanols are found mainly in some fruits (such as berries and apples) as well as in green and black teas.

Gunter Kuhnle, PhD, professor of food and nutritional sciences at University of Reading, UK, and leader of a study published in *Scientific Reports*.

happen every day, this monitor may not capture an episode. In this case, the patient may be advised to wear a different type of longer-term monitor (for example, a cardiac event recorder, mobile cardiac telemetry or Zio patch) for a longer period, such as two to four weeks.

Because some symptoms occur infrequently and/or are not due to cardiac arrhythmias, 30-day heart monitoring is sometimes done to help explain what the patient is experiencing.

When a woman has had a stroke from an unexplained cause, for example, wearing a heart monitor for 30 days can reveal if she is having episodes of atrial fibrillation, a type of heart arrhythmia that can lead to blood clots in the heart that can then travel to the brain and block blood flow.

The Truth About Life After Heart Failure

Clyde W. Yancy, MD, MSc, chief of cardiology, vice dean for diversity and inclusion and Magerstadt Professor at Northwestern University Feinberg School of Medicine in Chicago.

N ew treatment approaches are extending lives and providing hope for this common chronic condition.

Heart failure (HF)—also known as congestive heart failure—has traditionally been a gut-wrenching diagnosis because it gets worse over time and there is no cure.

Now, with new treatment approaches and a greater emphasis on lifestyle changes, people with HF are enjoying longer, more vital lives than ever before.

A caveat: Even as progress is being made, doctors acknowledge that there's an alarming trend in the rate of older adults affected by HF. About 6.5 million people in the United States (most of them age 65 or older) have HF.

While the older population has substantially increased in recent years, deaths from some types of heart disease, such as coronary artery disease, which leads to heart attacks, have declined. The number of people with HF, however, has increased. As a result, deaths from this condition have jumped by 38 percent, according to an important 2019 report published in *JAMA Cardiology*. Even though age is a leading risk factor for HF, cardiologists believe that getting more people to follow effective prevention strategies is the key to reversing this troubling trend.

Who Develops HF

The term heart failure may sound like your heart has stopped or is about to stop working, but it actually means that your heart has been weakened, making it harder for this life-giving organ to pump blood throughout the body.

HF can develop when the heart becomes damaged by any of a number of heart conditions, such as high blood pressure (hypertension), type 2 diabetes, ischemic heart disease (marked by a buildup of plaque in the coronary arteries), heart valve disease, and arrhythmia (an abnormal rate or rhythm of the heartbeat).

Over time, these conditions can cause your heart to enlarge or stiffen, slowing down the flow of blood throughout your body. This process can take days if an acute heart condition (such as heart attack) occurs, or it may take years or even decades when a chronic risk, such as hypertension, is present.

When the heart muscle is affected by these risk factors, the heart pumping ability is reduced and fluid builds up in your ankles, feet, and legs—a condition called edema.

Fluid may also back up in the lungs, leading to shortness of breath. Thus, the main symptoms of HF are shortness of breath, fatigue, and edema.

New Hope

Even though HF is irreversible once it develops, the prognosis is no longer so grim. In fact, more times than not, it is now hopeful.

The improved outlook is largely due to doctors' deeper understanding of when and how newer and older medications can be combined to fit the needs of individual patients. The older pharmaceutical stalwarts (including diuretics, ACE inhibitors, beta blockers, and digoxin) help reduce fluid buildup, ease shortness of breath and, by lowering blood pressure, ease strain on the heart and slow the heart rate—all of which help the heart beat stronger. Among the newer medications are *ivabradine* (Corlanor), which slows heart rate, and *sacubitril/valsartan* (Entresto), which relaxes blood vessels, making it easier for your heart to pump blood to your body. It may also reduce scarring (or fibrosis)—a benefit that, if confirmed, would be a new target for therapies. Both medications must be used precisely, and national guidelines have been established by professional societies.

When used correctly, both medications have been shown to reduce the risk for hospitalization due to HF (by 18 percent and 21 percent, respectively) compared with standard treatment alone. Entresto has been shown to lower the risk for death by about 20 percent. The combination of the legacy therapies and these new therapies—with more on the way—has fueled hope that the tide may be turning with regard to HF.

Surgeries and medical devices also are extending the lives of people with HF. These include heart bypass surgery if a blocked heart artery is causing HF, replacing a heart valve that causes HF, and implanting pacemaker and defibrillator devices to prevent dangerous abnormal heart rhythms associated with HF.

Left ventricular-assist devices (LVADs) are life-saving, implantable, mechanical devices that can help your heart pump. For advanced HF, LVADs can sometimes be used in place of a heart transplant. For the most severe cases, however, heart transplant is still an option.

Lifestyle Changes

If you already have been diagnosed with HF, controlling risk factors will also help you live longer. Many of these steps may sound familiar, but the key is doing them. The *JAMA* report states that the biggest areas of concern are type 2 diabetes, high blood pressure, and obesity.

Use the following strategies to reduce your risk for HF—and live better if you already have it.

• **Set up a reminder system that works for you to keep track of all your medications.** Take them as directed, but tell your doctor if the regimen is too complex, interferes with your rest, or makes you feel less well in any other way.

• **Stop smoking.** Period. Nicotine increases the risk for HF and worsens the condition in those who already have it.

• **Watch your weight.** Avoiding obesity is an excellent way to avoid HF. If you have the condition, following your weight closely serves as a barometer of how your overall system is doing. Excessive weight gain (or weight loss) in just hours or days is likely fluid, and can be an indication that your medications need to be adjusted. Weigh yourself at the same time each morning, and let your doctor know if you gain three or more pounds in one day or five or more pounds in one week. Find out how much you should weigh at CDC.gov/healthy weight/assessing/bmi.

• **Eat a heart-friendly diet.** This is a plant-focused diet that emphasizes vegetables and fruits with whole grains and lean proteins, such as skinless poultry, fish, and nuts.

Avoid fast foods, convenience foods, processed foods, trans fats, added sugars, and saturated fats.

If you have HF, your body is likely to retain water, and a high-salt intake will make you retain even more. Work with your team of providers for specific advice on a diet and lifestyle that will work for you.

• **Avoid or limit alcohol.** Over time, excessive alcohol weakens your heart, but it is difficult to know what is excessive for any given individual. People over age 65 with HF are generally advised to either avoid alcohol or limit their intake to a weekly total of no more than four drinks for men and two to three drinks for women. Ask your doctor what's right for you.

• **Stay active.** Bed rest used to be the advice for those with HF, but no more. Remaining active is therapeutic. Ask your doctor what activities are safe for you. Walking is an excellent choice for most people. Aim for 150 minutes of physical activity each week, ideally spreading it out so you get some exercise each day on most days of the week.

If you have HF and moderate exercise makes you short of breath, ask your doctor about cardiac rehabilitation, a medically supervised program of exercise training and counseling on heart-healthy living. The good news is that cardiac rehabilitation is usually covered by insurance.

• **Work with your doctor to get better control** of your blood pressure and your cholesterol. If you have HF, you may be asked to check your blood pressure every day.

• **Avoid NSAIDs.** There is good evidence that nonsteroidal anti-inflammatory drugs, such as *ibuprofen* (Motrin) and *naproxen* (Aleve), taken in high doses for an extended period of time, may damage the heart, increasing risk for HF or worsening it. *Acetaminophen* (Tylenol) is a better option.

• **Get your iron levels checked.** Iron deficiency and anemia are common in people with HF, and iron deficiency worsens HF. In HF patients with iron deficiency, iron supplementation has been shown to reduce hospitalization.

LVAD for Heart Failure

Marwan Jumean, MD, assistant professor in the department of advanced heart failure at McGovern Medical School, University of Texas Health and Science Center in Houston, Texas.

Today in America, about 350,000 people are approaching end-stage heart failure. In the past, their only hope for a long life was a heart transplant, but now there is another solution: a left ventricular assist device (LVAD).

An LVAD is a mechanical pump that is sewn into the bottom of the left ventricle. It draws in blood that has been returned from the lungs and sends it through a tube that runs outside the heart directly into the aorta. Batteries provide power to the portable system, which is worn in a harness, shoulder bag, or backpack. A driveline that powers the pump comes out through the upper belly and attaches to a controller that alerts the user if the power source is getting low. An LVAD will keep working no matter how weak the heart gets—even if there is no pulse.

New Use for an Old Tool

While this sounds like science fiction, the melding of man and machine, LVADs are not new. They've been used since 1984. Early LVADs were used only as a bridge until a heart became available for transplant. As LVAD technology improved, portable devices allowed patients to leave the hospital. Users felt their strength and stamina return. They could walk and breathe. They started returning to daily activities. That led to a new way of thinking about LVAD, not as a bridge but as a destination.

The one-year survival after placing an LVAD is almost 85 percent. At five years, it's 50 percent. LVADs are not yet better than heart transplants, but they are getting close.

A growing number of people are choosing destination therapy over transplant therapy.

Pros for the LVAD

The biggest benefit of an LVAD is that you don't have to wait for a heart transplant. It can lengthen and improve the quality of your life on its own. You may still have the option of a heart transplant, but you can also choose to just keep the pump. You may be eligible for the pump even if you are not eligible for a transplant. Hearts are given only to people with the highest chance of success, but the criteria for pumps are less restrictive. Furthermore, most transplant centers have an age cutoff of 70, while pumps can be used in people up to age 80 or even a bit older.

Cons of the LVAD

LVAD placement is major open-heart surgery. You have to be sick enough to need the pump, but healthy enough to survive the surgery. You will be on a heart bypass machine and in surgery for four to seven hours. After surgery, you will be in intensive care for four to five days and in the hospital for three to four weeks.

You need to be psychologically prepared to live with the knowledge that you are completely dependent on your pump and a power source. You will need to manage your pump, keep all your follow-up appointments, and take five to 10 medications daily.

Heart Failure Fundamentals

In a healthy heart, the left ventricle pushes oxygenated blood to the body through the aorta. Heart failure occurs when the ventricle loses its power to pump. As the heart loses the ability to keep the body supplied with blood, symptoms such as increasing fatigue and shortness of breath arise. Eventually, walking, climbing stairs, and other activities become difficult. Although medications can help for a while, heart failure gradually gets worse. There is no cure.

The risks while living with the pump are bleeding (you will need to be on blood thinners), stroke, right-sided heart failure, infection (you will need to keep your driveline area clean), and kidney or lung failure. You can return to many activities, but you can't swim, take a bath, jump, do strenuous exercise, or play contact sports. You also need to follow a healthy diet and avoid smoking and drinking.

Bottom Line

If you or a loved one has been diagnosed with heart failure, think about an LVAD sooner rather than later. If you wait too long, you could miss your window of opportunity.

Beware of Atrial Fibrillation After Any Surgery

David Sherer, MD, a retired physician, author and inventor. He is the lead author of *Dr. David Sherer's Hospital Survival Guide: 100+ Ways to Make Your Hospital Stay Safe and Comfortable*. He is a member of Leading Physicians of the World, and a multi-time winner of HealthTap's leading anesthesiologists award.

Atrial fibrillation, the most treated heart rhythm abnormality in the United States, is a worrisome and sometimes complex medical issue. It occurs when the atrial upper chambers of the heart's four chambers (2 atria or auricles and 2 ventricles) beat erratically and ineffectively. Patients who suffer this often describe a "skipping," "flip-flop" sensation or other unusual feeling in their chests and can complain also of fatigue, dizziness and lightheadedness. Some patients have no symptoms at all. Atrial fibrillation (abbreviated AF or A-fib), affects 2.7 million Americans and places people who leave it untreated at a five times greater risk of stroke and a doubled risk of cardiac-related death.

The traditional treatments for AF have been effective in lowering these risks, and they include medication, cardioversion (a non-invasive surgical option) and ablation (a more invasive surgical option). Many of the medications are structured to control the heart's ventricular rate, which often gets accelerated due to the spastic and disorganized activity in the atria. The atria in a normal heart conducts electrical impulses to the lower chambers, the ventricles, so that the heart beats in an organized and effective way. Cardioversion is an electrical shock to the heart designed to restore normal heart rhythm (also known as "normal sinus rhythm," named for the sinus node in the heart, the bundle of nerves that help regulate the heartbeat). Ablation is a surgical procedure formulated to electrically excise the abnormal focus of tissue that is causing the atria to go into spasm. It requires general anesthesia to accomplish that. Another less invasive option is a new technique that removes a part of the atrium, the "appendage," that is responsible for the faulty electrical signals. Finally, there is invasive treatment for AF, usually associated with other cardiac surgery.

But while AF alone is of concern, there has been increased attention paid to the presence of AF following surgical procedures, and this is something to look out for. *The Journal of the American Medical Association* (JAMA) has reported that after non-cardiac surgery, a number of patients present with a new onset of AF, which places them at a 2.69 increased hazard ratio for subsequent stroke or transient ischemic attack (the so-called mini-strokes). The National Institutes of Health in an older report (1995) found that between 0.4 percent and 26 percent of postoperative patients, depending on the study, developed AF. This postsurgical AF can be temporary or permanent. It requires monitoring and follow up to know which. And if permanent, it requires treatment.

Researchers postulated that there were a number of factors that contributed to that, including increased pain, increased sympathetic nervous system activity, low blood oxygen, low blood or plasma volume, too much acidity to the blood, abnormally low blood glucose, inflammation and other factors. That's why it is so important for doctors, nurses and the rest of the medical team keep these parameters as normal as possible in the immediate after-surgery period. It's also vital that patients and their loved ones inquire whether these abnormal factors are present.

The good news: If AF does not develop within days of surgery, most likely it will not occur because the contributing factors mentioned above will have abated. Some higher-risk patients may want to consider the advice in this new study presented at the American Heart Association's Scientific Sessions 2020 concerning 24-hour-a-day monitoring for 30 days after heart surgery (visit Newsroom. heart.org and search "patients at risk of atrial fibrillation may need additional monitoring").

So the next time you go in for surgery, particularly if you are older or have existing significant medical history (high blood pressure, heart disease, diabetes, inflammatory diseases or cancer, among others), have an advocate, family member, friend or other trusted person ask the staff if your heart rhythm has remained stable in the after-surgery period..

Say Goodbye to A-Fib

John D. Day, MD, an electrophysiologist at the Intermountain Medical Center Heart Institute in Salt Lake City, the immediate past Utah Governor of the American College of Cardiology, and a former president of the Heart Rhythm Society. He is recognized as an international thought leader on atrial fibrillation management. Dr. Day is coauthor of *The Afib Cure,* and the author of *The Longevity Plan.*

In the 1990s, a doctor would have been surprised to meet a patient under the age of 50 who had atrial fibrillation (A-fib), an irregular heart rate that occurs when the upper chambers of the heart beat chaotically and out of coordination with the lower chambers.

Now, we regularly see patients who are seeking treatment for A-fib in their thirties, and sometimes even their twenties. That's in no small part because of our poor diet and

exercise habits, increasing bodyweight, overstressed lives, and poor sleep.

While A-fib can increase the risk of stroke and heart failure, there's good news: You can reduce or even prevent A-fib episodes (arrhythmias) by following an anti-A-fib plan. Many of these strategies will sound familiar—get good sleep, quit smoking, lose weight—because they're the foundation of any healthy lifestyle. When it comes to A-fib, they can even help about 50 percent of people remain symptom-free even without taking medication.

Sleep Tight

Making wholesale lifestyle changes can feel daunting, so you might want to tackle one thing at a time. You'll soon see that each step can make the others easier. Let's look at sleep. Just one night of bad sleep can triple your risk of an A-fib attack the next day, but that's just the beginning. Sleeplessness can also make it harder to manage your weight, control your stress and have the energy to exercise—all key elements in an A-fib management plan.

Many people who struggle with sleeping well can benefit from the following practices. First, set a bedtime and a wake time with at least seven hours in between and stick to it. Don't stay up late and sleep in on weekends. Don't hit the snooze button. Sleep in a clean, quiet, and cool room with plenty of fresh air and no electronic devices. Limit caffeine to 100 milligrams per day and avoid it within six hours of bedtime. Avoid alcohol. While it may make you feel sleepy, it actually disrupts your sleep cycle, which decreases overall sleep quality and duration. In fact, unless you are feeling dehydrated, avoid drinking anything after dinner, and use the restroom before you go to bed. If you have trouble falling asleep, take a 104° F bath or shower and read something that relaxes you before bed. (Choose print or a non-backlit e-reader to avoid sleep-disruptive blue light.)

During the day, get some exercise. It promotes sleep and offers its own A-fib protections. Outdoor exercise is especially beneficial because you're exposed to natural light, which is vital to a strong sleep-wake cycle.

By practicing what's called good sleep hygiene, you'll feel more than rested. You'll likely be less hungry too. Studies show that people who sleep well eat about 522 fewer calories than people who are sleep-deprived.

Weight Management

There is no universal cause of atrial fibrillation, but if there's one characteristic that people with A-fib share more than any other, it is that they are overweight. Don't be discouraged if you have a lot to lose. In one study, my colleague and I showed that losing just 3 percent of a person's body weight, which could be as little as five pounds, increased the long-term chances of putting A-fib into remission.

If you are going to take the necessary steps to get your weight in check, however, you have to be 100 percent committed. Back-and-forth weight changes could be an additional A-fib risk factor.

What to Eat

A healthy diet is unquestionably important for losing weight and keeping it off. But "healthy" doesn't mean "low calorie." Diets that are based on counting calories don't work for most people. People can lose weight using almost any diet that regulates caloric intake, but that weight rarely stays off. So while these diets might be able to offer our hearts a temporary reprieve—and that's a start—it's not the secret to putting our metabolism into balance. Instead, look at the quality of your diet. Minimize or avoid added sugar and flour, eat lots of vegetables, and avoid processed and fast foods.

Next, weigh yourself every day. I've rarely seen a patient who hasn't successfully lost weight or kept it off by simply weighing themselves regularly. Why does this work so well? After seeing a bit of weight gain, people may exercise a little bit more the next day, or they may watch what they are eating more carefully. I've also had many A-fib

patients who have successfully maintained their weight loss through the use of a food journal. The key is accountability.

People who need to lose more than 100 pounds may want to consider weight-loss surgery. In a study of Swedish patients who were overweight, those who had bariatric surgery were 29 percent less likely to develop A-fib. I've even seen cases—quite a few, in fact—in which A-fib has gone into complete remission with bariatric surgery alone.

Exercise

Another way to maintain a healthy weight and a healthy heart is to exercise. Do something every day, even if it's just a little.

Your heart's atria are responsible for 20 to 30 percent of total cardiac performance, so A-fib can reduce your exercise capacity. The goal should be to do something that makes you breathe heavily and sweat a bit—if only for a few minutes each day. Research has shown that just a little strenuous exercise each day, like a five- or ten-minute jog around the block, can confer many of the same health benefits as much longer periods of vigorous exercise in terms of longevity and reduced risk of heart disease. Furthermore, several small bursts throughout the day can build up for more benefits.

Stress Less

It turns out that work stress really is bad for you. A study found that people who experienced negative job-related stress were 37 percent more likely to develop A-fib. Women were at particular risk with a 79 percent increased risk.

Stress comes from other sources, too, of course. Nowadays, news and the internet may top the list. What's the most common emotion you associate with consuming news content? If you said "anger," you should know that researchers have found that the likelihood of an atrial fibrillation episode goes up nearly six times following an experience with anger. By contrast, according to the same study, on the days you are feeling happy, your risk of an A-fib episode is decreased by 85 percent. To lower media-induced stress, cut back your time consuming it. You may even want to try a "social media fast," where you cut out all social media.

Yoga

To combine the benefits of both exercise and stress reduction, consider yoga. Dhanunjaya Lakkireddy, MD, a cardiologist from the University of Kansas Medical Center, has demonstrated that yoga can reduce a person's A-fib burden by 24 percent. It also lowers blood pressure, anxiety, and depression among patients with A-fib.

If stretches and poses aren't for you, consider other forms of mindful engagement like meditation, tai chi, prayer or nature walks. The key is turning distress into "eustress," a moderate state of stress that you can interpret as being beneficial.

Consider Ablation

For some people, early and aggressive lifestyle changes are enough to halt A-fib, but others may want to consider ablation. In a catheter ablation, an electrophysiologist uses catheters to damage the sinus node inside the heart that carries the signal that is causing the irregular heartbeat. In a fascinating study, researchers showed that by eliminating A-fib with an ablation, non-ablated, diseased areas of the heart were able to heal themselves over the following two years. This is nothing to rush into lightly but, for many people, it's a necessary treatment that should be discussed with a physician sooner rather than later.

Ablation is not a "cure" for atrial fibrillation—at least not by itself. You'll still need to optimize your lifestyle to keep A-fib in check in the long term.

Reducing the Need for Medication

Every case of A-fib is different, just like every person who experiences it. Some people can manage it just with the steps outlined above.

Others may follow this plan and still need some additional medications—but the odds are that taking these steps will likely lower the number and dosages of those drugs. That, in turn, will lower medication side effects, including things like the weight gain, low energy, and poor sleep that contributed to A-fib from the start.

Eliminating A-fib is an ambitious plan, but what you do right now to improve your health will set you up for future success.

Turn to Technology to Track Risk

To manage A-fib, you need to be in tune with your body, and technology is making that easier than ever. If you have A-fib, or if you are at risk of developing it, there's really no better investment than a quality smartwatch that will, at a minimum, be able to detect arrhythmias and record an EKG. While these devices are not 100 percent accurate (no matter what the marketers may tell you), they can still serve as powerful tools. Studies show that many people with A-fib experience episodes that they can't feel, so the smartwatch may be the only clue that something is amiss. Conversely, people may feel A-fib-like symptoms that turn out to be something else. Being able to check your wrist and then print out an EKG for your physician to review provides objective information that used to only be available in a hospital. They're also useful if you have episodes of A-fib that don't show up when you're at the doctor's office.

Positive Thinking Could Help Prevent a Stroke

The study "Positive Health Beliefs and Blood Pressure Reduction in the DESERVE Study" conducted by researchers at the New York University School of Global Public Health and published in *Journal of the American Heart Association.*

If you've had a stroke, blood pressure control is typically the coveted goal for preventing another stroke. But among those

Protein Helps Fight A-Fib

Recent finding: Postmenopausal women who ate 58 g to 74 g of protein daily—slightly more than the Recommended Dietary Allowance (RDA)—were up to 8 percent less likely to develop atrial fibrillation (A-fib), an irregular heartbeat that can lead to stroke or heart failure, than those who ate less. Just 10 g to 15 g more protein daily (equal to one cup of Greek yogurt or two eggs) than the RDA showed the positive results.

Theory: Metabolic effects such as improved insulin sensitivity may explain the benefit. More study is needed to determine whether the finding may also apply to men.

Daniel A. Gerber, MD, cardiovascular medicine fellow, Stanford University, California.

who do everything right—including taking prescribed medication, watching their diets and exercising regularly, about one-third of stroke patients still aren't able to reach their desired blood pressure levels.

Could something else help? Perhaps so, according to recent research conducted at New York University School of Global Public Health.

In a recent study published in the *Journal of the American Heart Association*, stroke survivors who said they believed they could protect themselves from a future stroke had a better chance of lowering their systolic (top number) blood pressure—a significant outcome because higher blood pressure is closely associated with increased risk for a future stroke.

Study details: Researchers asked 552 patients who were recovering from a mild/moderate stroke or a transient ischemic attack (TIA), commonly known as a "ministroke," if they believed the statement "I can protect myself against having a stroke." The study participants' blood pressure was measured at the start of the study and repeated one year later. A*mong the key findings...*

• **More than 75 percent of the study participants said that they believed in their ability to protect themselves against another stroke.**

• **Compared with patients who did not answer affirmatively,** the positive group had a 5.6 mm Hg greater reduction in systolic blood pressure, which is considered clinically significant, after one year.

• **Women stroke survivors with positive beliefs about their future stroke risk** were more likely than men to lower their blood pressure. Younger patients were more likely than older patients to lower their blood pressure.

• **Women who did not have a positive belief** were found to have slightly higher blood pressure after one year than at the beginning of the study.

Why beliefs matter: Positive beliefs about one's future health signal the presence of "self-efficacy" in an individual, which includes self-confidence and the motivation to follow stroke-management instructions by making necessary lifestyle changes, according to the researchers.

The findings also point to an effective risk-reduction management tool for doctors and patients. Based on the study, the researchers urge doctors to ask about a patient's belief in his/her ability to prevent a future stroke with medication and lifestyle changes.

When patients are well-informed about the importance of blood pressure control and the lifestyle approaches that reduce their risk for a future stroke, positive thinking can unleash the self-efficacy and confidence needed to make the necessary changes, the researchers explained.

Takeaway: If you've had a stroke, this study offers a powerful new endorsement for positive thinking!

Speech Therapy After Stroke Does Not Have to Be Rushed

Erin Godecke, PhD, is senior research fellow in speech pathology at Edith Cowan University, Joondalup, Australia, and leader of a study published in *International Journal of Stroke*.

When a stroke survivor loses the ability to speak, there's a perceived need to give intense therapy to help him/her recover communication ability as quickly as possible, and therapy often ends within 12 weeks. New research shows no benefit to this approach. While early intervention is important, spreading out therapy over many months may be better.

Restore Mobility and Sense of Touch After a Stroke

Study by researchers at Lund University, Sweden, published in *Proceedings of the National Academy of Sciences*.

It may be possible to restore mobility and sense of touch after a stroke. Scientists re-programmed human skin cells to become nerve cells, then transplanted those cells into the brains of rats that had suffered strokes. After six months, the transplanted cells had repaired the damage caused by the strokes.

Heavy Drinking Increases Waistline— and Stroke Risk

Linda Ng Fat, PhD, research associate, Institute of Epidemiology & Health Care, University College London.

In a study of 4,820 adults (ages 59 to 83) who retrospectively reported their drinking habits for each decade from age 16, those who drank the heaviest increased their waistlines by about 1.5 inches—and had nearly three times the stroke risk—as those who didn't drink heavily. Those who had stopped drinking heavily by age 50 had larger waistlines later in life by one-half inch. Having three or four drinks four or more times a week was considered heavy drinking.

Takeaway: Quitting heavy drinking at any age is beneficial.

Chapter 9

INFECTIOUS DISEASES

Put an End to UTIs

The first time you experience a urinary tract infection (UTI), it takes a doctor's visit and urinalysis to determine that microscopic bacteria are the cause of so much discomfort. But for people who experience recurring infections, the first signs of urgency, frequency, and pain are unmistakable.

If you experience so many UTIs that you've memorized your physician's phone number and only have to utter the words, "I have another..." to have an antibiotic prescription called in to the pharmacy, you're in good company. More than 25 percent of women will have a second UTI within six months and up to 70 percent will within a year.

Women have an anatomical disadvantage: A short urethra (about 4 centimeters long) gives bacteria a quick trip to the bladder, where infection can cause inflammation that leads to those telltale feelings of urgency and frequency. The bacteria can increase the acidity of urine, too, which can cause painful urination.

Sufferers may also experience discomfort or pressure in the pelvic and lower abdominal areas, and strong-smelling or cloudy urine.

Infection in the bladder is called cystitis. If the infection affects the kidneys (pyelonephritis), there may be pain in the back and sides, fever, chills, nausea, and vomiting. Infection can also affect the urethra (urethritis), which can cause burning when urinating. Untreated UTIs can lead to permanent kidney damage and life-threatening sepsis.

Causes of Chronic Infection

While simple anatomy raises the risk for women overall, some people have receptors on the bladder cells that make it easier for the bacteria to connect, leading to more frequent UTIs.

Women with pelvic floor dysfunction also have a higher risk as they may not be able to fully empty the bladder, creating a breeding ground for bacteria similar to that seen in men with prostate enlargement. Kidney stones can also increase the risk.

Antibiotic Resistance

The standard treatment for a UTI is a course of antibiotics, which should provide relief in one to three days. But for a growing number

---

Amin Herati, MD, an assistant professor of urology and assistant professor of gynecology and obstetrics at Johns Hopkins School of Medicine, Baltimore.

of people, antibiotics aren't working as well as they used to—if they work at all.

One-third of uncomplicated UTIs no longer improve with the combination medication *trimethoprim/sulfamethoxazole* (Bactrim), which used to be the standard of care. Furthermore, 20 percent of UTIs are resistant to five other antibiotics.

That means longer periods of discomfort and a higher risk of complications like kidney infections and sepsis, as physicians fight to find a drug that will work. Physicians are afraid that, one day, oral antibiotics won't work at all.

Prevention

A shrinking list of effective antibiotics makes it even more important to reduce the risk of developing a UTI in the first place. *Here are some science-supported strategies...*

• **Hydration.** Drinking more water is the simplest and cheapest preventive strategy. A study in *JAMA Internal Medicine* showed that women who drank 11 eight-ounce glasses of water per day had half as many UTIs over one year as women who drank an average of five glasses of water.

• **D-mannose,** an over-the-counter product, may prevent bacteria from latching onto cells. Some studies have found that it can be as effective as the antibiotic *nitrofurantoin* (Macrobid; which is generally no longer used) for preventing UTIs and *trimethoprim/sulfamethoxazole* for treating and preventing them. Research suggests that dissolving 1 gram (g) in water and drinking it twice a day can help prevent UTIs. For treatment, bump that up to 1.5 g twice daily for three days, and then once daily for 10 days. Alternately, you can double the dose and take it once daily.

• **Vaginal estrogen.** Menopause changes the vaginal pH, which can kill protective bacteria and encourage the growth of harmful bacteria. A topical estrogen cream can realign pH to support healthy bacteria. While there are no apparent side effects, vaginal

estrogen is contraindicated in women with thrombotic or cancer risk.

• **Prophylactic antibiotics.** At low doses, antibiotics stop bacterial replication, while at high doses, they kill the bacteria. People who are prone to chronic infections may benefit from daily low-dose antibiotics, such as *trimethoprim/sulfamethoxazole.*

• **Cranberry juice** has long been a staple in UTI prevention and care, but a recent study reported that it offered no significant protection over placebo. That's not the final word, though, and clinical trials continue to look at the potential benefits of much higher doses.

While there are no definite answers yet, pure cranberry juice is a low-risk intervention that's certainly worth a try. To avoid the high levels of sugar in juice, consider cranberry pills. Research suggests that cranberry supplements need to contain at least 36 milligrams of proanthocyanidins per daily dose to be effective.

• **Reduce the risk from sex.** Sexual activity makes it easier for bacteria to enter the urethra and cause UTIs for many women. To lower the risk, empty your bladder and gently wash the genital area before sex. Thoroughly rinse away any potentially irritating soap. Avoid diaphragms, spermicide, and non-lubricated condoms, all of which are linked to a higher risk of infection. Empty your bladder again after sex to help wash bacteria out of the urethra.

If you are prone to developing UTIs, your doctor may prescribe a single dose of an antibiotic to take after intercourse.

Phage Therapy: An Antibiotic Alternative

As antibiotic resistance increases, there is renewed interest in an old treatment for bacterial infections, including UTIs: bacteriophage therapy. A bacteriophage (or simply phage) is a virus that injects its DNA or RNA into a specific strain of bacteria. The DNA or RNA repeatedly replicates itself until the bacterium bursts and dies. Because each phage is matched with a specific bacteria, it doesn't cause collateral damage to beneficial bacteria or cells. The specificity of each phage can make it challenging for scientists to find just the right one, but researchers are finding success with cocktails that include multiple strains. While phage therapy is not currently approved by the U.S. Food & Drug Administration, physicians can submit a special request to the FDA's emergency investigational new drug program.

Better Probiotics Could Lead to Better Vaginal Health

Study titled "Exploring Potential of Vaginal Lactobacillus Isolates From South African Women for Enhancing Treatment for Bacterial Vaginosis," by researchers at University of Cape Town, South Africa, published in *PLOS Pathogens*.

Bacterial vaginosis (BV) is the most common vaginal condition in women ages 15 to 44. Besides causing uncomfortable symptoms, BV can increase the risk of sexually transmitted diseases (STDs) and complications in pregnancy. A new study from University of Cape Town in South Africa suggests that an improved probiotic could improve BV treatment and reduce risks and complications.

BV occurs when the normal "good" bacteria that live in the vagina, called *Lactobacillus* (LB), get overwhelmed by "harmful" bacteria species. Why this balance shifts is not known, but it is more common in women who are sexually active.

When LB are the dominant bacteria, they keep the acidity of the vagina high, which inhibits the growth of harmful bacteria. When the balance shifts to harmful bacteria, symptoms of BV develop, including vaginal discharge, odor, itching and burning.

The usual treatment is antibiotics, but BV comes back within six months in about half of all cases. Oral probiotic supplements for BV have been used to replace LB and improve treatment. Some studies show that probiotics help and reduce recurrence, alone or with antibiotics. However, studies have not found strong and consistent benefits.

The recent study, published in the journal *PLOS Pathogens*, found that although the commercial probiotics for BV have LB species, they rarely match the species actually found in a woman's vagina. The investigators isolated 57 LB species from vaginal secretions of 26 women. These LB species were compared to the LB species from available commercial probiotics. In a laboratory match up, actual LB species were much more effective at increasing vaginal acidity (lowering the pH) and inhibiting growth of harmful bacteria.

Five of the natural LB species were the safest and most effective. They were also resistant to *metronidazole*, a common antibiotic used to treat BV. This is important because they could be used along with the antibiotic and remain viable as the harmful bacteria were killed.

The researchers would like to see further studies that lead to development of new and better probiotics using the natural LB species. They believe this type of probiotic would be more reliable and could reduce BV complications of pregnancy like low birthweight babies and premature birth. It would also reduce STDs, including a reduction in the risk for HIV.

COVID-19 Symptoms Can Linger for Months

Jacob Teitelbaum, MD, holistic physician and author of numerous books, including *Real Cause, Real Cure* and *From Fatigued to Fantastic!* and is the creator of the app Cures A-Z. He runs the websites EndFatigue.com and Vitality101.com

COVID-19 has been a moving target since it was first identified. And just as we've learned that many parts of the body are points of attack during the active phase, we've found over time that many symptoms linger for weeks or months after tests to detect the virus come back negative. The good news is that a lot can be done to help you feel better.

The array of lingering symptoms suggests that patients develop a form of post-viral chronic fatigue syndrome/fibromyalgia, sometimes also referred to as myalgic encephalomyelitis/chronic fatigue syndrome (ME/CFS).

In fact, half of ME/CFS cases in general are triggered by infections. For instance, it occurs in about 40 percent of people who contract the SARS virus and up to 11 percent of severe cases of mono (Epstein-Barr virus, EBV).

Researchers are finding the same type of postviral fatigue can occur after COVID-19 with the addition of problems related to lung, heart and brain inflammation.

Why does this happen? Numerous infections can trip key "circuit breakers" in your body as they respond to the stress of the illness, and that leads to a cascade of symptoms.

Here are healing secrets from holistic physician Jacob Teitelbaum, MD, to help alleviate the most persistent post-COVID-19 symptoms. Because numerous systems are malfunctioning, there is no single "magic bullet." Rather, a large mix of natural and pharmaceutical treatments is needed to strengthen the system. Most can be discontinued six to nine months after the person has recovered from COVID-19.

Overwhelming Fatigue with Insomnia

These common lingering symptoms also are the hallmarks of ME/CFS. The paradox of having insomnia despite exhaustion tells you that you have tripped the "hypothalamic circuit breaker" in your brain. That is what distinguishes ME/CFS from other causes of fatigue. Anything that overwhelms your body's energy reserves can trip this circuit breaker. And this circuit breaker controls sleep, blood pressure, pulse and hormone function.

Meanwhile, low energy in your muscles causes them to get stuck in the shortened position. (That is also why your muscles go tight after a vigorous workout.) Persistent tight muscles then trigger chronic pain.

The end result? Insomnia, fatigue, widespread pain and brain fog. Countless other symptoms, including shortness of breath and palpitations, also are common.

Fortunately, our published research shows that all of these postviral ME/CFS symptoms are very treatable, with an average 90 percent improvement in quality of life. *The way to address these lingering symptoms is with a protocol that I developed to ease ME/CFS called SHINE, the acronym for…*

• **Sleep.** The goal is to get eight to nine hours of sleep each night. Because your sleep center isn't working correctly, however, you will need some sleep support. Chamomile tea at bedtime can help, along with 200 milligrams (mg) of magnesium… an herbal sleep blend (such as the Revitalizing Sleep Formula from Enzymatic Therapy)…and 5 mg of melatonin.* Also talk to your doctor about a low-dose prescription sleep aid such as *trazodone* (25 mg to 50 mg) or *gabapentin* (Neurontin/100 mg to 600 mg).

• **Hormones.** When your hypothalamus is affected, your entire hormonal system will be malfunctioning, despite normal blood tests. Feeling "hangry" (irritable when hungry) is a clue that you could need adrenal support.

Helpful supplement: Adrenaplex from Terry Naturally, which contains vitamins B-6 and C, adrenal extract and licorice root.

If you're tired, abnormally sensitive to cold temperatures and experience weight gain, you could need thyroid support. Supplements may help, such as Thyroid Care Plus (Terry Naturally), which contains iodine, L-tyrosine and selenium. If you have symptoms of low thyroid despite normal

*Check with a holistic doctor before taking any of the supplements mentioned in this article, especially if you take any medication and/or are being treated for another health condition. Dr. Teitelbaum has a financial tie to the SHINE D-Ribose and Recovery Factors supplements.

blood tests, you may need a holistic physician to get the necessary prescription for your thyroid.

• **Infections.** Though you may have been treated for COVID-19, you want to rule out other preexisting infections especially candida, or reactivation of other viruses (e.g., EBV and herpes simplex virus, HSV-1), which can contribute to your ongoing symptoms. Talk to a holistic doctor for proper evaluation and testing.

• **Nutritional support.** COVID-19 and secondary ME/CFS both trigger nutritional deficiencies (e.g., zinc) and result in increased nutritional needs (e.g., ribose, B vitamins and magnesium) to enhance energy production. A high-potency multivitamin with at least 50 mg of B complex, 200 mg of magnesium, 1,000 international units (IU) of vitamin D, 15 mg of zinc and 500 mg of vitamin C is recommended. Getting sunshine also is critical for optimal vitamin D production—aim for at least 30 minutes a day. *In addition, our research has shown that…*

• Ribose (preferably in the form of SHINE D-Ribose) increased energy by an average of 61 percent.

• Recovery Factors (RecoveryFactors.com), a unique serum-derived polypeptide, helped in 60 percent of cases with an average 69 percent increase in both energy and quality of life. This study was recently submitted for publication.

In general, your diet should be high in salt and protein to support adrenal function, and low in added sugars, which suppress immunity. Also, drink plenty of water.

• **Exercise.** Though you feel exhausted, a graduated increase in walking can help maintain conditioning. Start at a level that is comfortable, and increase by just one minute each day. Too much exercise can cause post-exertional malaise, a reaction that leaves you feeling as though you were hit by a truck, and it can last for days. If your exhaustion gets worse, that's a sign you're doing too much.

Coughing and Breathlessness

For most people, COVID-19 affects the lungs and heart to some degree, and that can lead to ongoing symptoms in your respiratory and cardiovascular systems. It's important to ramp up antioxidants to combat the damage done to these organs by the virus. In addition to a multivitamin high in antioxidants, take NAC (N-acetyl cysteine, 2,000 mg a day) to boost your respiratory system and the body's production of glutathione, the body's key antioxidant…and Clinical Glutathione (from Terry Naturally)—take one to two tablets dissolved under the tongue twice daily. This is the only glutathione that I use because it is highly absorbed and comes in the reduced form (most brands are already oxidized and therefore don't work).

Important: Use a fingertip pulse oximeter to check your oxygen saturation rate. A reading over 96 percent shows that you're getting enough oxygen, making significant lung or heart problems less likely to be the cause of the shortness of breath. If the reading goes down more than two to three percentage points (e.g., to 93 percent) during exercise rather than staying the same or going up a little, check with your doctor.

Breathlessness can come from heart issues, too. Your heart muscle can get stunned by COVID-19. The nutrients discussed above, along with coenzyme Q10 (200 mg), also markedly improve cardiac function. I also recommend a high-quality omega-3 supplement such as Vectomega (from Terry Naturally, one to two capsules daily).

Important: Check your blood pressure. Low blood pressure, or hypotension, is a major contributor to chronic fatigue. Adding adrenal support, drinking more water and adding salt to your diet helps.

GI Issues

If diarrhea, nausea and vomiting were among your primary COVID-19 symptoms, your gastrointestinal tract could now benefit from probiotics and 2 g of glutamine twice a day. Glutamine can help your intestinal lining heal faster. After six to 12 weeks, these supplements can improve intestinal function. In addition, I suspect candida overgrowth if you also have nasal congestion or sinusitis. Yeast grows by fermenting sugar, so a low-sugar diet and a good probiotic are especially important if these are present.

Loss of Smell and Taste

In other infections, these symptoms are thought to stem from inflammation around the olfactory nerve. But this is not the case in COVID-19. Rather, it is suspected that the loss of smell comes from zinc deficiency. Many viruses trigger the body to excrete zinc, which is critical for both immune function and the ability to smell and taste. Take 50 mg of zinc daily for one month to rebuild stores and then 15 mg a day for ongoing maintenance. This amount is usually present in a good multivitamin.

Once Exposed, the Immune System "Remembers" COVID Well

Marion Pepper, PhD, associate professor, department of immunology, University of Washington, Seattle, quoted in *The New York Times*.

New research on the human immune system's response to the coronavirus is encouraging. When the body encounters a virus, hordes of antibodies as well as immune cells called B cells and T cells that can recognize the virus appear and then wane as the threat dissipates. Studies of recovered COVID patients show that the body retains some of those cells. When those cells reencounter the virus, they recognize it and quickly fight off the threat. This bodes well for the continued effectiveness of current vaccines and treatments.

What We've Learned About Treating COVID-19

Joseph Feuerstein, MD, assistant professor of clinical medicine at Columbia University in New York City and director of Integrative Medicine at Stamford Health in Stamford, Connecticut. He specializes in family medicine, focusing on nutrition and disease prevention. Dr. Feuerstein is certified in clinical hypnosis, clinical acupuncture and homeopathy. He is author of *Dr. Joe's Man Diet*. StamfordHealth.org

More than 4 million people have died worldwide from the COVID-19 virus at press time. In the midst of an earlier resurgence, we spoke with Joseph Feuerstein, MD, who has been battling the virus on the hospital frontline and is a COVID-19 survivor himself.

In the beginning, when infection rates were exploding, we threw the kitchen sink at the virus to help sick patients—antibiotics… the antimalaria drug *hydroxychloroquine*… an HIV medication called Kaletra. Now, we have a much better idea of what improves outcomes, and new insights are constantly evolving best-care practices. *Here's what we've learned so far…*

•**Proning.** If you're sick enough to be admitted to the hospital, your oxygen-saturation levels are almost certainly low. Proning, flipping a patient onto his/her stomach, is a low-tech but extremely effective way of increasing the amount of oxygen that reaches the lungs. In this facedown position, gravity helps distribute oxygen more easily throughout the lungs. In a remarkable study, 25 patients who would normally have been put on ventilators were placed in the prone position instead. After just one hour, oxygen-saturation levels improved enough in 19 of the patients that they were able to avoid intubation at that time. Proning is helpful for hospitalized COVID-19 patients regardless of whether they are awake or have been placed on a mechanical ventilator.

•**Dexamethasone.** This powerful steroid, which helps reduce the inflammation that is common in severe COVID-19 cases, has been shown to reduce mortality by approximately one-third for patients on ventilators and by about one-fifth for patients requiring only oxygen. As with the other powerful treatments mentioned here, dexamethasone is for hospitalized patients with severe respiratory issues and difficulty maintaining healthy oxygen-saturation levels. It has long been used by doctors to treat certain cancers and cancer-related side effects, so it is very well-understood. It's also inexpensive.

•**Bamlanivimab.** Until late 2020, there weren't any truly effective treatments for patients with mild-to-moderate COVID-19. The recommendation was that you stay home, more or less battle through the symptoms, and hope for the best. In November 2020, the FDA approved the antibody treatment bamlanivimab to help milder symptoms from progressing to severe in high-risk patients age 12 or older. (As of April 2021, other monoclonal antibody therapies are available in combination with bamlanivimab.) The drug contains man-made antibodies that are similar to the antibodies of patients who recovered from COVID-19. Scientists think that these antibodies may help limit the amount of virus in the body and give the body more time to learn how to make its own antibodies. Bamlanivimab is administered in one dose via IV and works by blocking the virus's ability to enter healthy cells.

Exciting: In a *New England Journal of Medicine* study, 452 nonhospitalized adult patients with mild-to-moderate symptoms were randomly assigned to receive varying doses of bamlanivimab or a placebo. The majority of patients cleared the virus by day 11…but only 1.6 percent of those in the bamlanivimab group required hospitalization or an emergency room visit, compared with 6.3 percent of placebo-treated patients.

•**Antiviral drugs.** These medications that held so much hope have shown mixed-to-disappointing results in the studies. The injectable antiviral medicine *remdesivir*, orig-

inally developed to treat patients with Ebola and hepatitis C, was officially approved in October 2020 as the first drug to treat COVID-19 in hospitalized patients ages 12 and up to help speed up recovery time. That would reduce both health-care costs and risk for hospital-acquired infections. In one study, remdesivir reduced average recovery time from 15 to 10 days when compared with a placebo.

Hydroxychloroquine is another antiviral that causes continued debate within the medical community, with studies showing mixed results…some positive, some ineffective.

A study from the World Health Organization's global Solidarity trial was the largest on these medications. It included 11,330 adults from 30 countries hospitalized for COVID-19. Neither remdesivir nor hydroxychloroquine—nor the antivirals *lopinavir* and *interferon*—had meaningful beneficial effect on patients' mortality, need for ventilation or length of hospital stay versus patients who did not receive trial medications.

Supplements that can help reduce risk and severity. *For positive cases, in the hospital or at home, I recommend…*

•**Vitamin D.** 2,000 International units (IU) to 4,000 IU, depending on current blood level. Studies show a significant correlation between vitamin D deficiency and COVID-19 mortality. In one Spanish study, more than 80 percent of hospitalized COVID-19 patients were deficient in vitamin D.

•**Vitamin C.** 500 mg to 1,000 mg/day. Research suggests it has stimulating effects on multiple cell types of the immune system and antiviral effects.

•**Zinc.** 30 mg to 50 mg/day. Zinc prevents viral replication and has other antiviral properties.

But beware: If you take high doses for many months, it can cause a copper deficiency, so you need regular blood tests. The US recommended tolerable limit for zinc is 40 mg a day.

•**Melatonin.** 3 mg to 6 mg/day for its antiviral properties and anti-inflammatory effects on lungs, according to a review of studies on this hormone, which is more commonly known for its ability to help with sleep.

Beware: Don't take elderberry, quercetin or echinacea if you have COVID-19—these could stimulate the immune system in the acute phase, which would be dangerous for the progression of the virus.

On the horizon: Some research suggests that the antidepressant *fluvoxamine* (Luvox), typically used to manage obsessive-compulsive disorder, may suppress serious symptoms in COVID-19 patients. A November 2020 *JAMA* study found that when 80 patients took fluvoxamine within seven days of onset of COVID-19 symptoms, none developed the severe respiratory issues that could require hospitalization (versus the 8.3 percent of placebo recipients who did). The drug's anti-inflammatory properties may help prevent cytokine storms—the body's massive, sometimes deadly, inflammatory reaction to coronavirus and other infections.

Fever: To Treat or Not to Treat?

Paul A. Offit, MD, professor of infectious diseases, department of pediatrics, Children's Hospital of Philadelphia. He is also director of the Vaccine Education Center and professor of vaccinology at Perelman School of Medicine, University of Pennsylvania. Dr. Offit is the coinventor of the vaccine for rotavirus, the leading cause of severe diarrhea in children, and author of *Overkill: When Modern Medicine Goes Too Far.*

When the new coronavirus started traveling around the world, people were screened for fever to see if they might be ill with COVID-19.

That makes sense because fever is one of the first signs that your body is fighting an infection. But if fever is one of the body's natural defenses, is it wise to take medicine to lower your fever…or better to let your fever do its job?

Is It a Cold or COVID-19?

One way to tell is by the characteristics of the loss of smell and taste. COVID-19 patients typically notice a sudden loss of smell, can still breathe freely, tend not to have a runny or blocked nose and can't detect bitter or sweet tastes. The opposite is typical for a cold—difficulty breathing, blocked and/or runny nose and patients can taste (salt, sweet, sour, bitter, savory) normally.

Carl Philpott, FRCS (ORL-HNS), is professor of rhinology and olfactology at University of East Anglia, Norwich, UK, and leader of a study published in *Rhinology*.

What Does a Fever Really Mean?

Most people assume that fever means an infection is assaulting your body, but fever actually is a signal that your body is fighting infection. Although individual baseline temperatures can vary slightly, fever is generally defined as a body temperature above 100.4°F.* Your body expends a lot of energy with a fever. For roughly every two degrees Fahrenheit of elevated body temperature, your energy expenditure goes up by 12 percent.

Here's what happens: When a microorganism, such as a virus or bacterium, invades and attacks cells within your body, your immune system releases proteins (cytokines) that travel to your brain and reset your body's thermostat to raise your temperature. The increased temperature, in turn, ramps up production of antibodies and white blood cells that travel through your body to attack the invaders.

What many people don't realize is that lowering a fever with *acetaminophen* (Tylenol) or a nonsteroidal anti-inflammatory drug (NSAID), such as *ibuprofen* (Motrin) or aspirin, can do more harm than good. Dozens of studies in animals and humans show that when you interrupt your body's natural response by taking one of these drugs, your

*In older adults, fever may be present at a lower body temperature.

infection can cause symptoms that are more severe and last longer.

If you feel tired and uncomfortable while running a temperature, that means your body is using energy to produce a fever. These symptoms, including chills and body aches, are your body's way of telling you to stay in bed and conserve energy.

Important: Fever is often due to a bacterial infection that may require treatment, such as an antibiotic, so consult your doctor.

When a Fever Is Dangerous

For many people, fever can be frightening because they fear that a very high body temperature can damage the brain. This risk is real, but it depends on the cause of your fever.

A physiologic fever, which is caused by an infection, almost never causes brain damage. In fact, studies show that humans can tolerate very high temperatures, even as high as 106°F or 107°F, without damage.

Even febrile seizures, convulsions that can occur in children under age five when their fever spikes to 102.2°F or higher, do not cause brain damage or long-term problems, such as epilepsy or developmental delays.

An environmental fever is another story. This type of fever occurs when people are wearing heavy clothing or trapped inside a car during a hot, humid day, unable to dissipate heat through sweating. Environmental fever can cause heat stroke.

Older adults are at greater risk for heat stroke than younger adults because their bodies are less sensitive to temperature changes and they are more likely to become dehydrated. Taking certain medications, including laxatives, antihistamines and tricyclic antidepressants, also increases risk.

What to Do If You Have a Fever

While most fevers are due to common cold and flulike viruses, fever also can be caused by cancer and diseases that cause inflammation, such as rheumatoid arthritis and lupus, or by a reaction to drugs, such as certain an-

tibiotics. Let your doctor know about a fever that worsens, lasts for more than three days or keeps coming back.

Even though there are downsides to treating a fever, if your body temperature exceeds 103°F or is accompanied by other symptoms such as confusion, stiff neck, rash, severe pain or trouble breathing, call your doctor right away. While a physiologic fever doesn't cause permanent harm, the symptoms in this case may be a clue to a severe illness. *Otherwise...*

•**Drink plenty of fluids.**

•**Eat easy-to-digest foods,** such as soups. Your body needs energy to heal.

•**Get plenty of rest.**

•**Take a lukewarm bath.**

•**Apply cool washcloths.**

•**Stay home to protect others from any infection your body is fighting.**

Note: Fever can increase heart rate and breathing rate, so consult your doctor if you have concerns. Fever of 100.4°F or above in a young baby may be due to an illness that requires treatment—talk to a pediatrician.

MMR Vaccine Booster Could Improve COVID Outcomes

Paul Fidel, Jr., PhD, is associate dean for research, Louisiana State University School of Dentistry, New Orleans, and coauthor of a paper published in *mBio*.

Besides staving off its target diseases, the measles, mumps and rubella vaccine spurs a "nonspecific" immune response that experts think may dampen the lung inflammation and sepsis that often prove fatal in COVID-19 patients. Clinical trials and animal models are underway, but it is safe to get an MMR vaccine or booster, particularly for health-care workers/first responders and people in nursing homes.

Better Cleaning to Kill Germs

Roundup of scientists who study cleaning products, reported in *The New York Times*.

Spray a disinfectant long enough to wet the surface, then let it stay there. Follow specific label directions for how much time—same-brand products may have different contact times. If a product says the surface must be cleaned before product use, preclean any soil—germicides have to touch germs in order to work, and existing soil may block their action. If a wipe says it must be used for four minutes, that is the time from initial wipe to surface drying—not the time needed to do the wiping itself. It is OK to use one wipe for multiple surfaces as long as it remains wet, but it is best not to mix rooms—a wipe used on multiple bathroom surfaces should not then be used in the kitchen.

Be Careful When Using Potting Mix

CNN.com

Though rare, there have been cases over the years of people dying from diseases, such as Legionnaire's, contracted from potting mix. Potting mix is a combination of organic and inorganic materials, and the bacteria and fungi in the mix can thrive in the moist and warm conditions where it's stored.

Self-defense: Wear gloves when working with potting mix, and if you don't have gloves, thoroughly wash your hands immediately after. Wearing a mask while handling it also can help protect you, as some diseases, such as Legionnaire's, are airborne.

Disinfect Your Home After a Virus

Roundup of cleaning experts, reported at BHG.com

Focus on the bathroom, kitchen and shared surfaces in the bedroom. Clean areas the sick person spent time in and things he/she touched, including countertops, faucets, and cabinet hardware. Pay special attention to hard surfaces where germs can survive, such as TV remotes and door handles. Disinfect sheets, pillowcases and other bedding. Clean electronic devices, such as cell phones and tablets. Use the right products for each place—bleach for the bathroom, laundry sanitizer for clothing and bedding, and disinfecting wipes for many hard surfaces—be sure each surface stays wet for 15 seconds to kill germs.

5 Natural Ways to Repel Mosquitoes

Phyllis Kozarsky, MD, professor emerita of medicine in the division of infectious diseases at Emory University School of Medicine and retired medical director of TravelWell, a clinic that provides vaccinations and health services for individuals who are traveling internationally. She is a cofounder of the International Society of Travel Medicine. ISTM.org

Here are some nonchemical ways that you can ward off these bloodsuckers…

• **Fragrance-free products.** Mosquitoes may be attracted to scent, so use as many fragrance-free products as possible including personal-care products such as lotions and soaps, laundry detergents and fabric softeners and cleaning products. Don't wear perfumes or cologne.

• **Shower after exercising (with unscented soap).** Mosquitoes are attracted to damp, sweaty skin as well as to the carbon dioxide and lactic acid that our bodies secrete when we are active.

Too Much Salt Lowers Your Immune Defenses

Volunteers ate a high-salt diet—just over double the daily suggested limit of nearly six grams—equivalent to two regular fast-food burgers and fries every day. After one week, blood samples revealed a reduced ability to fight bacterial infections such as listeria and E. coli. And mice on a high-salt diet cannot defend as well against uropathogenic E. coli and listeria.

Best: Cap salt intake at six grams (about one teaspoon) a day.

Christian Kurts, MD, is director of the Institute of Experimental Immunology, University Hospital Bonn, Germany, and coauthor of the study published in *Science Translational Medicine.*

•**Turn on an outdoor fan.** Mosquitoes are notoriously bad fliers and will avoid breezy areas.

•**Dress to protect.** In addition to wearing as much clothing as you can tolerate in the heat, choose light-colored fabrics—particularly beiges and whites—because mosquitoes prefer dark colors.

•**Wear sneakers and socks instead of sandals**—mosquitoes love dirty, sweaty feet.

Fecal Transplant Better Than Antibiotics for C. diff Diarrhea

The study "Economic Evaluation of Faecal Microbiota Transplantation Compared to Antibiotics for the Treatment of Recurrent Clostridioides difficile Infection" led by researchers at the University of Birmingham, UK, and published in *EClinicalMedicine.*

Clostridium difficile (C. diff) causes a virulent bacterial infection that leads to inflammation of the colon and severe diarrhea. Those at highest risk for the illness include adults age 65 and older (especially those who live in nursing homes or have been hospitalized) and people who take antibiotics unnecessarily or have a serious illness or a weakened immune system. Tragically, C. diff infection sickens up to half a million Americans and kills nearly 30,000 each year.

Part of what makes the condition so dangerous is its tendency to strike more than once…it comes back in about 30 percent of people. Recurrent C. diff infection has traditionally been treated with an antibiotic—the most commonly used are *vancomycin* (Vancocin) and *fidaxomicin* (Dificid)—but recent studies show that transplanting gut bacteria from a healthy donor to restore the natural balance of the patient's gut microbiome is an effective alternative.

In fact, studies have shown that this treatment, known as fecal microbiota transplantation (FMT), has a better cure rate and a lower recurrence rate than antibiotics. However, many professional guidelines still recommend antibiotics as the first line treatment for recurrent C. diff infection despite the research showing that FMT is more effective.

Now: Researchers at the University of Birmingham in the United Kingdom have found that FMT is not only more effective at treating recurrent C. diff infection, but also is less costly than antibiotic treatment.

Study details: To analyze the effectiveness and cost of treatment for recurrent C. diff infection, the investigators used randomized controlled trials, observational studies and expert opinions focusing on patients over age 65 who were hospitalized due to the infection. Four treatments were compared—FMT administered by colonoscopy…FMT administered via a nasogastric tube, which is passed through the nose into the stomach…use of the antibiotic fidaxomicin…or the antibiotic vancomycin. The study, which was published in the online medical journal *EClinicalMedicine*, found that…

•**FMT by colonoscopy was slightly more effective than FMT by nasogastric tube but significantly more expensive.**

- **FMT by nasogastric tube was the least expensive treatment and more effective than antibiotics.**

- **Fidaxomicin was less effective and more expensive than either type of FMT.**

- **Vancomycin was the most expensive and least effective treatment.**

Based on these comparisons, FMT by nasogastric tube came out on top as a treatment option for recurrent C. diff infection due to its low cost and effectiveness.

Note: FMT also can be administered by other methods, such as an oral capsule or enema, but these options were not included in the study. For all delivery methods, FMT uses a stool sample from a donor who is screened for any health conditions that could be spread through feces. The donor's stool is emulsified, filtered and sometimes frozen to preserve healthy gut bacteria.

Bottom line: FMT is more effective—and less costly—than the two antibiotics most commonly used to treat C. diff infection. The researchers hope that this study may help change guidelines that continue to recommend antibiotics as a first-line treatment. The use of FMT also may provide long-term savings by cutting down on the number of days that C. diff patients must be hospitalized.

Can You Be Immune to Lyme Disease?

Andrew Rubman, ND, medical director of Southbury Clinic for Traditional Medicines in Southbury, Connecticut. SouthburyClinic.com He is author of the blog "Nature Doc's Patient Diary" at BottomLineInc.com.

***T**he patient:* "Tony," a 63-year-old landscape architect in Northwest Connecticut.

Why he came to see me: This robust outdoorsman contacted me to help evaluate his very unusual situation. Since moving to a very woodsy part of the state and being out in the forests and brush, both for his work

Eyeglasses Can Protect Against Viral Infection

Viruses enter the body through the nose, mouth and the surface of the eye. So always wear eyeglasses or sunglasses when going to the grocery store or any environment where the virus that causes COVID-19 could be present. Glasses do not fully protect the eye, since they do not seal around it. But they provide partial protection—and also help prevent you from accidentally touching your eyes, which could transport a virus to them from your fingertips. If you wear contact lenses, wear glasses over them...or stop wearing contacts and switch to eyeglasses.

If you do not need glasses for clearer vision, you can buy a nonprescription pair online or at many pharmacies.

University of California, Berkeley, Wellness Letter.

and his love of camping and hunting, he had been bitten quite frequently by ticks but he never felt any symptoms of Lyme Disease. Tony was concerned that an infection could be silently brewing inside him.

How I evaluated him: In our preliminary phone call, I told Tony to come in to the clinic the next time that he found a tick on himself. When he came in, I carefully removed the tick intact. Oddly, although it had definitely burrowed into his skin deeply enough to start extracting blood, there was no evidence of the swelling that characterizes successful "feeding." The tick appeared to be dead as well, which also was odd. I told him that we would send the critter into the State lab for analysis to see if it indeed was carrying the organism that causes Lyme Disease, *Borrelia burgdorferi.* We also discussed the testing available for evaluating possible infection and associated diseases that often go along as "co-infections" and sent a blood sample to a specialty laboratory known for extremely thorough evaluation beyond conventionally available screening, asking for evaluation relating to his contracting another tick-borne illness, Rocky Mountain Spotted Fever, as a youngster.

The test results came back from the State lab within a week and the specialty lab two weeks later. The State confirmed that the tick we removed from Tony arrived dead and indeed was carrying the Lyme organism. The specialty lab found no evidence of either current or past Lyme infection and did confirm the past exposure to the other tick-borne illness that he had so many years ago. I spoke to the lab director about Tony's situation and we decided that it was possible, in theory, for a certain "memory cell" that had been developed by his immune system to activate against the Lyme organism, providing actual immunity to the disease and killing the infected tick, but that this was the first time that he had seen any evidence of this.

The patient's progress: I shared my conversation with Tony and have mentioned his case with other physicians and continue to marvel at the power of the human immune system. Often we see that infections in the past to certain diseases may confer immunity to similar diseases that are present in our current environment. This may mean that many of us may not need certain immunizations to remain healthy, as Tony has certainly proved.

Best Humidifiers to Fight Viruses

Paige Szmodis, editor and reviewer for Hearst publications, including *Popular Mechanics*. Popular Mechanics.com

---

Did you know that the dry indoor air of winter might make it easier for airborne viruses to spread? Researchers have conducted experiments indicating that's possible.

One possible weapon: A humidifier.

Humidifiers add moisture to indoor air, weighing down virus particles and speeding their descent to the ground. Of course, humidifiers also provide relief for dry throats, noses, skin and lips.

However, buying a humidifier can be confusing. "Evaporative" humidifiers use a replaceable filter to wick water up from a tank while a fan blows the moist air through that filter out into the room. "Ultrasonic" humidifiers use high-frequency vibrations to convert water into a mist that a fan then distributes.

Ultrasonic humidifiers run the risk of over-humidifying and may create a "white dust" residue around the room if you fill the tank with unfiltered tap water.

Evaporative humidifiers require replacement filters, which adds to the cost. Another decision is whether you want a warm-mist option, which is available on some ultrasonic models.

Warning: Whatever humidifier you choose, clean it at least once a week and do not boost relative humidity in a room above 40 percent to 50 percent, or you could promote growth of mold and mildew.

We asked product reviewer Paige Szmodis to recommend some of the best humidifiers…

Best for a bedroom up to 400 square feet: Honeywell HCM-350 Cool Moisture Germ Free Humidifier is among the most reliable and easy-to-use evaporative humidifiers. Its 1.1-gallon tank has a handle for easy carrying and an opening wide enough for you to reach a hand inside for cleaning. It has parts that are dishwasher-safe…and it's large enough that it can run for up to 24 hours between refills. But like most evaporative humidifiers, it requires filters that should be replaced every month or two. $74.95. Replacement filters $13.95 each.

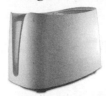

Best for large spaces: Levoit LV600HH Hybrid Ultrasonic Humidifier can humidify up to 750 square feet for up to 36 hours with its 1.6-gallon tank. This ultrasonic humidifier has an "auto mode" that uses a built-in sensor to automatically adjust humidity levels and avoid over-humidification. It has both cool- and warm-mist settings and a remote control. $89.99.

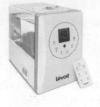

Best value: TaoTronics 4L Ultrasonic Cool Mist Humidifier is bargain priced and includes a humidity sensor to avoid over-humidifying, unlike many other low-cost ultrasonic humidifiers. It can humidify up to 320 square feet for as long as 30 hours on a 1.1-gallon tank of water. It has a filter, but that filter is reusable—soak it in a vinegar-water mix every month. $49.99.

Best for quiet in small rooms: Pure Enrichment MistAire Ultrasonic Cool Mist Humidifier is nearly silent—most other humidifiers create noticeable fan noise or humming. Its 0.4-gallon tank can humidify up to 175 square feet for up to 16 hours. Cleaning its tank is challenging, however—you have to reach inside with a special brush, which is included. $39.99.

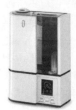

Best when you have a cold: Vicks VWM845 Warm Mist Humidifier doesn't just distribute warm, moist air. If you put Vicks Vapo-Steam cough-relief medicine in its "medicine cup," this ultrasonic humidifier will distribute that as well, providing additional relief for sore throats and coughs without the messiness of the well-known Vicks VapoRub balm. Its one-gallon tank can run for up to 24 hours and is easy to clean. $39.99.

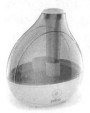

Six Ways You May Be Showering Wrong

Roundup of dermatologists and study findings reported at EverydayHealth.com.

• **Wrong temperature.** Too cold, and you'll be amped up afterward rather than relaxed.

Too hot, and your skin will be dry, dull and itchy. Go for lukewarm.

• **Wrong duration.** Standing there for too long causes your skin to lose oils and moisture. Make it five to 10 minutes, tops.

• **Wrong tools.** Poufs and washcloths, if you don't clean them regularly, are reservoirs for bacteria. Wash with your hands instead.

• **Wrong products.** Extra-strong cleansers can wreak havoc on your skin. Regular soaps will wash away COVID-19 and other germs just fine.

• **Wrong order.** Here's how your routine should go to keep you cleanest—shampoo, rinse, conditioner, soap the body, rinse the conditioner and body wash simultaneously.

• **Wrong time of day.** Showering only in the morning leaves you sleeping in whatever dirtiness you've collected throughout the day. Plus, a shower before bedtime has been shown to help bring on sleep.

Help for Fever Blisters

Alan M. Dattner, MD, a board-certified dermatologist and pioneer in integrating nutrition, holistic medicine, and dermatology. HolisticDermatology.com

The annoying appearance of fever blisters, those tiny, fluid-filled sores (often called cold sores), around the lip area are usually caused by a viral infection... and are never a welcome sight.

First, take a look at what could be causing the virus that causes fever blisters (herpes simplex) to flare up. When a fever blister goes away, the virus never leaves your body. It lies dormant in your nerves until something activates it. That activation could come from something as simple as eating too many arginine-rich foods, such as nuts grains, seeds, or chocolate. If you overindulge in any of these, take extra lysine before, during and after for a few days. One gram of lysine three times per day should work. Increase your dose if that is how much you take now. Since arginine promotes herpes reoccurrence but also supports the immune response, it is a good idea to take extra vitamins, herbs and supplements that support the immune system. This might include vitamins A, D and C and astragalus.

Hormonal changes and decreased immune function can trigger the virus too. Even your posture can affect viral activity by putting excess pressure on the sensory nerve *ganglia*, where herpes resides. A physiatrist, chiropractor or neurologist can test for such pressure and address it with exercise, posture correction or manipulation of the cervical spine in the neck or in the lumbar region.

If you have recurring cold sores, you may benefit from a trial of *valacyclovir*. I don't recommend taking it all the time, just when you start to feel that tingle. I also recommend taking a daily vitamin B supplement and 1,000 micrograms of sublingual B12 to support your nervous system. For some people, lemon balm as a tea or tincture can also be helpful.

Alcohol-Free Hand Sanitizers Protect Against COVID-19

Bradford Berges, PhD, is associate professor of microbiology and molecular biology at Brigham Young University, Provo, Utah, and leader of a study published in *Journal of Hospital Infection*.

The CDC recommends hand sanitizers that contain alcohol, but new lab testing shows that alcohol-free solutions containing benzalkonium chloride and other quaternary ammonium compounds destroyed the new coronavirus that causes COVID-19 just as quickly and effectively as those with alcohol. Alcohol-free sanitizers are easier on the skin and may be easier to find.

Rescue Dry, Chapped Hands

Kevin P. Cavanaugh, MD, dermatologist, Rush University Medical Center, Chicago.

Constant hand washing can be rough on the skin, leaving hands chapped and dry. What's the best for relief?

First, keep up the vigilant hand-washing! With or without the COVID-19 pandemic, hand hygiene is one of the most important weapons in our arsenal against germs and viruses.

After multiple daily washings, however, it's not unusual for our hands to feel like sandpaper or become raw and bleed. *But you can keep your hands clean—and soft and smooth…*

• **Opt for hand cream, not lotion.** Each time you wash your hands with soap or use a hand sanitizer (containing at least 60 percent alcohol), moisturize with hand cream. Lotions evaporate more quickly than creams, so they aren't as effective at repairing the skin's barrier.

Note: Let hand sanitizer air dry before applying hand cream.

• **Be prepared.** You'll want to wash or sanitize your hands after being in a public space. That's why it's smart to carry a small, travel-sized tube of moisturizer to use afterward.

• **Take care of skin cracks.** Frequent handwashing can cause the skin on your hands to crack and start to bleed. Apply a liquid bandage, which adheres to skin better than plastic or fabric bandages, up to twice daily to seal cracks and help them heal.

Good choice: New-Skin Liquid Bandage.

• **Go for some overnight TLC.** To penetrate the deeper layers of skin, apply an ointment, such as CeraVe Healing Ointment or Vaseline Petroleum Jelly, to your hands. Slip on a pair of cotton gloves, and wear them while you sleep. Your hands will thank you in the morning!

Humans vs. Virus: Curing Hepatitis C

David Sherer, MD, retired anesthesiologist, is author of *Hospital Survival Guide: The Patient Handbook to Getting Better and Getting Out.*

The curing of long-feared infection hepatitis C has been nothing short of a medical miracle and is a shining example of the adage that if you throw enough money and brain power at a problem you are likely to achieve great things. Hepatitis C, like hepatitis A and B, is a viral disease that affects liver function. The Baby Boom generation has been particularly hard hit with chronic hepatitis C infections, many of which were related to intravenous drug abuse and sexual transmission. But the numbers are creeping up in other generations too. It is estimated that the rate of acute hepatitis C illness that is self-limiting—meaning that a disease does not further develop into a serious medical issue—is in the minority and that 75 percent to 85 percent of people infected with the hepatitis C virus will go on to have chronic disease. Of those people with chronic disease a significant portion of them will develop serious sequelae (complications) such as scarring (cirrhosis), liver failure and even liver cancer.

Unlike hepatitis A and B, there is no vaccine to protect against hepatitis C but there are drug regimens that offer the chance of cure. A cure is defined in this sense as a sustained virologic response, where no virus is detected in your bloodstream three months after the completion of the treatment. The antiviral therapies used to cure hepatitis C are not without the potential for risk and side effects and must be carefully coordinated, depending on the specific nature of your disease and your general health, by your doctor and the team taking care of you.

You should always be mindful of the costs involved in the therapy and be in close contact with your insurer or health plan before and during treatment. According to the U.S. Department of Health & Human Services, an estimated 2.4 million individuals are living with hepatitis C...the number could be as high as 4.7 million since many do not know they have the virus. Most of these individuals can be cured, but at great expense. According to WebMD, one 12-week regimen cost $84,000. Another drug could average $23,600 a month for 6 months to a year of treatment!

So if you are in the high risk categories as explained above, it is time to talk to your doctor about getting tested and, based on the results, plan a course of action that might lead to the curing of a formerly incurable and serious condition. But do realize the financial, physical and emotional challenges that lie ahead. They can be substantial.

Another Strange Sign of COVID-19

Esther Freeman, MD, director of Global Health Dermatology, Boston, quoted in *The New York Times.*

Sore feet. Since the onset of the pandemic, dermatologists saw a spike in patients reporting chilblains—itchy, burning, red and purple lesions and swelling on the toes that usually result from cold and damp conditions. Most of these cases are among healthy children and young adults whose COVID infection was mild or even went unnoticed. Chilblains may signify a body's healthy immune response to the virus since they seldom appear in people with acute cases.

Chapter 10

NATURAL HEALING REMEDIES

Super Immune-Boosters Your Doctor Doesn't Know About

You probably already know about the immune-enhancing powers of zinc, vitamins C and D, and medicinal plants such as echinacea and elderberry. But several other powerful supplements exist that may decrease your chances of getting sick and help you recover faster if you do get sick.

Note: These supplements are generally safe in the amounts mentioned here, but discuss taking them with your doctor, especially if you are immune-compromised or taking medication.

Immune-Boosters for Everyone

• **N-acetylcysteine (NAC) is an amino acid that supports immunity directly.** Also, the body easily converts NAC into the antioxidant glutathione—more on glutathione later. NAC is well-tolerated, inexpensive and so effective against influenza that in one Italian study, only 25 percent of elderly people taking 600 mg twice daily throughout flu season exhibited flu symptoms, versus nearly 80 percent of those in the placebo group. Of those who did show symptoms, NAC significantly decreased the severity and intensity.

Daily dose: 1,200 mg daily, divided into two 600-mg doses. At the first sign of influenza or cold symptoms, increase to 3,600 mg to 4,000 mg daily for adults, divided into two doses a day, and continue until symptoms subside.

• **Probiotics.** For decades, naturopathic doctors have been saying a healthy gut, populated by beneficial bacteria, is necessary for a healthy immune system. This immune booster might not be as surprising as the others, but probiotics are so powerful and vital for a healthy immune system (the word probiotic itself means "beneficial for life") that they cannot go unmentioned.

Good bugs: While the cold virus and influenza are most certainly bad bugs, probiotics are the kind that are good for you. These

Mark A. Stengler, NMD, naturopathic medical doctor and founder of the Stengler Center for Integrative Medicine in Encinitas, California. He has served on a medical advisory committee for the Yale University Complementary Medicine Outcomes Research Project and is author of *The Natural Physician's Healing Therapies* and coauthor of *Outside the Box Cancer Therapies: Alternative Therapies That Treat and Prevent Cancer* and *Prescription for Drug Alternatives*. His newest book is *Healing the Prostate*. MarkStengler.com bacteria, which come in several strains, including *Lactobacillus, Bifidobacteria* and *Saccharomyces,* live in your gut and have many jobs, including regulating the immune system. In fact, about 70 percent to 80 percent of your immune system resides in your gut!

Supplemental probiotics taken regularly for preventive defense have been shown to decrease duration of the common cold in the elderly, adults and children.

Recent study: "A clear decrease" has been seen in numbers of Lactobacillus and Bifidobacterium strains in the guts of patients with COVID-19, according to an August 2020 *Frontiers in Microbiology* study.

Daily dose: Probiotics are measured in CFUs—colony-forming units, which represent the bacteria's potential to divide and reproduce. Aim for 20 billion CFUs a day. *You can get there via a combination of food and supplementation…*

• **Food.** When you consume probiotic-rich foods and beverages, such as kefir, yogurt, kimchee, sauerkraut, miso soup and other fermented foods, you bathe your gut in helpful bacteria. Kefir is especially good, as it has multiple strains of bacteria, whereas yogurt typically offers only one or two.

Try: Lifeway Kefir, with 12 strains and 25 billion to 30 billion beneficial probiotic CFUs per cup ($2.99 to $4.99 for 32 ounces). There also are dairy-free yogurts such as those with an almond, soy or coconut base that contain healthful bacteria.

• **Supplements.** When choosing a daily probiotic, look for one containing strains used in published human studies, such as *Lactobacillus paracasei* and *Lactobacillus plantarum.*

Try: Metagenics UltraFlora Immune Booster ($44.14 for 30 capsules).

Note: Some probiotics are stable at room temperature, but if a product's label says that it needs to be refrigerated, buy it only if it has been refrigerated at the store. This could help prevent some of the bacteria from dying on the shelf before you get the product home.

For an Even Bigger Boost

If you are immune-compromised with a chronic health condition or want to be more proactive, you also can add these supplements…

• **Glutathione.** Known as "the mother of all antioxidants," glutathione is one of the body's most powerful weapons against immune-damaging compounds. When viruses, bacteria or even toxins such as pesticides and heavy metals enter the body, the liver begins secreting glutathione to help neutralize them. Besides being worthwhile for those who are immune-compromised, taking glutathione preventively is beneficial to those who are exposed to a lot of toxins in the workplace, such as someone working in a hair salon or as a welder or painter, etc.

Powerful research: In a study published in *European Journal of Nutrition,* 54 healthy nonsmoking adults were given either 250 mg or 1,000 mg of glutathione every day for six months or a placebo. By three months, those receiving the larger supplement dose showed double the natural killer-cell activity, meaning that they were producing twice as many of these cells known for scavenging the bloodstream for bacteria, viruses and even cancer cells.

Created by a combination of three amino acids (cysteine, glutamic acid and glycine), glutathione also binds to free radicals—naturally occurring yet damaging by-products of daily living that contribute to cellular damage and premature aging.

Production of this important immune-system protector decreases with age and is compromised in individuals with chronic conditions such as obesity and type 2 diabetes, as well as in those who smoke. When levels drop, white blood cells are diminished, allowing viral and bacterial infections to thrive.

Daily dose: Glutathione is made by the body and also is found in small amounts in certain foods, including cruciferous veggies such as cauliflower and broccoli, asparagus, avocado, cucumber, green beans, apples and spinach. Most Americans consume only about 150 mg of glutathione per day through

Link with COVID-19?

A number of new studies have identified glutathione deficiency as a possible contributing factor to COVID-19 deaths in the elderly and people with chronic diseases. Higher levels of glutathione may protect against acute respiratory distress syndrome and cytokine storm—the massive flood of inflammatory cells into the body that can lead to death in COVID-19 patients—by inhibiting replication of the virus.

—Mark Stengler, NMD

the foods they eat, just half of the minimum daily amount recommended by most experts, making supplementation an excellent strategy. Try 200 mg/day to 250 mg/day for general immune support, or 250 mg twice daily if you're sick.

I like Healthy Origins Setria L-glutathione, the brand used in the *European Journal of Nutrition* study ($26 for 150 250-mg capsules).

Note: Although the label says to take this supplement with a meal, I think it is best to take it on an empty stomach so that it does not compete with other amino acids.

•**Beta glucan.** Derived from yeast or mushroom extracts, beta glucans are naturally occurring polysaccharides—chains of sugar molecules linked together—that activate the soldiers of your immune system known as macrophages. Once activated, macrophages gobble up viruses and signal the rest of the immune system to stand at attention. Various studies have shown that beta glucan supplementation reduces the number of symptomatic cold episodes…reduces upper-respiratory symptoms in colds and other infections…and reduces sleep difficulties caused by colds. In one study, 75 marathon runners between the ages of 18 and 53 took either 250 mg or 500 mg of a commercial form of beta glucan called Wellmune WGP, which is yeast-derived, or a placebo every day for four weeks post-marathon, a time when the immune system can become run

down from overexertion. Those in the beta glucan groups reported significantly fewer upper-respiratory symptoms, increased energy and better overall health compared with the placebo recipients. Beta glucan supplements also can help combat the immunosuppressive effects of daily stress.

Daily dose: Aim for 250 mg to 500 mg for prevention and treatment.

Try: California Gold Nutrition Wellmune Beta-Glucan, 250 mg ($26 for 90 capsules).

More from Mark A. Stengler, NMD

If You Catch a Cold... Pelargonium

Should you catch a cold, you can give Pelargonium sidoides a try. This South African plant, known as umckaloabo, effectively relieves cold symptoms, sinusitis, sore throat and bronchitis. It is available in syrup, drops, powder and chewable tablets.

Try: Nature's Way Umcka ColdCare Soothing Hot Drink Packets in Lemon flavor ($10.99 for 10 packets)…Nature's Way Umcka Cold-Care Cherry syrup ($15.99 for four ounces)… or Integrative Therapeutics V Clear EPs 7630 Original Flavor syrup ($16 for four ounces). Follow package directions for dosing.

After a COVID-19 Infection: Healing Your Brain and Body

Laurie Steelsmith, ND, LAc, medical director of Steelsmith Natural Health Center in Honolulu, where she has a busy private practice, and is an associate clinical professor at Bastyr University. She is coauthor of three books—*Natural Choices for Women's Health, Great Sex, Naturally* and *Growing Younger Every Day.* DrSteelsmith.com

---

Chances are, your health, along with the wellness of your loved ones, has been on the forefront of your mind for well over a year—and that may be putting it mildly. How could it not? The pandemic that's swept the globe has, as of writing this, infected 176 million people and taken 3.8 million lives, placing the strength of our bodies to withstand such a rampant illness above everything else.

For a good reason, too: The "novel" coronavirus is truly novel. Scientific papers are published nearly daily, with each new piece of information showing how new COVID-19 is, operating like no other pathogen we have ever known. And yet what we do know is that the virus can wreak widespread havoc, impacting the lungs, kidneys, liver, GI tract, and our ability to cope peacefully and contentedly with life.

We also know that, in some people who have recovered from a COVID-19 infection, they have won the war—so to speak—but are left feeling tired, moody, and depressed, just as they may be experiencing alterations in their ability to concentrate or sleep.

If you are one of the millions who has been infected with COVID-19 and are feeling the same, you're likely searching for ways to mend your brain and body as compassionately and expediently as possible. While effective vaccines for COVID-19 now exist, there is no cure or treatment for lingering symptoms. So here are a number of ways you can nourish yourself back to health. *Here are four pillars that may help you along the way...*

1. Establish Foundational Health

Whether I'm treating someone with COVID-19 or estrogen dominance, I treat my patients from their scalp to their toes. Meaning, I don't want to just mitigate or help treat the dominating symptoms, but encourage full-body—and mind—health.

The key to this? Eating wisely, exercising often, sleeping restfully, hydrating always, dealing with life's challenges smartly, detoxifying regularly, and thinking well.

A brush with an infection—or an all-out battle—is often an ideal time to honestly assess where you are in these terms. Do you need to add more vegetables to your plate? Move your body more frequently? Give up your nightly glass of wine for the sake of a better night's sleep? Drink more water? Decompress on daily stresses, and pay special mind to your emotional and mental health?

As you work on restoring your body, make sure that you prioritize diet, manageable exercise and mind/spirit health. Healing starts with holistic health, and lifestyle changes, both big and small, can help you achieve this.

2. Rebuild Tissues from Inflammation and Oxygen Starvation

When a person infected with COVID-19 (or SARS-CoV-2, as it's officially called) projects virus-filled droplets—say, through a cough or a sneeze—and someone else breathes them in, the virus enters the nose and throat where it can then gain entry into the cell through its receptor, called ACE2. These receptors are found throughout the body. The virus then takes over the cell, makes multiple copies of itself, and invades other cells. If the immune system is incapable of fighting off this initial wave of trespassers, COVID-19 makes its way down the windpipe and into the lungs, where it can turn fatal.

For some, COVID-19 may initiate an inflammatory or cytokine storm—an overzealous immune response that does more harm than good. For others, it may result in damage to the heart and kidneys. Some may experience the whole range of symptoms; others may have only a dry cough, for example, or body aches. For others still, the virus may eventually lead to mood changes such as anxiety, depression, fatigue, and insomnia. Some people have reported post-traumatic stress disorder (PTSD) symptoms.

No matter how COVID-19 affected your body—from aches to heart or kidney damage—one of the unifying complications of COVID-19 is that it can cause both oxygen deprivation and systemic and specific inflammation.

To nurture yourself towards wellness, the inflammation and oxygen deficit your body has gone through must be addressed. *First, I would urge you to take anti-inflammatory healing herbs and supplements...*

• **Curcumin**—the main active ingredient in turmeric—has tremendous antioxidant and anti-inflammatory effects; I recommend 1,000 mg three times daily for six to eight weeks.

• **Cordyceps sinensis** has long been used in Traditional Chinese Medicine to soothe the lungs, and present-day research demonstrates that it may be "a useful approach for COPD therapy," the National Institutes of Health reports. I would recommend 1,000 mg three times a day for six to eight weeks.

To bring your kidneys back on line, consider a low-protein diet (protein is a lot of work for the kidneys), hydrate with minerals (Jigsaw, for example, has a good electrolyte powder that you can toss into your water), or drink celery juice—it's high in the nutrients your body needs for wellness, including potassium, folate and Vitamins A, K and C. Note that the juice is more concentrated than eating the vegetable and most people can't eat enough celery to reap its full range of benefits.

Additionally, IV nutrient therapies can help rebuild your immune system and support damaged tissues. Also known as Myers Cocktails, these therapeutic concoctions, administered intravenously, are chock-full of essential vitamins and nutrients, including vitamin C, magnesium (which your blood needs for energy) and B-complex. Another option is to get intravenous infusions of glutathione—the potent antioxidant that supports immune function and regenerates vitamins C and E. It also aids in detoxification and inflammation.

After an infection of any kind, the liver needs to be given some TLC too. Operating as your body's waste system—detoxification starts with your liver—its health is imperative to recovery and wellness. You can urge it towards restoration through diet (think: beet greens, lemon, dandelion greens, and dandelion root tea) and by using castor oil packs. (Place a castor oil pack on your abdomen near your liver, which is located underneath your diaphragm on the right-hand side of your body, apply a heating pad on top of it, and rest for 20 minutes.) This can encourage the liver to "get moving," and may help accelerate the toxin-elimination process.

Also, given that COVID-19 does a number on the lungs, increasing oxygen utilization is paramount to healing your body and regaining your energy. To this end, hyperbaric oxygen therapy could work wonders, in that it helps increase oxygen concentration in the tissues and fortifies the body's immune system. Another option for post-COVID patients who have the resources is an Exercise With Oxygen Training device. Also known as an EWOT, it helps your cells absorb more oxygen when you exercise, thereby putting you on the path towards recovery.

COVID-19 can also infect a person through the GI tract because it is rich in ACE 2 receptors. Roughly 20 percent or more of patients have diarrhea, while others have reported vomiting, abdominal pain, and a loss of appetite. To get your intestines back on track, turn to probiotic foods (such as yogurt and miso), eat pomegranate, drink green tea, take a probiotic supplement, and fuel up on foods high in quercetin—an antioxidant, found in many grains, fruits, and vegetables (including apples, onions, kale, and spinach), that increases gut microbial diversity.

Remember: the more varied your intestinal garden, the healthier you will be.

Lastly, I would urge you to consider acupuncture and/or acupressure. The ancient technique works with the body's own healing mechanisms to promote overall wellness. We don't know exactly how acupuncture works, but we do know that people have had great benefit from acupuncture treatments for a wide range of conditions. It has been used for thousands of years in Traditional Chinese medicine. If someone is weak, tired, and exhausted after a massive flu or illness, such as COVID-19, acupuncture could help to restore the body. Acupuncture is done by a licensed practitioner who puts small needles into acupuncture points which are on meridians, or highways of energy, in the body. There are acupuncture treatments designed specifically to help with boosting Qi—the vital force—or for emotional issues like anxiety.

3. Support Your Adrenals

Your adrenal glands—which sit like little party hats on top of your kidneys—are responsible for a number of critical bodily functions, from releasing sex hormones to impacting our physical energy. After an episode as challenging as a viral infection, especially one of COVID-19's magnitude, your adrenals may be fatigued. Why? Because your adrenals respond to stress, such as stress of an illness, by pumping out hormones like cortisol and adrenaline, effectively burning out the glands and leaving you worn out.

To repair your adrenals and rediscover your energy, you should aim to eat three meals and two snacks, made up of whole foods, daily. Now is not the time to fast, or eat light—your body needs nutrients to repair itself, and your blood sugar and cortisol (stress hormone which is released when you fast) needs to be kept at an even keel. At the same time, avoid all sugar, including high-glycemic fruit, such as watermelon, raisins, dates and bananas, and foods with hidden sugars, including white rice, white bread and fried foods—all can ravage your immune system.

In addition, take 500 mg of pantothenic acid (vitamin B5) twice a day for six weeks, then taper off to 500 mg once a day for one month—the vitamin has been shown to improve stress resilience in animal studies. Ginsengs are also the gold stars when it comes to repairing the adrenals, and should be taken according to your constitution or body type. A good measure of this? Your tongue. If your tongue is red, dry and thin—and you have relapsing fevers—take American Ginseng. If your tongue is pale and coated in white, take Panax Ginseng. For each, take 500 mg twice a day for six to eight weeks.

4. Nourish Your Emotional Health.

As mentioned, increasing evidence reveals that those who have been infected with COVID-19 are at risk for a slew of emotional complications—not just because of the trauma it can cause (it's nerve-wracking to be one of the virus's victims) but also because the virus literally impacts the brain: As *Psychology Today* reports, "There is some evidence that coronavirus does attack the brain. According to a paper by Adbul Mannan Baig, 'the brain has been reported to express ACE2 receptors that have been detected over glial cells

and neurons, which makes them a potential target of COVID-19' and patients have had it reported in the cerebral spinal fluid." In addition to neurological manifestations, people who have been infected with COVID-19 have experienced panic attacks (especially at night), crippling anxiety (isolation from others, in this case, can be harmful) and the post-viral blues.

To diminish these symptoms, introduce movement to your life again. You may be feeling too weak for a long run, but even a leisurely walk can increase positive brain chemicals. In addition, moving your body is associated with a healthy immune response.

The mood-boosting and adrenal-supportive herb called rhodiola, meanwhile, helps fight fatigue and may reduce the symptoms of depression. (The recommended dose is 100 to 170 mg of the herb in a standardized form containing 2.6 percent rosavin.) The supplement SAMe—or S-adenosyl-methionine—is another safe bet for managing the symptoms of depression. It boosts neurotransmitter synthesis along with Vitamins B12 and folate. I recommend 800 mg, taken in the morning with food, for six to eight weeks.

Above all, rest. Jumping immediately back into life may be tempting, but you need to give yourself the time, space, and permission to convalesce. You have survived something huge. Honor that.

Restorative Yoga Is the New Power Yoga

Caren Baginski, author of *Restorative Yoga: Relax. Restore. Re-energize.* She has been teaching yoga and meditation since 2009 and is trained in yoga nidra as well as restorative and vinyasa yoga and soon will complete her certification in yoga therapy. You can subscribe to her YouTube channel, which offers free restorative yoga videos. CarenBaginski.com

I f you've ever taken a yoga class, you know the routine. You move through a series of postures, stretching and twisting and building strength and flexibility. At the end of each session, you lie in Savasana (Corpse Pose), tired but feeling good.

Restorative yoga is different. It doesn't involve moving. You don't even stretch. Instead, you get into each pose and stay still for five minutes or so, focusing on your breath in a mindful way. As your body gradually realigns itself during the pose, your breathing and heart rate slow. You calm down and experience the same deep well-being, only with a lot less effort. Restorative yoga may feel passive, but it's more like active relaxation—and the perfect antidote to your busy, super-scheduled life.

Restorative Yoga Basics

There are four essentials to restorative yoga…

• **Stillness.** Rather than push yourself to the edge, you settle into a pose and let your body open up, taking all of the tension out of the muscles so that they are free to relax. To help in the process, props are used to gently hold your body in that particular pose. You can buy yoga-specific ones or simply use items that you already have.

• **A dimly lit practice space.** When you withdraw from sensory overload, it's easier to rediscover your body's natural rhythm. Create this environment by turning down the lights, drawing the shades and/or using an eye covering during practice.

• **A quiet space.** Noisy environments can increase the body's stress-hormone levels. Opt for silence, which relaxes the brain even better than soothing music or nature sounds.

• **Staying comfortably warm.** Your body will naturally cool down as you stay still. You may want to keep your socks on and cover up with a blanket as you practice.

3 Restorative Poses

Practicing for 20 minutes a day will help train your body and your brain to become calm more easily. Some poses may compress the abdominal region, so make sure you have not eaten for at least two hours before you get on your mat to allow food to digest. To practice these poses, you'll need a yoga mat, two to three blankets, a yoga strap (or belt or scarf), two yoga bolsters or regular bed pillows and an eye covering (such as an eye pillow or washcloth). Many people choose to practice in the evening to wind down before bed, but experiment and see what works best for your routine.

Legs Up the Wall: This pose helps ease tired leg muscles, reduce swelling in the legs, lower blood pressure and decrease stress.

1. Preparation. Fold one blanket into a large square, and place it on a mat that is set

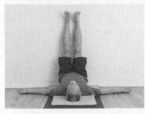

perpendicular against the wall. That will cushion your hips. Take another blanket, fold it into a slightly smaller square and place it in the middle of the mat to provide support for your head. Have your eye covering nearby. Set a timer for 10 minutes.

2. Sit on your left hip with your back against the wall and legs tucked away from your mat. Plant your hands on the mat in front of your body, thread the left arm under the right one to help you tuck and roll until your legs are up against the wall. Your goal is to lie on the floor with your legs up the wall and your back/pelvis area flat on the floor (shown above).

3. As you look upward, set your ankles, knees and hips in a line. Relax your feet with toes neither pointed nor flexed. If your legs are splaying outward, take your strap or scarf, tie it around your calves and corral your legs so that they are hips' width apart but in a straight line.

4. Put on your eye covering, or simply close your eyes. Open your arms in a V-shape by your sides, palms up. Breathe fully into your abdomen and lungs for three rounds of breath, using your exhalations to relax your face, lips and finally your whole body.

5. Rest in silence, breathing naturally. If your legs tingle or feel numb, bring the soles of your feet together in a butterfly shape and lower your legs until the feeling returns. Then place them against the wall again.

6. When you're ready to get out of the pose, wiggle your toes. Bend each knee one at a time, and slowly walk your feet down the wall. Once you can reach your legs comfortably, slip off the strap if you're using one.

7. Rest with your knees bent and feet against the wall. Slide your legs down from the wall, lift one arm over the head, slip off the eye covering, and slowly roll to that side. Rest on your side in a fetal position for as long as necessary.

8. Roll into a seated position on the blanket, and take a moment to reflect on how you feel.

Mountain Brook: This gentle backbend opens up your chest and shoulders, improves breathing and eases tension in the throat while boosting a low mood.

1. Preparation. Fold two blankets into skinny rectangles as wide as your yoga mat, and stack them on top of each other on one-third of the mat. Take the third blanket, 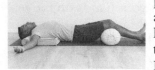 place it four inches away from the blanket stack and toward the top of your mat. Roll it up halfway or all the way to support your neck. Place the bolster near the bottom of your mat. Set a timer for five minutes.

2. Sit in between the bolster and the blanket stack, and drape your legs so that your knees are over the bolster and your legs are flat on the mat.

3. Lie back, placing your shoulder blades on top of the blanket stack but making sure your lower back isn't touching the stack at all. Rest your neck on top of the roll.

4. Extend your arms, palms up, into a T-shape in the space between the blankets. Your chin should be slightly higher than your forehead, but if that's uncomfortable, change the roll so that your chin and forehead are level. Make any adjustments necessary to become fully comfortable. Your hips will be grounded on the floor.

5. Close your eyes and visualize your body as a mountain brook, flowing over the props. Breathe in fully through your nostrils, counting to four. Breathe out slowly through your nose, counting to eight. Keep breathing at a comfortable pace, with the exhales longer than the inhales.

6. Begin to breathe naturally and just be still in the pose.

7. Guide yourself back by breathing deeply in and out. Bending one knee at a time, anchor your feet on the bolster. Roll the bolster away from your body until your feet touch the mat. Gently slide the blanket roll to one side so that your head rests upon the mat.

8. Pull your knees inward and roll onto one side, using one arm as a pillow to cradle your head. Rest for a few seconds. Inhaling, use your hands to push yourself up slowly to a comfortable seat. Observe how you feel after this pose.

Supported Side Lying Stretch: Like all restorative yoga poses, this two-sided stretch calms the nervous system, reducing stress and inflammation. And because this pose affects the digestive organs—the liver, gall bladder, spleen and stomach—it's particularly good for improving gut health. After all, when you're angry or anxious, you definitely feel it in your stomach!

1. Preparation. Fold the blankets into two thick double squares, and stack them on 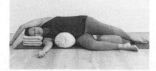 top of each other to support your head at the top of your mat. Place the round bolster in the middle of the mat and the flat bolster at the bottom. Set a timer for three minutes.

2. Sit in between the round and flat bolsters. Lay with your left hip on the floor, your right leg on top of the flat bolster, and place your left leg in front of the bolster at the edge of your mat.

3. Hold onto the round bolster with your right hand as you inhale, wedging the bolster into your waist. Exhale, sliding your left arm forward, palm up, as you lie on your side. The blankets should be supporting your neck and head. Make sure the top of your head lines up with your shoulder, hip and right foot.

4. Your right arm can rest against your hip. Or for more opening, send your right arm over your head so that your right bicep rests against your ear and your hand touches the floor. (If your hand can't reach, place a blanket or block under it for support.)

5. Close your eyes. Inhale fully. As you exhale, release all effort in your body. Breathe naturally, and rest in silence.

6. When you are ready to switch sides, return your right hand to the space next to your left hand. Press against the floor, inhale and lift up slowly sideways. Turn away from the round bolster, and keep turning to come to the other side. Repeat the pose on this side, again setting the timer for three minutes.

7. Once complete, sit up slowly into a comfortable seated position. Place your hands to your heart, with your right hand stacking on top of your left hand. Close your eyes, and connect with your heartbeat. As you take deeper breaths, feel the expansiveness in your waist, ribs and chest. Thank yourself for taking this time to support yourself in self-care so that you may continue to be a support for others.

Photos of yoga poses: © DK: Jimena Peck

Morning Light May Speed Healing After Mild Concussion

A jolt to the head can upset the body's internal clock, causing headaches, sleep problems and mental fogginess.

Promising: 30 minutes of exposure to blue light, such as sunlight, every morning for six weeks can reset that inner clock and help return sleep to normal. Since the brain repairs itself during sleep, this could mean faster recovery from a concussion.

William D. "Scott" Killgore, PhD, is professor of psychiatry, medical imaging and psychology at University of Arizona College of Medicine, Tucson. His study was published in *Neurobiology of Disease*.

Natural Cure for an Abnormal Pap Smear

Andrew Rubman, ND, medical director of Southbury Clinic for Traditional Medicines in Southbury, Connecticut. SouthburyClinic.com He is author of the blog "Nature Doc's Patient Diary" at Bottom LineInc.com

---

The patient: Elsie, a married woman in her late 40s taking good, preventive care of herself.

Why she came to see me: She has been a patient for many years and chose to have my "go to" gynecologist in town perform a routine gynecological exam. The Pap findings were characterized as "ASCUS," or atypical squamous cells of uncertain significance—mildly abnormal cell changes that may be solely due to inflammation or the very beginning of pre-cancerous changes, or a combination of both. The condition may be treated in a number of ways by conventional physicians and naturopathic physicians, either separately or working in tandem.

How I evaluated her: Elsie and I had a thorough discussion about cellular pathology and the effects of inflammation on cell division—the more prolonged and intense inflammation is, the more frequently cells divide and the more probable the disorganized division that characterizes cancer becomes. After careful consideration of her options offered by both me and the gynecologist, she decided to use natural interventions initially and schedule a follow-up exam in three months with the gynecologist to include a specialized direct microscopic evaluation of areas of her cervix in question with a device called a colposcope. If after the colposcopy and a follow-up tissue sampling the tissue was still exhibiting the dysregulated changes, ablation or deeper removal of the tissue would probably be advised by the gynecologist.

How we addressed her problem: I provided her with a probiotic powder and specialized vaginal suppositories containing botanical extracts in a cocoa butter base designed to normalize the microbial environment in the area and help shed the disturbed tissue that were underlying the inflammatory changes seen. This treatment would be continued daily for at least one month, discontinued for a month, and reinstituted again for a month, and then followed up with a repeat Pap and considered colposcopy. This therapy has a two-fold benefit of potentially "curing" the tissue by exfoliating the atypical cells, quenching the inflammation and, at the very least, "unmasking" any remaining pre-cancerous changes that may have been lurking under the surface.

The patient's progress: At the three-month follow-up with the gynecologist, Elsie showed entirely normal tissue both by repeat Pap test and the additional colposcopy.

Natural Therapies That Ease Parkinson's Symptoms

Michael Edson, MS, LAc, a licensed acupuncturist, certified herbalist and qi gong teacher based in Yonkers, New York. He is the author of *Natural Parkinson's Support: Your Guide to Preventing & Managing Parkinson's.* NaturalEyeCare.com

If you or a loved one has Parkinson's disease (PD), you want to do everything possible to control the brutal symptoms, such as tremors, stiff muscles and anxiety.

Until recently, the standard treatment regimen mainly paired powerful medications, such as *carbidopa/levodopa* (Sinemet) and *pramipexole* (Mirapex), with exercises to ease symptoms.

Now: More people with PD are adding gentle, nondrug therapies to the mix. Essential oils and acupuncture are two safe options with a growing body of evidence—and clinical success—to support their use alone or in combination as a complement to PD treatment. *For example...**

Essential Oils for Tremors, Anxiety

When using essential oils, nonmotor symptoms, such as anxiety, often improve within a few days. Tremors may require a few weeks of regular use before showing improvement.

• **Frankincense.**

Scent: Spicy, woodsy.

Helps with: Tremors.

In PD, nerve cells in the brain that produce dopamine, a neurotransmitter that regulates many motor and cognitive functions, progressively die off, leading to tremors. In a 2019 animal study published in *Avicenna Journal of Phytomedicine,* frankincense was shown to have anti-inflammatory and antioxidant properties that protected dopamine-producing neurons, improving the motor impairments of PD.

• **Bergamot.**

Scent: Citrus.

Helps with: Anxiety and agitation.

Perhaps due to its nonsedating, analgesic effects, bergamot essential oil is used to relieve anxiety and agitation in people with PD. Researchers also are investigating bergamot's ability to control agitation in patients with dementia.

How to Use Essential Oils for PD

To get the most benefit from essential oils, they are best applied to the skin of the person with PD. This combines the calming, therapeutic qualities of touch with the benefit of inhaling the healing scent. Even though up to 96 percent of newly diagnosed patients with PD have lost some degree of their sense of smell, essential oil is still beneficial because the oil's healing compounds not only penetrate the skin but also are still inhaled,

*Consult your physician before trying these therapies—especially if you have a chronic medical condition such as high blood pressure.

even if the scent is not as strong as it would be to a healthy person.

What to do: Add a few drops of your essential oil to one ounce of a carrier oil (such as almond, olive or coconut oil), and massage it two to three times a day into your or your loved one's neck, temples (being sure to avoid the eyes), arms, legs and/or soles of the feet...use a diffuser...or, with agitated or aggressive patients, add the drops to a cotton ball and discreetly pin it to the upper half of his/her shirt so that it's inhaled.

Important: Do an allergy test before full application. Apply a small amount of the diluted oil to an area of skin, and check for an allergic reaction after 24 hours. (Allergic reactions can, in rare cases, occur several days later.) Never ingest an essential oil. If you want to use more than one essential oil, wait at least three minutes between oil applications.

Good essential oil brands: Rocky Mountain Oils...dōTERRA...and Plant Therapy.

Acupuncture

Acupuncture is based on a system of energy pathways, called meridians, through which life force, or qi, flows. When these pathways become blocked, pain, illness and degeneration can develop, according to traditional Chinese medicine (TCM). By inserting ultra-thin, stainless-steel needles along various meridians, acupuncturists strive to rebalance the flow of energy to restore health—or, in the case of PD, improve symptoms.

Scientific evidence: In a study published in *CNS Neuroscience & Therapeutics* involving 519 patients with PD, acupuncture improved motor symptoms, such as tremor, rigidity and slowed movement, and "markedly improved" nonmotor symptoms, including sleep problems and depression, according to research. When acupuncture was used with levodopa, the medication was more effective.

With acupuncture, nonmotor symptoms often improve within one to six treatments, while tremors and other motor symptoms may require about a dozen treatments.

To find a licensed acupuncturist, consult the National Certification Commission for Acupuncture and Oriental Medicine, NCCAOM.org.

Let Nature Be Your Medicine

Nadine Mazzola, certified guide and director of New England Nature and Forest Therapy Consulting. NatureandForestTherapy.org

If these stressful times tempt you to binge on hours of Netflix, you're not alone. But there's a much healthier option. With a Japanese practice known as "shinrin-yoku" (*translation:* "forest bathing"), you can melt away the pressures.

Why head outdoors? One good reason: Americans typically spend approximately 90 percent of their time indoors.

A city park is pleasant, but it's not the same as a forest or any area that's dense with vegetation and wildlife. When Japanese researchers compared people who took leisurely forest walks with those in urban environments, the forest group had 12.4 percent lower levels of the stress hormone cortisol and 5.8 percent lower average heart rates.

For the uninitiated, there's "forest therapy," in which a trained guide helps clients to slow down (a three-hour session is ideal) and use their senses to experience natural landscapes, explains Nadine Mazzola, a certified guide and director of New England Nature and Forest Therapy Consulting. The guide will encourage you to listen closely to the sounds of birds and other creatures...notice the way the sunshine illuminates the colors of leaves and rocks...and enjoy the subtle scents carried by the wind. To find a guide near you, visit the Association of Nature & Forest Therapy website, NatureandForestTherapy.org.

Note: When outdoors, be sure to practice any "social distancing" that may be in effect due to COVID-19.

Irritable Bowel Syndrome Eased by Walking

College students "mildly affected" with IBS reduced the severity of their symptoms from a five to a four (on a scale of one to seven—with anything above five indicating severe symptoms) simply by walking. Those who walked 9,500 steps a day had 50 percent less severe symptoms compared with those who walked 4,000 steps.

Study by researchers at Graduate School of Health Science, Saitama Prefectural University, Japan, published in *PLOS One.*

Stopping Inflammation Is More Important Than Ever: 9 Ways to Reverse Chronic Illness, Prevent Infection and More

Jacob Teitelbaum, MD, board-certified internist, holistic physician and nationally known expert in the fields of chronic fatigue syndrome, fibromyalgia, sleep and pain. Based in Hawaii, he is author of numerous books, including *Real Cause, Real Cure, The Complete Guide to Beating Sugar Addiction* and *The Fatigue and Fibromyalgia Solution,* as well as the phone app *Cures A–Z.* Vitality101.com

Medical experts have known for years that many serious medical conditions tie back to chronic inflammation. That includes the most significant and dangerous conditions in modern life, such as cardiovascular disease, cancer, asthma, diabetes and autoimmune diseases including rheumatoid arthritis, lupus and inflammatory bowel disease. Chronic inflammation also makes you more vulnerable to acute viruses, such as the common cold, flu and COVID-19 that has taken over the globe.

Isn't it time that you actually do something to bring your body back into balance? You don't need medication to do that! *Here*

are the most important lifestyle changes you can make to help you feel great for years to come...

●**It's all about the food.** Nutrient-filled foods help your body work at its best while "junk" foods make your body angry and inflamed, just as bad fuel gums up the engine of your car. Start by increasing your intake of colorful produce, seafood and nuts, which contain antioxidants and other nutrients that keep inflammation in check. Even a handful of blueberries on your morning cereal and three to four servings of salmon or tuna each week can have a dramatic effect. The Mediterranean diet, which focuses on colorful fresh vegetables and fruit, healthy oils and nuts, is an ideal model for reducing inflammation.

On the other hand, get rid of refined carbs including sugar and white flour. Having sweets, fruit juices and soft drinks, with their high levels of sugar (even natural sugar) and high-fructose corn syrup, are like throwing gas on a fire when it comes to creating inflammation in your body. Also nix trans fats such as those found in Crisco, margarine and processed foods, all of which can contribute to inflammation.

Vegan and vegetarian diets are great choices for reducing inflammation, but if you're having meat, opt for grass-fed beef, which is higher in omega-3s, instead of inflammation-fueling grain-fed beef.

Warning: Preparation methods are also important. Fast-food fried fish has lost most of its omega-3s. Some good news? Certain dairy products, such as yogurt, are associated with decreased inflammation.

●**Watch the alcohol.** A landmark *Lancet* study found that both nondrinkers and heavy drinkers had higher levels of C-reactive protein, an inflammation marker associated with cardiovascular disease, than people who drank moderately. (Moderate drinking is no more than one drink per day for women and no more than two drinks per day for men.) Red wine offers the most potential benefits. Although people who have one or two drinks a day live longer than teetotalers, there are numerous other ways to get these benefits without the alcohol. So have it if you can enjoy it in moderation.

• **Increase your omega-3 intake.** Most people don't get enough omega-3 fatty acids, the anti-inflammatory polyunsaturated fats that have been shown to help prevent or treat cardiovascular disease, Alzheimer's disease, arthritis, cancer and more. Your body cannot produce its own omega-3 fatty acids, so it all must come from your diet. Oily fish such as salmon, tuna, sardines, herring and mackerel all are good choices—or consider taking a daily fish oil supplement.

Tip: When you're choosing a fish oil supplement, look for one that is all omega-3. Most fish oils contain other oils that you don't need.

*One I like:** Vectomega from Terry Naturally. Algae-sourced omega-3s can be effective if one is vegetarian.

• **Take some curcumin.** A chemical found in the golden-hued curry spice turmeric, curcumin is a noted anti-inflammatory. However, unless you eat curry a few times a day, you likely won't get enough of the compound, and it is notoriously hard for your body to absorb and reap the benefits of curcumin if it's not taken in combination with a fat. Curcumin supplements that add back some of the turmeric oil are much easier for your body to use and digest.

One I like: CuraMed from Terry Naturally.

• **Nutritionally optimize your own immune function.** The key nutrients for your immune system are zinc (15 mg a day), vitamin A (2,500 international units/IU a day), vitamin D (1,000 IU a day) and vitamin C (200 mg to 500 mg a day). But don't subscribe to a "more is better" approach. For example, doses of vitamin A over 8,000 IU a day can trigger birth defects.

Note: Use the retinol version of vitamin A (the type found in fish oil) for optimal results.

*Dr. Teitelbaum receives consulting fees for some of the supplements mentioned in this article and donates the money to charity.

Two multivitamin supplements I like: ViraPro from Terry Naturally, and the Energy Revitalization System vitamin powder from Enzymatic Therapy—both offer optimal amounts of zinc, selenium and vitamins A, C, D and E.

• **Reduce your body's chemical load.** Chemicals in your environment can trigger your immune system and cause inflammation. When you have the option, choose natural household products that can do the job—or at least reduce your use of chemicals.

Examples: If you need to use insecticide to deal with a bug problem in your home, try to spray it just on the outside of your home or buy a natural one. Choose natural cleaners instead of chemical-laden ones. Skip the air freshener, dryer sheets and scented candles.

• **Get out in the sunshine.** The vitamin D your body produces from a little time in the sun also has been shown to help boost immunity. Pair it with a little moderate exercise—such as a walk or a bike ride in the park—and you'll get even more benefits.

• **Get good sleep.** We all know we should be getting seven to nine hours of sleep every night, but how many of us actually do? People who consistently get too little sleep have increased inflammation activity in their bodies. This is no surprise—even in short-term studies, researchers found higher levels of inflammation markers such as white blood cells. Try to get the amount of sleep that leaves you feeling your best.

• **Tune out the stressors.** Stress plays an important role in developing chronic inflammation. When you feel safe, your immune system is at ease, and that eases inflammation. But if your body is feeling threatened constantly, your immune system goes into overdrive. Try to tune out things that make you feel fearful—such as the news, for instance—and focus on the things that make you feel happy and safe.

Helpful: Meditation, yoga and breathing exercises all can help you feel less stressed.

Chronic Indigestion Relieved with Acupuncture

Andrew Rubman, ND, is medical director of Southbury Clinic for Traditional Medicines in Southbury, Connecticut. SouthburyClinic.com He is author of the "Nature Doc's Patient Diary" blog at BottomLineInc. com.

The patient: Xian was a 36-year-old male construction worker in the Chinese city of Guilin who was having stomach complaints.

Why he came to see me: Perhaps better stated, why I came to see him. I was consulting and lecturing in Guangxi Province, PRC and was invited to attend rounds at the Acupuncture Hospital of Guilin. Xian was one of the patients who came to the clinic. Through my translator, I found that Xian's issues involved chronic indigestion and that conventional medicine in China had found no ulcers or negative findings in his colonoscopy. He had found traditional acupuncture and moxibustion (treatment using smoldering mugwort to heat areas of the body and warm needles) suited him well. Although my translator remained with the group during Xian's treatment, I preferred to communicate with the Chinese physicians with gestures and have them explain to the patients in Mandarin what we were thinking and what treatments would be provided. I felt that this novel approach would intrigue Xian and also show deference to my Chinese colleagues.

How I evaluated him: Using my skills in Chinese medical diagnosis and treatment taught to me as a component of my naturopathic medical education, I performed an energetic evaluation using palpation, examination of the face, eyes, lips, tongue and mouth. Further, and perhaps most importantly, I assessed the wrist pulses on each arm. The area on the wrist around where most people feel their pulse, above the joint with the hand on the "thumb side," can be used to identify and discern three discrete locations, each having a deep and superficial character-

istic. Thus 12 pulses all together are used to determine imbalances and conditions within the context of traditional Chinese diagnoses.

How we addressed his problem: By letting my colleagues closely observe what I was evaluating and "communicating" my findings through my gestures and expressions with each of the 12 pulses, we were able to decide on where to place the acupuncture needles and where to burn the moxa (mugwort) over specific spots on his belly. I was offered the opportunity to place the needles into Xian but deferred to the senior physician who was on rounds with the group as a sign of respect for his station. All of my observations and suggestions were appreciated and guided the therapeutic applications.

The patient's progress: After the visit to the hospital concluded and pleasantries were exchanged, the physicians had the translator express their appreciation for my participation in the rounds, their delight in my chosen method of communication with them, their appreciation of my training in their art and perhaps most importantly, the fact that Xian loved the attention and greatly benefitted from our ministrations! Xian commented that he appreciated my participation in his assessment and guidance in his treatment and how he felt that this session was particularly effective.

Curcumin Effective for Ulcerative Colitis

Study titled "Novel Bioenhanced Curcumin with Mesalamine for Induction of Clinical and Endoscopic Remission in Mild-to-Moderate Ulcerative Colitis," by researchers at Department of Gastroenterology, Asian Institute of Gastroenterology, published in *Journal of Clinical Gastroenterology.*

Curcumin is an active ingredient in turmeric, a spice from the ginger family that has become a popular supplement for pain relief. Turmeric has a long history of use in traditional Indian and Chinese medicine to treat many disorders, including digestive conditions. One area where curcumin may have a significant benefit is as an add-on therapy for the chronic condition ulcerative colitis (UC), an inflammatory bowel disease that causes ulcers in the colon and rectum. Symptoms include pain, diarrhea, fatigue, fever and weight loss.

Important recent finding: Patients with mild to moderate UC who take curcumin experience significant improvement, according to research from the Asian Institute of Gastroenterology. The study is reported in the *Journal of Clinical Gastroenterology*. In clinical studies, researchers have had limited success determining the effectiveness of curcumin, since it's not easily absorbed into the bloodstream. Researchers have been developing biologically enhanced curcumin to overcome that limitation.

The study: Sixty-nine patients with mild to moderate UC were equally divided into two groups. One group received curcumin twice per day along with a standard UC medication, *mesalamine*. The other group received mesalamine along with a placebo. Neither the patients nor the researchers knew which patients received the curcumin (known as a randomized double-blind placebo-controlled trial). Mesalamine is an anti-inflammatory drug often used as front-line therapy for mild to moderate UC.

The researchers looked at three outcomes—clinical remission (symptom-free), endoscopic remission (ulcer-free on colonoscopy) and clinical response (improvement of symptoms). *These were the key findings...*

•**At six weeks,** the curcumin group had a clinical remission of about 44 percent and an endoscopic remission of 35 percent compared with no remission in the placebo group.

•**At six weeks,** clinical response was seen in about 53 percent of the curcumin group compared with about 14 percent in the placebo group.

•**After three months,** 56 percent of the curcumin group were in remission, and over 80 percent of them remained in remission at

six and 12 months, compared with no remissions in the placebo group.

The researchers conclude that curcumin as an add-on therapy was superior to a placebo. Their finding supports earlier studies. A 2016 study reported in the journal *Clinical Gastroenterology and Hepatology* found over 50 percent of patients given curcumin along with mesalamine achieved remission compared with no remissions in a placebo group. Both studies found curcumin to be safe as well as effective.

Charcoal: A Versatile Treatment

Jamison Starbuck, ND, is a naturopathic physician in family practice in Missoula, Montana, and producer of *Dr. Starbuck's Health Tips for Kids*, a weekly program on Montana Public Radio, MTPR.org. She is a past president of the American Association of Naturopathic Physicians and a contributing editor to *The Alternative Advisor: The Complete Guide to Natural Therapies and Alternative Treatments*. DrJamison Starbuck.com.

Medicinal-grade activated charcoal (AC) is a versatile, effective, and safe treatment for a variety of conditions. AC is made from wood, coconut shells, or other natural fibers that have been burned at a very high temperature and then "activated" by creating holes and crevices to increase the surface area.

It works as a medicine because it is adsorptive, which means it draws things to itself, such as chemicals, drugs, viruses, and bacteria. It is also inert, which means that it will not enter your bloodstream but will pass through your intestines and leave via stool—taking attached substances with it.

AC is commonly used in emergency rooms (ER) as a treatment for many types of poisoning and overdose. But while it's very effective, it should never be used for poisoning at home. The necessary dosage is extremely high, and there is no guarantee that a product purchased for home use has the same strength as that used in the ER.

There are some home uses, however, that are quite safe as long as you use medicinal-grade AC purchased over-the-counter from a pharmacy or vitamin store. Never ingest charcoal briquettes or charcoal sold for fish tanks, water filters, and other commercial purposes. They can be toxic.

• **Intestinal gas and diarrhea.** Several studies show that AC reduces excessive intestinal gas accumulation, according to the European Food and Safety Authority, which gives a green light to its use. It also appears to have an anti-diarrheal effect. In 2018, researchers reported in *Current Medical Research and Opinion* that it is a suitable treatment that offers fewer side effects than other anti-diarrheal medications.

For an acute bout of painful gas or diarrhea, I recommend taking three to four 250-milligram (mg) charcoal capsules with an 8-ounce glass of water. Repeat in 30 minutes or after every bowel movement as needed for up to 24 hours. Do not use charcoal on a daily basis because it can interfere with the absorption of nutrients and medications. Don't take it within two hours of taking medication, as it may make some medications ineffective.

• **Insect bites.** Relieve the pain, swelling, or itch from bee stings, spider, and fly bites with a charcoal poultice. Open a charcoal capsule into a bowl and add a few drops of water to make a paste. Apply the paste to the bite or sting. Cover with a bandage and leave it on for a few hours. Wash away the charcoal with cool water and repeat if needed. Because it is inert, it will not be absorbed by the skin.

• **Splinters.** Charcoal can help bring a stubborn splinter up and into view where you can remove it with tweezers. Make a poultice as you would with insect bites.

• **Poison ivy.** Mix a tablespoon of charcoal into 8 ounces of water. Soak the affected area in the slurry or pour the slurry over the poison-ivy lesions and cover with plastic wrap for 30 minutes. Repeat as needed.

Face Rash Cured from the Inside Out

Andrew Rubman, ND, is medical director of Southbury Clinic for Traditional Medicines in Southbury, Connecticut. SouthburyClinic.com He is author of the "Nature Doc's Patient Diary" blog at BottomLineInc.com

The patient: "Loretta," a nationally known TV anchor.

Why she came to see me: I was delighted to have an office visit from a media personality I watched regularly on television. I was aware of the fact that for many months a persistent rash on her right cheek had been concealed during her broadcasts quite effectively by the station's makeup artist—still noticeable to my trained eye. A colleague of hers at the Manhattan-based network who has been a patient of mine urged her to come up to my clinic in Southbury, Connecticut, as her rash, while not getting worse, was not getting better despite the treatments from some of "New York's finest" dermatologists.

How I evaluated her: After exchanging pleasantries, we carefully reviewed the history of Loretta's rash as well as her diet, lifestyle and challenging events like relationship or employment changes. Her prior diagnoses and treatments ran the gamut from psoriasis to atopy (a kind of immune-related dermatitis) and topical corticosteroids to "biologics" typically used for autoimmune diseases, the latter she had ardently refused to take.

I explained how quite often the skin mirrored internal issues and treating chronic conditions required both external and internal interventions. What I saw during our first visit presented like a chronic "zymotic" condition (characterized by an overgrowth of yeast and/or fungus) with a minimal contribution of normal surface bacteria.

How we addressed her problem: Since Loretta's job was inherently stressful and she was a "young" 58-year-old woman, I convinced her to take a digestive enzyme formula to not only enhance her system's ability to extract nutrients from her meals, but also to help her liver bind and remove substances that may not have been sufficiently exported via the stool and instead were ending up being "excreted" into her skin.

I also explained that improving the function of her large intestine and its resident microbiome quite often will have a direct impact on the health and resilience of the skin. We discussed and agreed upon an improved diet that included cutting down on hurried commissary fast food, giving up French fries and basing her meals around a large, fresh garden salad with healthy protein and carb "toppings"...a regime of digestive enzymes and immune-enhancing supplements...and naturally derived topical applications for her skin, all of which would gradually improve the outward appearance while addressing the underlying causes of her skin rash.

The patient's progress: Two weeks after our initial appointment, Loretta and I had a video check-in. She reported improvement in both digestion and the appearance of her skin, confirmed by her makeup artist and clearly visible to me as well. Within a month's time the chronic problem on her face was virtually gone. We do stay in touch with periodic consults, but I reminded her that as I see her frequently on television, she can't hide from my scrutiny!

Finding Natural Relief for SIBO

Laurie Steelsmith, ND, LAc, medical director of Steelsmith Natural Health Center in Honolulu, where she has a busy private practice, and is an associate clinical professor at Bastyr University. She is coauthor of three books—*Natural Choices for Women's Health, Great Sex, Naturally* and *Growing Younger Every Day.* DrSteelsmith.com

---

The patient: "Clara," a 39-year-old mother of two.

Why she came to see me: Clara came into my office complaining of intestinal distress, primarily in the form of excessive gas production and alternating constipation and diarrhea.

How I evaluated her: Clara and I began our work together by covering her personal and medical history. "Hardly a fanatic" about her health, as she put it, she nonetheless strived to take care of herself by refraining from alcohol and taking Spin classes four times a week. As the mother of two young children, her time away from work was spent chasing after her daughter and son, who she "never had a problem keeping up with" until she started to not feel well.

Three months earlier, however, she experienced a bout of food poisoning. While it resolved itself within a few days, shortly thereafter she began experiencing a host of symptoms that not only depleted her energy but also caused her incredible intestinal discomfort. In addition to the gas, constipation and diarrhea she initially described, I learned that she suffered from acid reflux, nausea, intestinal bloating and stomach pain, as well as bouts of exhaustion and the blues. Clara had tried a number of "remedies" aimed at mitigating her stomach troubles, including snacking on saltine crackers, drinking ginger ale, avoiding cruciferous vegetables and lentils, following the BRAT diet (bananas, rice, applesauce, toast) and using Alka-Seltzer. These, unfortunately, provided her only a modicum of relief.

To get to the root of her intestinal discomfort, I asked Clara to conduct a breath test from the comfort of her home. The test, called The Lactulose Breath Test for SIBO, gathers a three-hour illustration of intestinal gases that are produced by resident bacteria. As I explained to Clara, when bacteria digest food, they produce gasses that travel through your intestinal walls, into your bloodstream, and ultimately to your lungs, which one then breathes out. Samples from this breath test reveal the amount of hydrogen and methane gas being exhaled, which shows that bacteria are fermenting as well as how much gas they are generating.

What my evaluation revealed: The results from Clara's breath test confirmed what I suspected: She was suffering from Small Intestinal Bacterial Overgrowth. The condition, also known as SIBO, describes imbalanced bacterial growth in one's small intestine.

This means that, in the simplest terms, one has too much bacteria growing where it shouldn't be. These bacteria aren't necessarily a pathogen, or "bad bacteria." It just shouldn't be thriving in the small intestine. When it does set up house there, it can create systemic inflammation and the release of lipopolysaccharides (LPS), which can lead to fatty liver disease, fatigue, symptoms of bladder pain (called interstitial cystitis), joint pain, migraines, skin rashes, mood changes (such as depression and anxiety), acne rosacea, and even restless leg syndrome.

There are a number of reasons why people develop SIBO. Food poisoning—such as in Clara's case—is one of them. Other causes include adhesions after abdominal or intestinal surgery and medications such as opiates, antibiotics, and antacids (or proton-pump inhibitors). Diet and excessive alcohol can also contribute to SIBO. Some people have autoimmune conditions that could contribute to it as well, such as scleroderma and Crohn's disease. Furthermore, SIBO can develop in those who have had a traumatic brain injury, immune suppression, or who are immune compromised. Other possible contributors include having Parkinson's disease, Ehlers-Danlos Syndrome, hypothyroidism, diabetes, parasites, and Lyme or other tick-borne diseases. Having a biotoxin illness related to mold exposure could also contribute to the development of SIBO.

As I told Clara, the constipation and diarrhea she was frequently experiencing from the condition was the result of the gases the bacterial overgrowth was producing—gases that were damaging her migrating motor complex, which helps keep stools moving through the intestines at a steady rate. I also explained that, because the health of one's

microbiome (the microbial world living in a person's intestines) has a direct effect on one's mood, SIBO can contribute to fatigue and depression—the very tiredness and "blues" she was experiencing.

How I addressed her problem: We took a multi-pronged approach to Clara's recovery. *Known as the "5Rs" in natural medicine, it consisted of the following...*

1. Remove.

To remove the overgrowth of bacteria from Clara's microbiome, I urged her to take these botanicals: 500 mg of Berberine (from Golden Seal root) three times a day and 100 mg of oregano oil three times a day. I also prescribed an antibiotic called Rifaximin (550 mg three times a day for 21 days). Additionally, I encouraged her to take what's known as a biofilm buster. Consisting of ingredients such as bismuth, lipoic acid and black cumin seed, this "buster" does precisely what its name implies: It helps break up the "house" the bacteria is residing in inside one's intestines.

In addition, I encouraged her to remove foods that feed unfriendly bacteria. These are known as high FODMAP foods, which stands for Fermentable, Oligosaccharides, Disaccharides, Monosaccharides, and Polyols. The list of high-FODMAP foods include processed foods that contain high-fructose corn syrup, sorbitol and other artificial sweeteners...fruit juices...agave and honey... and condiments such as jam, jelly and relish.

What's more, I asked Clara to "remove" her Standard American Diet. Also called SAD, this diet has an excess of sugar, refined carbohydrates, saturated fats and trans fats— many of the foods she was also giving her children.

2. Replace.

After the first step was complete, I asked Clara to replace her typical diet with low FODMAP foods that are unprocessed and organic whenever possible.

I also urged her to replace her poor eating habits with healthy habits. This meant that, instead of snacking off her children's plates while cleaning up after meals, she would have to sit down and eat—preferably in a serene environment—and thoroughly chew her food. I suggested that she eat three meals per day and avoid snacking in between, which would allow her small intestine to fully empty before she consumed more food. I encouraged her to drink warm lemon water before meals (this "primes" the stomach for digestion by increasing stomach acidity) but to abstain from drinking copious amounts of liquids while eating, as fluids can dilute digestive juices. To further support healthy digestion, I recommended she take digestive enzymes with meals and a carminative, or "anti-gas," tea comprised of fennel and caraway seeds.

3. Re-inoculate.

Next, I encouraged Clara to introduce her microbiome to more of what she needed: Good bacteria. To this end, I urged her to take small amounts of probiotic foods such as kimchee and sauerkraut, and supplement with probiotics (50 billion organisms) with high amounts of lactobacilli and bifidobacteria. Good bacteria need healthy food to eat so I also encouraged her to eat foods high in prebiotics, which help friendly bacteria flourish. These foods include Jerusalem artichoke, cabbage, leeks, chicory root and garlic. After eradicating the undesirable overgrowth of bacteria in her small intestine, she is now able to tolerate some of the forbidden FODMAP foods and prebiotics. Taking "friendly" flora supports a healthy biome and regularity, which in turn can help prevent a recurrence of SIBO.

4. Repair.

As I explained to Clara, her chronically irritated gut wall had led to what's often called leaky gut syndrome. To repair it requires not only the first three steps in the "5R" process but also supplements that organically foster a more resilient gut mucosa. I prescribed one scoop per day of a product called GI Revive. This consists of a blend of ingredients including L-glutamine, N-acetyl glucosamine, Aloe Vera, slippery elm and zinc carnosine,

and works towards naturally encouraging a healthier gut.

5. Rebalance.

I made it clear to Clara that there is life after SIBO—and that a person can prevent it from becoming a chronic condition by cultivating a life that supports health on all levels. With this in mind, I encouraged her to practice self-care, continue going to her Spin classes (and engaging in other forms of exercise), find ways to quiet her mind and relax her body, and eat the best food around.

The patient's progress: Within three months, Clara was feeling healthier than she ever had. By practicing the "5Rs," her symptoms subsided to the point that intestinal distress of any kind was infrequent. Her commitment to whole, organic foods transformed her family meals from chicken nuggets on the run to home-cooked, creative dishes that incorporated nutrient-rich foods—and longer, more satisfying dinners with her husband and children. As for that energy to keep up with her kids? She had it in spades.

Acupuncture Before Surgery Lessens Pain

Brinda Krish, DO, is an anesthesiology resident at Detroit Medical Center. Her research was presented to the American Society of Anesthesiologists.

When 106 veterans underwent surgery for hip replacement, gallbladder removal and other common problems, researchers gave one group "battlefield acupuncture," in which tiny needles are inserted at trigger points on the ear, before their procedures. After surgery, those patients required one-third to one-half as many opioids and reported significantly less pain and much higher satisfaction compared with the control group.

No-Hassle Natural Therapies for Varicose Veins

Jamison Starbuck, ND, is a naturopathic physician in family practice in Missoula, Montana, and producer of *Dr. Starbuck's Health Tips for Kids*, a weekly program on Montana Public Radio, MTPR.org. DrJamisonStarbuck.com.

Purple, blue and red. The more veins I see, the more I say, "This aging I do dread." Writing medical poetry amuses me and helps me cope. In this case, with my varicose and spider veins. I'm not alone, though. It's estimated that about half of adult women have these unsightly veins. Men can have them, too, but develop them much less often.

Some veins are closer to the surface of the skin than arteries, so when they become stretched or damaged, they can look like reddish-purple spider webs (spider veins)… or bluish-purple bulging cords (varicose veins). Spider veins are small, dilated blood vessels that are painless. They most often show up on the face, chest or legs or in places where one has suffered an injury or had a surgery. Fortunately, spider veins don't cause symptoms.

Varicose veins are wider and longer than spider veins and most often appear in the lower legs and ankles. The primary cause is a malfunction of the valves inside the veins, which leads to a buildup of blood. When the pressure is more than the thin vein wall can handle, bulging occurs. Varicose veins can be painless, or they may ache and cause a painful heaviness that's fatiguing. Varicose veins don't cause blood clots, but people who have a lot of them may have a higher incidence of clots due to an unhealthy vascular system.

These vein issues often are blamed on pregnancy, obesity and jobs that involve a lot of standing, but the latest research finds that inflammation, poor circulation and genetic vulnerability are the most common causes of spider veins and varicose veins. Even if you undergo surgery, laser treatment or saline injections, called sclerotherapy, you need to improve blood vessel health, enhance circulation and reduce inflammation or problematic veins will return. *What I advise to help prevent and treat varicose veins and spider veins…*

•**Walk, ride a bike or swim every day.** Gentle exercise that uses the leg muscles helps move blood out of veins in the lower legs. Exercise doesn't reduce existing vein problems, but it does prevent more from developing. If your varicose veins hurt, elevate your legs above your abdomen for five minutes after exercise and/or consider wearing compression stockings.

•**Take supplements that support healthy blood vessels.** I recommend 100 mg of CoQ10…400 IU of vitamin E…1,000 mg of vitamin C…and 300 mg of magnesium citrate daily. Take these nutrients with food.

Note: Always check with your doctor before starting a new supplement.

•**Eat an anti-inflammatory, blood vessel–beneficial diet.** This means one-half cup of dark-colored fresh or frozen berries daily and plenty of foods rich in vitamin K, such as kale, chard, brussels sprouts and broccoli.

Important: If you take a blood thinner such as *warfarin* (Coumadin), be careful about consuming vitamin K–rich foods. Check with your doctor.

•**Take botanical medicines that promote circulation and blood vessel health.** I usually prescribe a tincture containing equal parts of horse chestnut, hawthorn, linden and ginkgo. A typical dose is one-quarter teaspoon of the mixture daily, taken in two ounces of water, away from meals.

Caution: If you are taking prescription heart medications, check with your doctor before using these herbs.

Bye, Bye Baker's Cyst: No Cortisone, Drugs or Knee Surgery

Andrew Rubman, ND, is medical director of Southbury Clinic for Traditional Medicines in Southbury, Connecticut. SouthburyClinic.com. He is author of the "Nature Doc's Patient Diary" blog at Bottom LineInc.com

The patient: "Randolph" is an active retiree in his late 60s who had been troubled with rheumatism in his left knee, which was uncomfortably swollen.

Why he came to see me: Randolph wanted to inquire if there were any "more attractive" solutions to heal his knee other than draining fluids and taking drugs, which he was averse to.

How I evaluated him: I reviewed the medical records from Randolph's primary care doctor and rheumatologist and discussed the findings with him. Other than the bothersome knee, he had no other sites of rheumatic arthritis and all his bloodwork came back entirely normal, including a negative "RF" finding. That made me suspect of his rheumatism diagnosis. While the X-ray of his knee showed some fluid accumulation, there were none of the changes that one would expect from an advancing autoimmune disease like systemic rheumatoid arthritis. That made me even more skeptical of his rheumatism diagnosis.

How we addressed his problem: I explained to Randolph that much of the immune dysregulation that may prompt the array of autoimmune pathologies, like rheumatoid arthritis, scleroderma, lupus, Grave's disease, etc. starts in the gut, particularly in the large intestine. So, I worked with him on improving his diet—increasing raw and lightly cooked food, fruits and veggies, and dark berries…and decreasing fried and grilled meats and processed foods. I prescribed supplements to enhance gastrointestinal func-

tion as well as prebiotics and probiotics to improve his microbiota (intestinal bacteria).

After a month on the regime, his knee improved remarkably but he developed a "lump" behind the knee, off to one side. A simple X-ray proved this to be a Baker's cyst (named after William Morrant Baker, a 19th-century London surgeon who first described it) that had been produced by the knee's joint capsule in an attempt to remove the excess synovial (joint) fluid. I told him that topical applications containing certain botanical extracts assisted by phonophoresis (ultrasound) could enable the cyst to dislodge completely and move to the surface.

The patient's progress: Sure enough, the cyst rose to directly under the skin after a few treatments and then ruptured to the outside (like a big pimple), draining the encased fluid that had been bothering his knee. After this, he reported feeling completely better and shared the story with his other physicians. I think that we were all equally wowed by this resolution and the body's ability to participate in healing.

Calming the Pain of Chronic Tendonitis

Jamison Starbuck, ND, is a naturopathic physician in family practice in Missoula, Montana, and producer of *Dr. Starbuck's Health Tips for Kids*, a weekly program on Montana Public Radio, MTPR.org. DrJamisonStarbuck.com.

"**O**uch! I can't believe this still hurts. It's been so long!" Those were my patient's words as I asked her to flex and turn the wrist she had sprained three months ago, words common in patients suffering with tendonitis.

Tendonitis is inflammation in a tendon, the fibrous cords that attach muscles to bones and other body structures and move the bone or the structure. Tendonitis is generally caused by either acute injury, such as a sprain or strain, or chronic inflammation, such as arthritis, fibromyalgia or failing to heal well from an acute injury. An injured tendon usually takes four to eight weeks to heal. That healing can be helped along nicely with rest, ice, limited gentle movement, Arnica topical applications three times a day, and large doses of vitamin C (1,000 milligrams [mg]) and bioflavonoids (500 mg), each three times a day with food. (If you experience loose stools or diarrhea from the vitamin C, cut back your dose.)

It's trickier to effectively care for chronic tendonitis or acute tendonitis that isn't getting better. Conventional medicine offers daily nonsteroidal anti-inflammatory drugs like *ibuprofen* (Advil, Motrin) and sometimes steroid injections. These medicines help with pain, but they are rarely curative, so I prefer a different approach.

• **Reduce inflammatory foods from your diet.** That means that coffee, alcohol, sugar, processed preservative- and dye-rich foods, and fried foods need to go. You don't have to become a vegan, but if you want to reduce inflammation and pain, limit meat intake to no more than 6 ounces a day.

• **Drink 70 to 90 ounces of water each day.** Water delivers nutrients to tendons, and it helps remove pain-inducing waste. Try to drink most of your water away from meals for optimal benefit.

• **Eat lots of beta-carotene-rich foods.** Beta-carotene converts to vitamin A inside the body. Vitamin A is known for its ability to reduce inflammation and promote elasticity in blood vessels and muscle tissue. But unless you like eating liver, it can be hard to get vitamin A directly from food. Instead, eat lots of carrots, sweet potatoes, dark leafy greens, cantaloupe and squash.

People with chronic tendonitis often have calcium deposits on the tendon fibers that cause pain and limit mobility. With chronic tendonitis, limit calcium supplementation to no more than 300 mg per day. Take 1,000 micrograms of B12, 2,000 mg of vitamin C, and 1,000 mg of bioflavonoids daily. Research indicates that supplementation with these nutrients may reduce calcium deposi-

tion on tendons, decrease inflammation and increase flexibility.

My favorite botanical medicine for chronic tendonitis is Boswellia serrata, which you can find in tablets and capsules. It's often combined with another popular and effective anti-inflammatory botanical, turmeric. Because formulations vary, your best bet is to follow the manufacturer's recommendations for dosing.

Excellent Health Benefits of Chamomile

Laurie Steelsmith, ND, LAc, medical director of Steelsmith Natural Health Center in Honolulu, where she has a busy private practice, and is an associate clinical professor at Bastyr University. She is coauthor of three books—*Natural Choices for Women's Health, Great Sex, Naturally* and *Growing Younger Every Day.* DrSteelsmith.com

Mother Earth doesn't just supply us with the air we breathe and the stunning sunsets we see. The plants she produces provide us with heaps of health benefits, from turmeric's brain-boosting properties to echinacea's immunity-enhancing qualities.

Chamomile doesn't just fall under this category of healing plants. The herb epitomizes it. There are two different types of chamomile—German and Roman, with the former being the more potent of the two and the one used most often for therapeutic applications. Thanks to the flavonoids, sesquiterpenes and antioxidants it contains, it's traditionally been used to treat everything from rheumatic pain to ulcers. Now, chamomile is gaining even more ground as a large body of research shows its varied benefits. *Whether you choose to drink chamomile tea, take a chamomile supplement, use chamomile essential oil, or invest in a topical treatment, here are nine ways the herb may bolster your wellness…*

1. Improves sleep. Savoring a cup of chamomile tea before bed is a common habit for many—and not just for the earthy, apple taste it offers (indeed, "chamomile" goes back to the Greek word, khamaimëon, or "earth apple"). Chamomile contains apigenin, an antioxidant that binds to certain receptors in your brain that help decrease restlessness and induce sleep.

2. Reduces premenstrual symptoms. Bloating, cramping, mood swings—we women are well-aware that PMS can do a number on us. Fewer of us, however, may know that chamomile can be used to mitigate its symptoms. A systematic review of chamomile's benefits, published by the *Journal of Pharmacopuncture*, demonstrates that chamomile's anti-inflammatory, anti-spasmodic and anti-anxiety effects renders it a stellar remedy for alleviating abdominal and pelvic pain, as well as period-related anxiety and irritability. Drink as a tea, one cup twice a day from mid cycle until the period starts. One of my favorites is Organic Chamomile with Lavender tea by Traditional Medicinals containing not only chamomile but two herbs that soothe the nervous system, lavender and lemon balm.

3. Relieves eczema. Atopic eczema—a dermatological condition that causes the skin to become red, itchy, and inflamed—is often treated with hydrocortisone cream. Data published by the National Institutes of Health show that chamomile is roughly 60 percent as effective as 0.25 percent of the over-the-counter remedy. While additional research is needed to evaluate the true efficacy of chamomile's effect on eczema, present findings show that it may be a promising alternative option. You can reap its skin-soothing benefits in a topical treatment or use chamomile essential oil. How? Dilute with a carrier oil, such as coconut and jojoba, and add to warm bath water or your favorite body lotion. Alternatively, you can make a hot compress by soaking a towel or cloth in warm water, adding one to two drops of diluted chamomile oil, and then applying it to your skin.

4. Helps inflammatory conditions. While acute inflammation helps keep you alive—the process is your body's first line of defense against injuries, toxins and infections—chronic inflammation tells a different story, and may result in tissue damage, gastrointestinal distress and skin issues. Chamomile may aid in these consequences. Studies have shown that chamomile inhibits Helicobacter pylori, the bacteria that causes stomach ulcers, while its anti-spasmodic effects can help relax the abdominal aches frequently associated with gastrointestinal inflammatory disorders. The herb can also help with inflammation of the skin. Approved by the German Commission E for wound and burn therapy, one of chamomile's active constituents, *levomenol*, has anti-inflammatory and naturally-moisturizing properties that can diminish the signs of photoaging, reduce pruritis (itchy skin), and improve skin texture and elasticity.

For gastrointestinal issues, drink the tea (a few cups a day) or take chamomile as a supplement (900 mg/pill, two pills three times a day). For topical issues, the tea can be applied topically by soaking a wash cloth in a warm cup of tea and then apply the compress to affected tissue. Or have a lovely chamomile soak by adding six bags of chamomile tea to your bath water. You could also use the bulk herb—which is less expensive—by pouring two cups of chamomile flowers into your bath. A bath provides a special experience with chamomile flowers keeping you company.

5. Osteoporosis. While further studies are needed before chamomile can be considered for clinical use in the treatment of osteoporosis, research on the topic demonstrates great potential: In one study, chamomile extract was shown to stimulate osteoblastic cell differentiation, the NIH reports. Translation? It may help protect bones that are prone to depletion due to age and the loss of estrogen. Take chamomile as a tea and drink a few cups a day.

6. Aids in digestion. Chamomile is chockfull of health-boosting properties, including compounds, called *sesquiterpene lactones*, that urge the pancreas to produce the digestive enzymes your body needs to break down food. What's more, stress-related gastrointestinal issues that thwart proper digestion can be helped by chamomile's naturally calming effects. Drink a cup of chamomile tea after meals to support your digestion.

7. Lowers anxiety. That soothing effect isn't reserved just for sleep or your stomach. Chamomile can help diminish anxiety, period. One study, published in the journal *Phytomedicine*, found that chamomile extract lessens symptoms of general anxiety disorder (GAD). Harvard Health seconds this and suggests it can be a safe and effective alternative remedy for anxiety. (Do note that chamomile is not recommended if you're taking *warfarin, clopidogrel*, and other blood thinners.) Drinking a few cups a day of chamomile tea on a daily basis can soothe your nerves.

8. Boosts oral health. Chamomile's antiseptic properties make it a boon for your oral health by heading off infections, protecting your teeth and gums, and warding off gingivitis. It can also help relieve the discomfort of toothaches. "Administering" it is simple too. All you have to do is swish chamomile tea around in your mouth before drinking it.

9. Bolsters Immunity. Immune health is your health—and chamomile can be used to encourage it. Why? Because the herb boasts a number of phenolic compounds—acids with tremendous antioxidant activities that can help rouse the action of leukocytes and T-cells (cells responsible for safeguarding you against infections and toxins). You can use chamomile tea on a daily basis to support your immunity, or you can take it as a supplement. Most supplement products contain 900 mg of German chamomile extract. Take 900 mg twice a day.

Sip a cup of soothing tea and protect your health while you're at it? Now there's a(nother) reason to start stocking chamomile in your pantry!

Chapter 11

PAIN RELIEF FOR WOMEN

When Menopause Causes Arthritis...How to Ease the Pain and Get Back to Life

The patient: "Serena," a 49-year-old marketing manager.

Why she came to see me: Serena came to my health center because of joint pain. Her knees and hips often ached when she woke up, but it was her hands and fingers that were troubling her the most. What started as occasional discomfort in her hand joints progressed to the point that she found daily tasks such as typing, cooking and carrying bags of groceries painful. She wanted to get to the bottom of her discomfort—and to find out if there was anything she could do to treat it naturally.

How I evaluated her: I began my evaluation of Serena with an in-depth discussion about her medical and personal history.

Serena had arrived in Hawaii shortly after college and loved every aspect about it: the tropical climate, the people and the bounty of outdoor activities. Up until a year before she came to see me, she spent almost all of her non-work time outside—stand-up paddling, surfing, hiking and kayaking.

Her athletic leanings organically fostered a healthy lifestyle. A self-proclaimed flexitarian, she ate what she pleased but aimed to eat organic as often as possible. She'd been in a long-term happy relationship since her early 30s, did not have children and had an overall positive outlook on life.

Given how much she relied on her body for the sports she relished, she was keenly sensitive to every change she experienced—including the pain in her joints, which had started out gradually and increased over time. She hadn't been injured, or changed her diet, or done anything more physically taxing than usual. That said, her period, which used to arrive "every month on the dot," had become almost non-existent in the last year—her last period was at least seven months earlier.

In addition to the joint pain she described when she first came in, she was experiencing night sweats, insomnia and weight gain. Most disconcerting of all, she hadn't been able to enjoy the sports she so loved since her joint

Laurie Steelsmith, ND, LAc, medical director of Steelsmith Natural Health Center in Honolulu, where she has a busy private practice, and is an associate clinical professor at Bastyr University. She is coauthor of three books—*Natural Choices for Women's Health, Great Sex, Naturally* and *Growing Younger Every Day.* DrSteelsmith.com

251

pain started and was feeling "flat" about life itself. She had also been, she admitted, "feeding her feelings," which caused her to put on 15 pounds and brought her down further.

To determine the cause of Serena's joint pain, I conducted a full physical exam, a set of X-rays and blood tests to rule out autoimmune conditions that could be associated with joint pain. Further, I ordered a hormone test to assess her levels of estrogen, progesterone, testosterone, DHEA and thyroid hormones.

What my evaluation revealed: Serena's physical exam revealed what was obvious: She was in good health, with admirable blood pressure and blood sugar levels. Her X-rays, however, revealed cartilage loss, which is indicative of osteoarthritis, also known as degenerative joint disease, that causes pain, swelling and stiffness in the joints. Significantly more common among women than men, it typically impacts the knees, hips, hands and fingers—the very places that were concerning Serena the most.

Additionally, Serena's hormone test demonstrated that her estrogen levels were low. I was quick to assure Serena that this was entirely normal at the age of 49. Women's natural supply of estrogen begins to decline as they move into menopause. This "era," if you will, is accompanied by plenty—hot flashes, night sweats, weight gain, headaches and mood swings, most of which she was also experiencing. And yet what few know or discuss is the direct link between declining estrogen levels and joint pain.

Why does this happen? In part, this occurs because in order for estrogen to exhibit its effects—those rushes of confidence and happiness we women commonly feel a week after our period, when estrogen levels are high—the hormone must bind to an estrogen receptor. Two types of estrogen receptors exist, what's known as "ERa" and "ERb." The first exists in a half dozen places, including the uterus, the ovaries and the mammary glands. The second receptor, which is just as ubiquitous, exists, among other places, in the brain, the liver, the blood vessel walls and the synovial fluid—a viscous solution that surrounds joints and helps protect cartilage against damage generated by friction during movement. During PMS, perimenopause or menopause, this synovial membrane thickens due to the natural decline in estrogen production. For a woman still menstruating, this may cause her to feel heavy during PMS (that bloat we know). For a woman whose days of menstruating are nearing their end, it can result in joint discomfort. What's more, estrogen impacts the structure and function of other musculoskeletal tissues and affects collagen content. Waning estrogen levels also spur inflammation, leading to the pain and discomfort from which Serena was suffering.

How I addressed her problem: While there is no cure for osteoarthritis, it carries with it two pieces of good news: First, estrogen-related osteoarthritis does not worsen over time. In fact, as a woman's hormone levels find equilibrium after menopause, pain may fade. Second, its symptoms, from aches to swelling, can be moderated through a combination of lifestyle changes, hormones and supplementation.

To address the first, I urged Serena to return to her healthier weight, as joints bear the brunt of the pounds we carry. Also, excess weight creates more systemic inflammation in the body. To this end, I urged her to not only adopt a tweaked diet that included more satiating clean protein and antioxidant-rich vegetables, but to also adopt exercises that would help her deal with the hormone fluctuations she was going through and the deflation she was experiencing.

Within this, though, I encouraged her to find exercises that didn't put repetitive stress on her wrists and hands. Sadly, this meant avoiding the paddling and kayaking she enjoyed. Repetitive actions, such as typing, can "overwork" one's joints and increase joint pain. Swimming provides a low-impact, full-body workout without stressing out one particular area. Yoga, meanwhile, has been shown to diminish pain and improve physical function and joint stiffness.

We then discussed estrogen replacement therapy. While Serena was nervous that the treatment would increase her risk of breast cancer, I explained that her family history, as well as her overall health, put her in a low-risk category. I also provided her with data showing that estrogen replacement therapy may help mitigate joint pain. I started her off with bio-identical hormones from a compounding pharmacy consisting of two types of estrogen: estradiol and estriol, mixed together in a ratio of estradiol 20 percent/estriol 80 percent, at a dose of 1.25 mg. This was mixed in a cream base that she applied to her vulva each night when she also took a bio-identical progesterone pill (100mg).

When it came to supplements, I recommended that Serena take 1,000 mg of curcumin per day. Curcumin, a major active component of turmeric, was shown, in one study, to be as effective as OTC pain relievers. I also encouraged her to take 500 mg of magnesium glycinate per day, as low magnesium has been associated with increased osteoarthritis-related pain. Optimal amounts of magnesium, meanwhile, may improve sleep quality, while poor sleep can exacerbate joint pain and ultimately lead to depression. In addition, I recommended she take 1,500 mg of glucosamine sulfate and 400 mg twice a day of wild yam root extract. Technically known as diosgenin, wild yam root extract has been found to decrease menopausal symptoms and to inhibit inflammatory mediators, thereby reducing pain.

Lastly, I recommended that she omit nightshades from her diet. Belonging to the same family as belladonna (yes, the ancient form of poison), nightshades include tomatoes, tomatillos, potatoes (sweet potatoes are fine—they're not nightshades), eggplant, peppers and goji berries as well as pepper-based spices like paprika and cayenne. While perfectly palatable to many, some people—myself included—are highly sensitive to the alkaloids (or toxic compounds) in these plants and may experience joint pain after consuming them.

The patient's progress: Eight weeks after Serena started her recovery, she returned to my office with a grin. Ten pounds lighter—"back at my fighting weight," she joked—and with a newfound love for long-distance swimming, she felt stronger than she'd been at 40. While her osteoarthritic pain emerged when it rained or when she "overdid it" while playing outside, for the most part she was symptom-free and thrilled to have full range of movement in her hands. Most of all, though, she felt happy again, which made any pain she did encounter all the easier to handle.

Got Painful Hand Arthritis? Get Relief Without Drugs

Carole Dodge, OTR, CHT, who supervises the occupational hand therapy program at University of Michigan Health System in Ann Arbor. She specializes in osteoarthritis, rheumatoid arthritis, joint replacements and traumatic hand injuries. She is also director of the Michigan Medicine Hand Fellowship program.

The hands often bear the brunt of this "wear and tear" arthritis. The good news is, there are plenty of under-the-radar nondrug strategies that can ease the pain of hand arthritis.

Beyond the Pill Bottle

Many people don't know about the approaches that follow because they're not heavily advertised and few doctors talk about them. While the benefits may be temporary, these tactics can be used as often as desired—with no downsides. *Among the best nondrug therapies to relieve hand OA…*

•**Arthritis gloves.** Gentle compression from arthritis gloves, which are not the same as those used for burns or lymphedema, eases pain and lessens OA swelling. The gloves can be worn all day and night, if needed, for pain relief—even in the summer, since they are lightweight. *Good products…*

• Norco Compression Gloves. A soft, nylon-and-spandex blend, these gloves are sold individually for left and right hands and come in two fingertip styles (full-finger and tipless for easy smartphone use) and wrist lengths. A built-in wrist slit makes them easy to slide on, and they're sold in three sizes. The soft compression gets raves from patients who've tried them for symptom relief. *Cost:* $9.95 each.

• IMAK Compression Arthritis Gloves. Endorsed by the Arthritis Foundation, these mostly cotton, part spandex gloves are breathable, flexible and have open fingertips. Sold in three sizes. *Cost:* About $20 a pair.

• **Splints and braces.** These devices, known as orthotics, provide more structure than arthritis gloves and can stabilize the entire hand or just individual knuckles…and are particularly useful for arthritis affecting the base of the thumb. *Good product…*

• Comfort Cool Thumb CMC Restriction Splint. This splint supports the arthritic thumb while offering flexibility and freedom for the fingers. It's made of spongy, thin neoprene and lined with terry cloth for softness against the hand and wrist. Since it's pliable, it can be trimmed if desired. It should be worn during the day when performing activities that increase pain. *Cost:* About $26.

• **Paraffin baths.** Paraffin baths are an easy way to get moist heat deeply into the soft tissues of the hand and joints. Paraffin should be heated to 120°F to 130°F. After dipping your hand(s) in warm paraffin, wrap the hand in a plastic bag and place in an oven mitt or towel, keeping it still for 15 to 20 minutes. The paraffin then peels off easily. Paraffin gives immediate relief that lasts about two hours. *Good products…*

• GiGi Digital Paraffin Bath. A somewhat pricey but highly effective option, the GiGi has a quick-melt feature with an easily adjustable digital temperature control. The oversized steel tank also has a see-through and spill-resistant lid. *Cost:* About $155 (including eight pounds of paraffin).

• HoMedics ParaSpa Plus Paraffin Bath. This lower-priced product has a light to let you know when the wax is ready for use, along with a locking safety lid. You can monitor the temperature with a meat or candy thermometer. *Cost:* $39.99 (including three pounds of paraffin).

• **Topical pain relievers.** To avoid the potential side effects, such as upset stomach and stomach ulcers, of oral nonsteroidal anti-inflammatory drugs (NSAIDs), many doctors recommend topical treatments for hand OA—especially capsaicin cream, which uses the key ingredient in chili peppers to help block pain messages to nerves. Over-the-counter arnica and Biofreeze are other good topical products. Ask your doctor for advice.

• **Hand therapy.** Hand therapists are specially trained to teach strategies that will enable you to use your hands with less achiness and stiffness. The therapy usually involves four visits, including evaluation of self-care, management of assistive devices, orthotic fabrication and management, and instruction in a home exercise program. Many health insurers cover hand therapy. To find a qualified hand therapist near you, consult the Hand Therapy Certification Commission website at HTCC.org.

Arthritis Drugs Linked to Depression

Study titled "Introduction and Switching of Biologic Agents Are Associated with Antidepressant and Anxiolytic Medication Use: Data on 42,815 Real-World Patients with Inflammatory Rheumatic Disease," by researchers at National and Kapodistrian University of Athens, Greece, published in *RMD Open: Rheumatic & Musculoskeletal Diseases.*

An estimated 1.3 million individuals suffer from rheumatoid arthritis, and 75 percent of those afflicted are women. In addition to severe pain, depression and anxiety often occur with rheumatic disease…all of which are difficult to treat.

Latest development: A recent study out of Greece finds that people with inflammatory rheumatic joint disease who start or switch to biologic drugs are more likely to be taking an antidepressant or anti-anxiety medication. This is the first study to show a link between the use of biologic drugs and the use of medication for depression or anxiety.

Biologic drugs are newer anti-inflammatory drugs used to treat rheumatic diseases such as rheumatoid arthritis, psoriatic arthritis and ankylosing spondylitis. Biologics are started when a conventional disease-modifying antirheumatic drug (DMARD) is not effective. Patients may switch from one biologic to another if treatment is still not effective.

Rheumatic disease often leads to depression or anxiety, and depression may make the disease worse, creating an endless loop. Researchers from the National and Kapodistrian University of Athens, Greece, wanted to find out if patients who started a biologic drug, or switched from one biologic to another, were more likely to eventually take medication for depression or anxiety. Their study was published in the journal *RMD Open: Rheumatic & Musculoskeletal Diseases*.

The research: Using data from the Greek Government Center for Social Security Services, the researchers identified nearly 43,000 patients with rheumatoid arthritis, psoriatic arthritis or ankylosing spondylitis between 2016 and 2018 who were taking a DMARD or biologic drug. *Compared with patients who did not start or change biologics…*

• **Patients starting a biologic** were about 25 percent more likely to be taking an antidepressant and 18 percent more likely to be taking an anti-anxiety medication.

• **Patients switching biologics** were about 50 percent more likely to be taking an antidepressant and 16 percent more likely to be taking an anti-anxiety medication.

The researchers cite three possible explanations for the link between biologics and mood disorder drugs. First, having a rheumatic disease may cause depression and anxiety due to pain, disability and loss of social activities. Second, depression or anxiety may make rheumatic joint disease worse. Third, depression or anxiety may increase a patient's perception of pain. This may increase the reported pain scores that doctors use when deciding to start or switch biologics.

Takeaway: The researchers conclude that doctors should consider how mood disorders may affect rheumatic disease before deciding to start or switch a biologic. Worsening of joint symptoms may be due to a mood disorder. Managing a mood disorder may reduce the need to start or change medications.

Ease Your Pain With These Soothing Self-Massage Tools

William G. Oswald, DPT, clinical instructor of rehabilitation medicine at NYU Grossman School of Medicine in New York City.

Are you relying on muscle relaxers to ease pain? A study from University of Pennsylvania found that prescriptions for these drugs—often handed out along with opioids—have skyrocketed in recent years…even though their benefits are largely unproven and their use has been linked to falls, accidents and addiction.

Self-massage is a safe, soothing and convenient nondrug alternative to relieve muscle pain and return range of motion. It also is effective at dissolving trigger points, those localized nodules of tight muscle that develop as a result of trauma, stress, overuse, fatigue or simply from failing to warm up properly before exercise. Applying pressure relaxes the compressed muscles and increases blood flow to the area, bringing relief.

Your hands alone can't always penetrate muscle fibers as deeply as you'd like, and it's hard to reach certain areas, such as the center of your back. That's where self-massage tools come in. In fact, it's great to have a toolbox of these aids for the large muscles of your legs and trunk as well as your neck, hands, feet, head and even your fingers.

Vibrating Foam Rollers

Foam rollers usually are used for larger areas of tightness, such as the thighs, hips and calves. A new generation of these massage 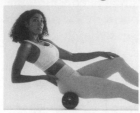 tools—with built-in vibration—has elevated the results you can get. The vibration allows you to go deeper without the added discomfort that actual deep-tissue massage can cause.

To use: Lie over the roller so that your own body weight creates pressure on the area you want to work. Roll back and forth in a slow, controlled way.

Product pick: The cordless and rechargeable Vyper 2.0 from Hyperice ($199*) is especially compact and can easily fit in a gym bag or suitcase.

Massage Sticks

These batonlike massagers are much shorter, thinner and firmer than foam rollers and 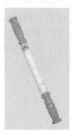 are made of very dense foam and rubber, usually with a line of nubby segments or beads that roll. They're often about 18 inches long, so they're very portable, but they do require more elbow grease than a foam roller because the pressure is coming from the exertion of your hands and arms rather than the weight of your body. One benefit over a foam roller is that you can more easily vary the amount of pressure you exert. Massage sticks can be used on the neck, thighs, calves and shins.

To use: Position the center of the stick on the area you want to ease, and use both hands to slowly roll the stick back and forth. For comfort, look for a massage stick that has contoured grips at the ends.

Product pick: The Stick muscle massager ($42).

*All prices in this article reflect recent prices from major online sellers.

Percussive Therapy Devices

These very popular handheld products, which look like an electric drill, are a favorite in professional sports locker rooms. 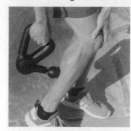 They deliver short-duration pulses (about 40 per second) deep into soft tissue to relieve pain. One theory is that trigger points can stem from a lack of circulation, so increasing blood flow to these areas through the percussive action can help with recovery. On their own, percussive devices can reach deeper into the muscle than vibration devices, plus you can further increase the depth of penetration by exerting additional pressure with your hand. Speed and intensity are adjustable on the device, which has different heads for different parts of the body. The open-handle design lets you work just about anywhere on the body, although it will be more relaxing—and more fun—if you can snag a friend to help you with harder-to-reach spots such as your back or hamstrings.

To use: Apply the device head directly to a tight spot, and hold it in place for 30 or so seconds before moving to another area or resting and then repeating on the same spot. You also can use a circular motion over a wider area for a massagelike effect. Just beware of applying too much pressure, which could damage capillaries and cause bruising. Do not use on your face, neck or throat. Also avoid using percussive therapy devices if you are on blood thinners, at risk for blood clots or have a condition that affects the blood vessels such as peripheral artery disease.

Product pick: Theragun ($299 and up).

Massage Balls

These handy hard rubber balls come in many designs—smooth, nubby (great for feet!) and even with built-in vibration. Some deliver heat, while others, such as T Spheres ($30 and up), offer the addition of aromatherapy, which can be relaxing when you're stressed and in a state of chronic pain. Massage balls

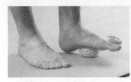

can provide more specific direct pressure similar to that of a percussive therapy device but not as expensive.

To use: A massage ball can apply pressure by rolling it with your hands on your neck, arms and legs. You also can lean onto the massage ball against the wall for your shoulders and back. You can roll on the ball on the floor for your lower back, thighs and feet.

Acupressure Massagers

These mats and pillows have raised areas with hundreds to thousands of small plastic

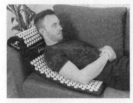

points in a set pattern. The acupressure points create pressure on trigger points and all over your body, stimulating circulation.

To use: Using one is as easy as lying down on the mat and putting the pillow under your neck or placing the mat over a chair and sitting on it for a few minutes at a time. The instruction booklet typically shows different positions to target different spots on the body.

Product pick: ProsourceFit has a variety of acupressure mat and pillow sets that have a cotton or linen base ($24.99 and up).

Specialty Massagers

These inexpensive tools can be part of your full-body arsenal to relax and feel better

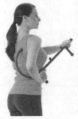

faster.

For the back: The Thera Cane Massager ($29.95) looks like a coat hook with six treatment balls placed along its length. It's great for hard-to-reach areas of the back.

For the head: A head/scalp massager, widely available with 12 or 20 metal "fingers," or spindles, is a tool for relaxation, and some people find it also brings headache relief. Choose a model with a tiny rubber bead at the end of each spindle for smoother action and less hair tangling. Simply move it up and down over your skull for three or four minutes at a time (various manufacturers, about $8 and up).

For the fingers: For a fun way to relax, try acupressure rings (various manufacturers, about $7 for 12). Each finger has acu-

pressure points that connect to different points on the body, which the rings stimulate when you twist them on your fingers.

More from William G. Oswald, DPT...

How to Relieve Muscular Pain Points

No matter what self-massage tool you use, the general principles for releasing trigger points are the same. Apply pressure directly to areas of pain—the trigger points—one at a time. This pressure will feel painful at first, but when you take off the pressure, the pain will start to subside. How long you maintain the pressure is unique to you. It can be a matter of seconds or up to a few minutes. Sometimes, it's simply the amount of time you can tolerate. You can rest and then reapply the pressure. Just keep in mind that a total of 10 to 15 minutes per spot per session is the limit, just as it is when applying ice or heat. You won't achieve more relief by doing it for any longer.

Relieve Your Neck Pain

Mitchell Yass, DPT, specialist in diagnosing and resolving pain. To learn more, check out Dr. Yass's YouTube channel. His most recent book is *The Yass Method for Pain-Free Movement: A Guide to Easing Through Your Day Without Aches and Pains.* MitchellYass.com

Neck tightness is a common annoyance that can ruin your entire day… and night. Short-term fixes such as pain-relieving medication, massage and chiropractic care don't address the real cause. Most neck pain is rooted not in the cervical spine, but in the muscles of the upper trapezius region that support the shoulder and arm complexes. Being glued to the computer or constantly checking your cell phone causes them to overwork and eventually shorten and strain—you actually can see the distance between your ear and shoulder shrink!

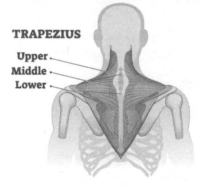

TRAPEZIUS
Upper
Middle
Lower

To protect your shoulders and allow for normal neck motion and function, you want to strengthen the opposing muscles to the levator scapulae and upper trapezius muscles at the back and sides of the neck and upper spine. Specifically, you want to strengthen the lower trapezius, the muscle that runs from the shoulder blade to your mid-back. All it takes is two progressive resistance exercises. They can be done with weights or resistance bands (available at sporting-goods stores and online) as shown.

For each exercise: Perform three sets of 10 repetitions with one minute rest between sets, three times a week, always with a day of rest in between.

Start with a resistance equal to an exertion level of eight out of 10 (10 feels as if you are overexerting, and 0 feels as if you are doing nothing). Stay at this level until muscles adapt and grow, and the exertion level feels like five out of 10. This is when you increase the resistance until it feels like an eight out of 10 again. Do this by using a heavier weight or by grabbing higher on the band or switching to a band that has a stronger tension.

Instructions here are for bands, but use the same positioning and movement if you are using weights.

Lower Trapezius

Sit in a sturdy chair, and lean back slightly, at about a 20-degree angle. Secure one end of

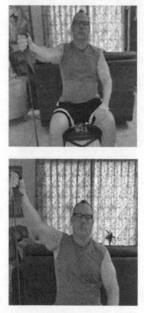

the resistance band to a chair leg at your right foot, and hold the other end of the band in your right hand. Your arm should be at a 45-degree angle, midway between your chest and your side, hand at eye height and elbow just unlocked. Keep your arm straight, and raise it to about a 130-to-140-degree angle (elbow is about level with your cheek). Return to start. Repeat all reps and sets. Then repeat on the left side.

Lat Pulldown

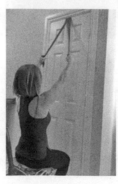

Use a door anchor specifically designed to work with resistance bands to attach the center of your band to the top of a closed door. Sit in a sturdy chair, leaning back at about a 30-degree angle. Hold one end of the band in each hand with arms nearly straight, elbows just un-

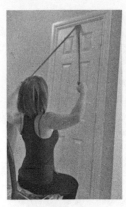

locked. Pull down the band, keeping arms wide and bringing elbows just below shoulder level and slightly behind the line of the shoulders—the shoulder blades should squeeze together. If the elbows drop lower than shoulder level, you're using the wrong muscles. Return to start.

Exercise photos courtesy of Mitchell Yass, DPT
Illustration: GettyImages

Breakthroughs in Migraine Relief

Alexander Mauskop, MD, founder and director of the New York Headache Center (NYHeadache.com), and a professor of clinical neurology at SUNY Downstate Medical Center. His scientific papers have appeared in *Headache, Neurology, The Journal of Pain* and many other medical journals. He is the author of the books *The Headache Alternative* and *What Your Doctor May Not Tell You About Migraines.*

U p to 40 million Americans suffer from migraine headaches, 75 percent of them women. Symptoms can include throbbing head pain, nausea, vomiting, sensitivity to light and sound, fatigue, and dizziness.

Sobering statistic: According to the World Health Organization, migraine is the second-leading cause of disability, with only back pain causing more downtime.

To prevent or relieve migraines (which can strike as often as every couple of days), doctors prescribe two types of drugs—preventive, to stop attacks before they start; and abortive, to stop attacks once they've begun.

Preventive Drugs

Preventive drugs have plenty of problems. None of them were developed specifically to prevent migraines. Drug by drug, each was accidentally discovered to block migraines—

Beware Uncommon Symptoms of Jaw Problems That Lead to a Temporomandibular Joint Disorder (TMJ)

Lesser known signs: Headaches...painful earaches or feeling stuffed up with trouble hearing...neck pain...discomfort when swallowing.

Surprising causes—beyond tooth grinding and clenching: Poorly adjusted orthodontia and dental restorations...trauma, such as whiplash or an upper-body sports injury...cracking your neck...nail biting... chewing on only one side.

Jeffrey Bassman, DDS, is director of the Center for Headaches, Sleep & TMJ Disorders in Davenport, Iowa. |BassmanTMJ.com

---

which means they deliver a host of unwanted side effects. *These problematic drugs originated for a variety of conditions...*

• **Beta-blockers,** such as *propranolol* (Inderal) and *timolol,* are usually prescribed for hypertension. Common side effects include fatigue, lightheadedness, shortness of breath and, in migraineurs, low blood pressure.

• **Anti-seizure drugs,** such as *topiramate* (Topamax), are used for epilepsy. They can cause memory loss, osteoporosis, and hair loss. They can also cause birth defects—a big risk for premenopausal women.

• **Antidepressants,** such as *amitriptyline* and *nortriptyline* (Pamelor), can cause insomnia, weight gain, and loss of libido, as well as distressing withdrawal symptoms if you suddenly stop taking the medication.

• **Botox** is best known as the anti-wrinkle drug. For migraines, the dose is five to six times higher than that used for cosmetic purposes. It's injected once a month in the back of the head, in the neck and in the shoulders. Botox is the safest and most effective of the preventive drugs, but the U.S. Food and

Drug Administration (FDA) has approved it only for chronic migraineurs who have 15 or more migraine days per month.

Because of the many downsides, only 20 percent of migraineurs who are prescribed preventive therapy stay on the drug long term.

New Development

Twenty-five years ago, scientists discovered that a chemical called calcitonin gene-related peptide (CGRP) is released in the brain during a migraine. CGRP's exact causative role in migraines isn't yet understood, but it may stimulate the sensory nerves that cause or contribute to the pain.

After decades of research by drug manufacturers, with hundreds of millions of dollars invested, six CGRP-blocking drugs were approved by the FDA in 2019 and 2020. They're proving to be reasonably effective and mostly safe in preventing migraines. About 30 percent of people who try them get good results—with one out of five of those experiencing dramatic relief (75 percent to 100 percent reduction in migraines), and one out of two experiencing a 50 percent reduction.

So far, CGRPs have been used by more than 300,000 migraineurs, with very few side effects. For some people, they work when no other drug does.

Here's what you need to know about this new class of drugs and how they might work for you or your loved ones…

Current Options

There are currently four preventive CGRP drugs on the market, with a fifth likely to be approved within the year. There are also two migraine-abortive CGRPs.

The injectable preventive CGRPs. Three drugs, *fremanezumab* (Ajovy), *erenumab* (Aimovig), and *galcanezumab* (Emgality), are self-administered by a push-button device where you don't have to see the needle. Aimovig and Emgality are injected once a month. Ajovy is injected either once a month or as a triple dose once every three months.

Sometimes, the results are cumulative: The second treatment is more effective than the first, and the third treatment is even better.

The three drugs have slightly different mechanisms of action. Aimovig blocks the CGRP receptor on cells, whereas Ajovy and Emgality block CGRP itself. While none of these drugs consistently works better than the others, in about 10 percent to 20 percent of cases, Ajovy or Emgality might work better than Aimovig. If you're taking a monthly drug, try it for at least three months before giving up on it.

Warning: Some people develop constipation on Aimovig. In about 100 cases, the constipation was so severe that surgery was necessary to resolve the problem. If you have constipation, don't take this drug.

• **The intravenous preventive CGRP.** *Eptinezumab* (Vyepti) is delivered intravenously at the doctor's office once every three months. This might be the right drug for you if you don't like injecting yourself and because there's only one treatment every three months.

• **The oral abortive CGRPs.** *Rimegepant* (Nurtec) and *ubrogepant* (Ubrelvy) stop a migraine that's starting. They are prescribed only if the gold standard for abortive drugs— the triptans, such as sumatriptan (Imitrex)— have failed.

• **An oral preventive CGRP.** Atogepant is a migraine-abortive drug that has not yet been approved by the FDA. It is currently in phase 3 clinical trials and may be FDA-approved sometime in 2021.

Here's the rub: These drugs are very expensive—around $600 per treatment. Currently, they're covered by insurance only after every other preventive drug has failed.

A Different Type of Drug

• ***Lasmiditan* (Reyvow).** This new migraine abortive drug was approved by the FDA in December 2019. Like the triptans, it works on serotonin receptors: Triptans work on 1B and 1D receptors, while Reyvow works on 1F.

Why this matters: Reyvow doesn't cause vasoconstriction of blood vessels so, unlike Imitrex, it's not contraindicated for people with cardiovascular disease.

If you have cardiovascular disease, don't respond to a CGRP abortive drug, or have side effects from a triptan, this may be the abortive drug for you.

Caution: Reyvow can cause drowsiness. Don't drive a car for eight hours after taking the drug.

Non-Drug Options

•**Nerivio** is a new, FDA-approved electro-stimulator that eased migraine pain in two out of three people who tried it in a clinical trial. Placed under the upper arm for 45 minutes at the first sign of a migraine, it generates a low-level electrical current that activates nerve fibers to block pain messages from reaching the brain.

A prescription product, it should be covered by insurance, but check with your provider. Many patients find it very effective when combined with an abortive drug such as Imitrex, and some find the device useful on its own to abort a migraine. You can find out more about the Nerivio device at Theranica.com (see also page 263).

•**Allay Lamp.** This non-prescription lamp was invented by Harvard-based migraine researcher Rami Burstein, PhD. Knowing that migraineurs are affected by light, he studied each color in the spectrum, first in rats and then in people, to see which worsened migraine and which made it better. He discovered that green light was the only color that eased migraine—and created the green-generating Allay Lamp.

How to use it: When you feel a migraine coming on, go into a room, close the shades, turn off all other sources of light (including your smartphone, computer, and TV screens), and spend an hour or two with the Allay Lamp turned on. (It provides enough light to read or work.) The lamp costs $149. You can learn more at AllayLamp.com.

Yoga Improves Migraine Treatment

Study titled "Effect of Yoga as Add-on Therapy in Migraine (Contain), A Randomized Clinical Trial," by researchers at All India Institute of Medical Sciences, New Delhi, published in *Neurology*.

A new study suggests that adding yoga to the usual migraine treatments can significantly reduce the frequency and intensity of migraine attacks. Migraine headaches are common and they can reduce the quality of life for people who suffer from them. Medications to prevent migraine attacks only reduce migraines in about 50 percent of migraineurs.

Researchers from the All India Institute of Medical Sciences enrolled 114 migraineurs into the new study. Participants ranged in age from 18 to 50 and experienced four to 14 headaches per month.

Half of the migraineurs were randomly assigned to a group that received the usual medical and lifestyle treatments for migraine. These treatments included drugs such as the beta-blocker propranolol and the antidepressant *amitriptyline*, along with lifestyle counseling on sleep, diet and exercise. The other group got the same treatment along with yoga. The yoga treatment included one month of yoga instruction three days a week, followed by two months of self-yoga practice five days a week. Yoga therapy included breathing, relaxation and using yoga postures.

Over the three months of the study, the migraineurs in both groups were evaluated for the number of headaches they had, how severe the headaches were, by how much headaches impacted daily life and how much medication they needed to take. *These are the key findings...*

•**Headaches improved in both groups,** but the yoga group had better improvement in frequency, intensity and quality of life, and they had less need of medication.

• **Frequency of headaches decreased by 48 percent in the yoga group** compared with 12 percent in the usual-treatment alone group.

• **The number of migraine pills decreased by 47 percent in the yoga group** compared with 12 percent in the usual-treatment group.

The researchers are not sure why yoga improves the usual migraine treatments. Yoga may increase blood levels of nitrous oxide, a gas that may reduce migraine attacks. Yoga may also relax muscles in the neck and shoulders. Tense muscles may be a migraine trigger.

The researchers conclude that adding yoga to the usual migraine treatment is both safe and inexpensive. It is estimated that migraine accounts for about $15 billion in lost productivity and medication costs in the US. Adding yoga to migraine treatment could save a lot of money and go a long way to improving the quality of life for migraineurs.

What to Take for a Tension Headache— No Drugs Needed

Trupti Gokani, MD, board-certified neurologist and founder of the Zira Mind and Body Center in Glenview, Illinois. Her special interests include alternative approaches to headache management and women's issues. ZiraMindandBody.com

Its trivial-sounding name seems to imply that the problem is "just stress"…but the viselike pain of a tension headache can make you truly miserable and significantly disrupt your day. Popping a painkiller is not a great solution because such drugs can have nasty side effects, including increased risk for gastrointestinal bleeding, blood pressure problems and liver or kidney damage.

So what can you take when a tension headache grabs hold? Integrative neurologist Trupti Gokani, MD, founder of Zira Mind and Body Center, Glenview, Illinois, suggested trying any or all of the following options. Products are available at health-food stores and/or online. *Consider taking…*

• **A few bites of food or a big drink of water.** If hunger or dehydration is triggering your headache, the pain may disappear once you assuage your body's basic needs. Just about any healthful food will do…but stay away from known headache triggers such as processed meats, aged cheeses, red wine and anything with monosodium glutamate.

• **Butterbur supplements.** Though various supplements may prevent headaches when taken regularly, butterbur works best to help halt a headache you already have. This anti-inflammatory herb should be taken as soon as you feel the pain coming on. Try the brand Petadolex (Petadolex.com), which contains a purified form of butterbur free from liver-damaging pyrrolizidine alkaloids. Or consider Zira Nourished Mind by Pure Balance, a product Dr. Gokani helped develop, which contains Petadolex and other headache-relieving ingredients (available at Shop.ZiraMindandBody.com).

Caution: Do not use butterbur if you are pregnant or have liver disease.

• **Some whiffs of an aromatherapy remedy.** Finding the right scent may require some experimentation because aromas work differently with different people.

Options to try: Essential oil of lavender… basil…or clary sage.

To use: Sprinkle three drops of the desired essential oil onto a tissue or handkerchief and take a sniff every few minutes… or sprinkle three drops onto a hot or cold compress and apply to your forehead until the pain lets up.

• **A moment to ask yourself why you have this headache.** A tension headache usually has an underlying trigger.

Consider: Do you need a break from your computer screen? Are you working in a poorly lit room? Maybe a short walk or a chat with a friend will relieve whatever stress you're under.

High-Tech Help for Migraine Pain

Brian M. Grosberg, MD, director of Hartford Health-Care Headache Center, Ayer Neuroscience Institute, and professor of neurology at University of Connecticut School of Medicine, Farmington. He is principal investigator of a study on the Nerivio published in *Headache: The Journal of Head and Face Pain.*

Medications have helped many people impacted by migraines, but now there's a new FDA-approved non-drug treatment that offers relief. It's a wearable electric-stimulation device for people who prefer nondrug relief...don't get relief (or enough relief) from treatments such as triptans or non-specific migraine medications...or experience unwanted side effects from those drugs. Called Nerivio, it also can be used in tandem with medications for greater pain relief.

Unlike earlier stimulation devices that are placed on the head, Nerivio goes on the upper arm and can be discreetly covered by clothing. It works by delivering electrical stimulation to the peripheral nerves in the arm. This relays pain-sensitive information to the brain, triggering the release of chemicals to reduce the pain signals from migraines.

Important: Start treatment as early as possible, but always within 60 minutes of migraine headache or aura onset.

Participants who wore the armbands in a recent clinical trial experienced relief lasting up to 48 hours after the treatment.

Through an app on your smartphone, you set the intensity level yourself. It should feel strong but comfortable and not painful. Available by prescription, each armband delivers 12 45-minute treatments and costs $99. (There are no rechargeable versions yet.)

Note that Nerivio is not for people with chronic migraine.* Also, the device is not recommended for anyone with a severe heart condition, uncontrolled epilepsy or any implanted medical device.

*Defined as having a migraine at least eight days a month and a total of at least 15 headaches a month for more than three months.

Green Light Reduces Migraines

Laurent Martin, PhD, department of pharmacology, and Mohab Ibrahim, PhD, MD, department of anesthesiology, led a study published in *Cephalalgia.* Both are at University of Arizona, Tucson.

When 22 chronic migraine patients were exposed to green light-emitting diodes (LEDs) for one to two hours daily for 10 weeks, the average number of headache days per month dropped from 22 to nine. Patients also reported significantly improved quality of life and no negative side effects. This appears to be a safe, drug-free way to reduce migraines. The green LEDs used in the study had 525-nanometer wavelengths, eight watts and a 120-degree beam angle.

Surprising Migraine— Dry Eye Connection

Richard M. Davis, MD, associate professor, Kittner Eye Center, University of North Carolina at Chapel Hill.

Patients with migraines were 20 percent more likely than people without migraines to also have dry eye disease, according to a 10-year study of nearly 73,000 patients. The association was highest for older patients—men age 65 and older were nearly twice as likely to have chronic dry eye, and women in that age group were 2.5 times as likely. Inflammation, which plays a role in both conditions, may be the common link. While the study didn't prove that inflammation from dry eye causes migraine attacks, treating dry eye might improve migraine symptoms.

The Role of Cannabis in Pain Management Is Unclear

Alexis Cooke, PhD, MPH, is a postdoctoral fellow in psychiatry at University of California, San Francisco. Her study was published in *International Journal of Drug Policy.*

Among 295 legal users who were surveyed on their pain levels, health trajectories and frequency of use, daily cannabis use among those with severe pain was associated with decreased health over a year.

Unknown: Whether more frequent users had more severe health problems to begin with or certain conditions respond better to medical marijuana than others.

Sit Smarter and Prevent Pain

Shani Soloff, PT, CEO and founder of Stamford Physical Therapy in Stamford, Connecticut, and The Posture People, a national ergonomics consulting firm.

Having the perfect workstation on the job is essential to prevent issues such as back and neck strain and the resulting pain. How you sit at home is just as important, especially if home has become your new workplace. It is very easy to get lax about good positioning when you're working in the dining room, reclining on the couch, eating in the kitchen or lounging in bed. *Here's how to sit smarter and comfortably to remain pain-free...*

For Knee Arthritis, PT Beats Steroid Injections

Osteoarthritis patients received either physical therapy (PT) or cortisone injections. One year later, the PT group's pain and disability level was significantly better. Steroid injections seem easier than PT, but risks include infection, cartilage loss and bone fractures. And after the initial appointment, most PT patients walked better while injection patients had to rest for 72 hours.

Gail Deyle, DSc, professor of physical therapy at Brooke Army Medical Center, San Antonio, Texas, and leader of a study published in *The New England Journal of Medicine.*

●**Find your most supportive chair.** Whether you're sitting at a desk for most of the day or just to pay bills, sit in a chair that allows your knees to bend with feet supported on the ground. If your feet don't reach the ground, use a foot stool. Your thighs should be fully supported by the chair seat. The chair is too shallow if it ends at mid-thigh... too deep if your calves touch the edge. Better leg support means better back support.

●**Support your back**—whether you're sitting on an upright chair, the couch or a cushy chair. If the seat is deeper than the length of your thighs, place a pillow behind your back to fill the space. For extra lumbar support, place a folded towel or lumbar back cushion in the small of your back.

Beware: Low-backed couches and chairs do not provide adequate back support.

●**When in bed reading or watching TV,** put a small pillow beneath your knees to maintain a small bend—keeping your legs out straight strains the low back.

●**Get up and move before you feel discomfort.** Once an hour is typical, but if you know that you'll start feeling stiff sooner, move sooner. Adopt new habits that drive movement such as using an upstairs bathroom when you're downstairs and vice versa.

•**Change position whenever you change activity.** Rather than go from sitting to sitting—for example, from working at your computer to reading on the couch—spend at least a few minutes standing up and/or walking in between activities.

Prevent Gas, Pain and Intestinal Bloat

Roundup of experts on gastrointestinal discomfort, reported at Prevention.com.

Eat slowly so you swallow less air during a meal. Practice meditation or mindful breathing to reduce anxiety and stress, which are linked to increased gas. Exercise at least 30 minutes three to five times a week—workouts help move food through the gastrointestinal tract more quickly, reducing gas and bloating. Cut back on gluten—this can help even if you do not have celiac disease. Keep a food journal so you know if you become particularly uncomfortable after consuming specific foods or food combinations. Limit certain foods—some healthy, high-fiber foods can cause gas and bloating, such as beans, peas, cabbage, onions, broccoli, cauliflower and prunes.

---

8 Stretches That Ease Your Aches and Pains

Karl Knopf, EdD, director of fitness therapy and senior fitness for the International Sports Sciences Association and retired director of adaptive fitness at Foothill College in Los Altos Hills, California. He is author of *Stretching for 50+* and *Foam Roller Workbook*.

Overcoming the many aches and pains that come with living a long and active life can't be achieved simply by luck.

As we age, we lose muscle mass and our muscles become tighter and less flexible, especially if they're not exercised well. Add to that poor posture, injury and diseases such as osteoarthritis, and muscles can fall prey to inflammation, spasms and misalignments. Tight muscles get tighter, and weak muscles get weaker. The secret to successful aging: Stay flexible.

Many older adults I meet don't see the importance of flexibility work until they are hunched over and in constant pain, looking and feeling older than their years.

In addition, I meet people who don't think that stretching is beneficial—and find it outright boring—and believe that they'll get more benefit by spending their time doing cardio and resistance exercises. The truth is that daily stretching is as important as regular aerobic exercise (five days a week) and weight training (two to three times a week).

Stretching Tips

It's easy to sneak stretching into your life. Simply incorporate stretches into your normal routine or while working at your desk... watching TV...or between sips of tea while you read. *But stay safe...*

•**Warm up your muscles before you stretch by walking around for a few minutes first.**

•**Don't bounce through stretches.** Instead, hold steady, extending slightly on the outbreath, but push only as far as comfortable.

•**Hold stretches for at least 30 seconds or as tolerated,** not to one minute unless otherwise noted for individual stretches below.

You're unlikely to notice immediate changes in your flexibility and range of motion, but if you keep up with daily stretching, you'll notice subtle changes. It will be easier to bend over and tie your shoelaces...you'll feel less stiff when you get out of bed in the morning...and you'll have an easier time getting in and out of the car.

The following are effective but simple exercises that can improve posture, prevent injuries and target the most common sites of aches and pains...

Neck: The Turtle

This exercise reverses aches associated with sitting in front of a computer for hours a day and pushing your head forward. You can do it standing or sitting. Just be sure to keep your neck and back in alignment. The focus of the exercise is to pull the head back, which stretches the neck muscles.

1. Pretend you're holding an apple under your chin, or keep your chin parallel to the floor. Inhale deeply.

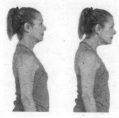

2. Exhale through your lips while pushing your chin forward.

3. Inhale through your nose, and slowly return your head to the neutral position you started with. Repeat as many times as you like to loosen up your neck.

Shoulders: The Zipper

This exercise loosens the shoulder muscles. You can do it standing or sitting. As you become more flexible, you can eliminate the strap and try to grab your fingertips instead.

1. Hold a strap in your right hand, and raise your arm above your head. Bring your right hand down behind your head. Grab the end of the strap with your left hand.

2. Raise your right hand up as high as is comfortable, lifting the left hand along with it. Hold. Perform two times on each side.

3. Pull your left hand down to also bring your right hand down. Hold. Perform two times on each side.

4. Switch sides and repeat.

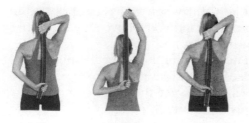

Lower Back: Seated Knee to Chest

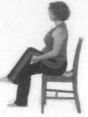

This exercise stretches the lower back and gluteus maximus muscles and has been shown to improve blood flow and relieve muscle tension.

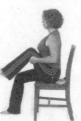

Sit with proper posture in a stable chair, and place your feet on the floor...or lie on the floor. Clasp both hands beneath your left leg.

Bring your left knee toward your chest. Hold, feeling the stretch in the gluteal region. Release the knee, switch sides, and repeat.

Standing Hip Flexor Stretching

Sitting for much of the day, as a lot of us do, can lead to tight hip flexors—the muscles that support the hip joints. To loosen them up, stand behind a sturdy chair with your hands on the back of it. Slide your right leg

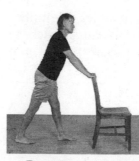

back a comfortable distance. Gently tuck your tailbone under and press your hips forward while keeping your rear heel down. When you can feel the stretch in your upper leg/hip region, hold.

Do two more times. Then do three repetitions on the other side.

Legs: Seated Hamstring Massage

The hamstrings—the areas on the back side of the thighs that connect to both the hips and the knees—are prone to tightening up and are common areas of injury and pain. This exercise massages the area to boost blood flow and calm muscle tension.

Sit in a sturdy chair, and place a foam roller under one thigh...or, if you prefer, lie on

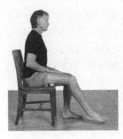

the floor. Slowly and gently roll and press your leg along the roller. Hold the roller there for five to 30 seconds. If you notice a particularly tense area, return to it. Repeat with the other leg.

Wrists: Seated Wrist Stretch

With all of the computer work and driving we do, our hands and wrists are prone to tightening up and cramping. This exercise targets both the wrists and the forearms.

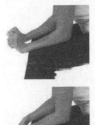

1. Sit in a chair, and rest your forearms on your thighs with your wrists dangling just beyond your knees. Make loose fists with your hands, and slowly lift your knuckles toward the ceiling. Hold.

2. Lower your knuckles slowly toward the floor. Hold.

Repeat this exercise as many times as feels comfortable.

Feet: Arch Rocks

Many people have trouble with foot cramping, stiffness and tightness as they age. This exercise helps to loosen the arches to relieve that discomfort.

1. Sit in a chair with both feet on a foam roller.

2. Slowly roll your feet forward and then back to massage the bottom of your feet. If you feel particular areas of tension, apply additional pressure and concentrate on those areas.

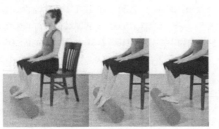

Hands: V-W Stretch

This exercise targets the hands and fingers and can be helpful for wrist strain. While the instructions are for sitting, it also can be done standing.

1. Sit with proper posture in a stable chair. Rest your hands on your thighs, palms facing down. Squeeze all your fingers together.

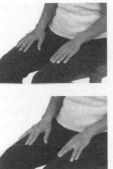

2. Separate one finger at a time, starting with the little finger, then the ring finger, until you've separated all your fingers. Squeeze your fingers together, and repeat.

To increase the challenge: Hold your arms straight out in front of you. Instead of just separating your fingers, try to make a V and W with them.

To make a V: Spread your little finger and ring finger away from your index finger and middle finger.

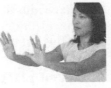

To make a W: Put your ring finger and middle finger together and separate the little finger and index finger from the group.

The Four-Step Plantar Fasciitis Plan

Colin Dombroski, PhD, a Canadian certified pedorthist who has managed over 6,000 cases of plantar fasciitis since 2002. Dr. Dombroski runs SoleScience (SoleScience.ca) and is an adjunct research professor at Western University in London, Ontario, Canada. He is the author of the book *The Plantar Fasciitis Plan*, available on Amazon.

The plantar fascia is inelastic connective tissue that runs the length of the foot and supports your arch. If you stand or walk on hard floors all day, wear the wrong shoes, or simply have a body mass index over 30, the fascia can develop tiny tears that lead to inflammation and pain.

As you rest your foot in your sleep, or by sitting for a while, the fascia shortens. When you stand, it lengthens, which makes it prone to developing more tears. So while it feels like you can just push through that morning pain, you're actually reinjuring the fascia.

To get rid of plantar fasciitis pain for good, the first step begins before you even get out of bed.

Step 1. Reduce morning pain

To reduce both pain and the risk of reinjury, set your alarm a few minutes earlier so you can complete this series of simple exercises before your feet hit the floor...

• **Write the alphabet with your foot.** Sit at the edge of the bed with your knee extended. Pretend that you're holding a pen with your toes and trace each of the letters of the alphabet in the air. This will stretch the foot and ankle.

Next, cross your foot over the opposite knee and use your hand to gently pull your toes back toward your shins to relieve muscle tightness. You can also wrap a towel under your foot and pull on that. Hold the stretch for 10 seconds and repeat three times.

• **Sit on the edge of the bed and place a tennis ball, foam roller, or a similar object under the arch of your foot.**

• **Roll it back and forth for about two minutes.** Any time that you're sitting for more than 30 minutes, repeat these stretches.

Once your foot is stretched and before you get out of bed, put on your most comfortable, supportive shoes (not slippers). This will distribute your weight over the arch of the foot and help prevent additional tearing.

Step 2. Evaluate your activity

Plantar fasciitis can be deceiving. You may feel perfectly fine while you're being active, only to be struck with pain after you've finished exercising and are resting. The trick is to reduce your activity just enough to prevent the pain from kicking in. If you know that your plantar fasciitis acts up after the 18th hole on the golf course, try ending your game a few holes earlier and see how you feel. A good rule of thumb is to reduce activity by 20 percent to see if it makes a difference. If you can't find a comfortable level of activity for even short periods of time, try other types of exercise, such as bicycling and swimming. But don't stop moving. Inactivity can cause the plantar fascia to stiffen. You may need to experiment with the activity.

Step 3. Choose your shoes

There is no single shoe that is the best choice for people with plantar fasciitis, but there is one type of shoe everyone should avoid: One that is worn out. I've met many patients who have been running in the same shoes for three years or who work on their feet all day in shoes that are no longer supportive.

If you see uneven wear on the soles of your shoes, it's a sure sign that it's time to get new ones. But you can't always see the whole story. Generally, shoes lose their support after a year. Athletic shoes can wear out much faster. If you're a long-distance runner, for example, you should replace your sneakers as often as every three months. Likewise, if you stand at work all day and wear the same shoes when you get home, you should probably replace your shoes more often than you have been.

When choosing new shoes, the first criterion is comfort. A good-quality shoe feels different on different types of feet, so you need to find the one that feels best to you. It's a great idea to go to a running store or a traditional shoe store with professional employees who can assess your foot mechanics and suggest options that are made to work with your type of foot. When it's time to buy, you usually get what you pay for. A $35 pair of sneakers isn't the bargain it looks like: You'll end up paying in other ways down the road.

Step 4. Try OTC solutions

If you can't find just the right shoe, there are many over-the-counter products that may help. For example, if you're working all day in steel-toed boots and you can't find a comfortable fit, something like a gel heel cup or insole can reduce pressure, provide support, and make you more comfortable. The objective is to be as comfortable as possible so you don't compensate by walking differently. Turning your foot to the side to reduce plantar fasciitis pain can quickly turn into knee pain. Whatever cushioning device you use, be sure to put it in every pair of shoes you wear.

If orthotic therapy is not effective, you might want to try night splints to prevent shortening of the fascia while you sleep.

A nonsteroidal anti-inflammatory drug, such as aspirin, ibuprofen, or naproxen, can also help relieve pain and inflammation. These simple strategies can resolve pain in most patients, though it may take some time. If you still have pain after six months of following this plan, you may be a candidate for additional treatments, such as physiotherapy or custom orthotics.

Suffering from Sciatica?

Start physical therapy (PT) right away if you're suffering from sciatica. Patients whose lower-back pain extends into their legs often are told to remain active and monitor the condition. But when researchers randomly assigned 220 such patients to either take that wait-and-see approach or immediately begin PT, by week four the PT group reported less pain and that difference continued for the entire year of the study.

Julie Fritz, PT, PhD, is associate dean for research at University of Utah College of Health, Salt Lake City, and leader of a study published in *Annals of Internal Medicine*.

Debilitating Sciatica Relieved in 10 Minutes

Andrew Rubman, ND, is medical director of Southbury Clinic for Traditional Medicines in Southbury, Connecticut. SouthburyClinic.com. He is author of the "Nature Doc's Patient Diary" blog at Bottom LineInc.com.

The *patient:* "Bonnie," a professional dancer in town for a series of performances.

Why she came to see me: This event occurred when I was in my residency in naturopathic medical school in Oregon. I was helping to support myself by working with the Stagehands Union (Local 28 of the IATSE) as a union member, and was notified by the director of the nationally renowned ballet company that I had been working with during their local stay that one of their lead ballerinas had come down with sudden excruciating sciatic pain. I offered to see her the following morning, knowing that she was supposed to perform that evening and for the next few days in our city.

How I evaluated her: During my examination, I found that there was a slight, but obviously significant, misalignment of a joint where her hip met her sacrum, causing a nerve that ran from her hip down into her foot—the sciatic nerve—to feel "like it was on fire." Because of her profession and extreme athletic activity, the area was extraordinarily developed and thus the tissue surrounding the joint and the point of exit of the nerve from her hip was involved in a debilitating spasm.

How we addressed her problem: In order to reduce the joint misalignment, or *subluxation,* I used a combination of physical therapy and parenteral (injection) techniques including electro-acupuncture, phonophoresis (using ultrasound to move botanical extracts through the skin into underlying tissue) and trigger-point injections where I would introduce a 1 percent buffered lidocaine solution into the areas surrounding the affected area around the hip joint (the posterior superior iliac spine) and the musculotendinous junction areas of the piriformis muscle that had swollen and was impinging against the sciatic nerve. She appreciated the detailed explanation as she told me that ballet dancers were quite aware of physical anatomy and she was curious as to the cause of her pain.

After allowing the local anesthesia to take hold and the physical medicine to further relax the area, I performed a series of quite aggressive adjustments causing her hip to move slightly back and into proper alignment with her sacrum. I thanked her for allowing me to "twist her up like a pretzel" and she forgave me, saying that it was her own fault for being so flexible!

Note that not all states allow naturopathic doctors to give injections. I would not have been able to provide this level of relief if Bonnie came to see me in my office in Connecticut today.

The patient's progress: After allowing her 10 minutes of hot packs to allow her to settle out, she got off the table, did some rather astounding and seemingly unnatural bending of her torso and legs and broke out into a broad smile announcing to me that I had "cured her."

Counting Down Can Keep Pain in Check

Study of 20 volunteers by researchers at Ludwig-Maximilians-Universität, Munich, Germany, and University of Oxford, UK, reported in *eLife*.

Recent study: Volunteers who were exposed to painful cold were asked to handle it in one of three ways—by counting down from 1,000 by sevens…thinking of something beautiful or pleasant…or persuading themselves that the feeling was not really too bad. Those who counted down reported feeling the least pain of all the groups—as much as a 50 percent reduction in perceived pain intensity. The high level of concentration required to count down by sevens was able to distract significantly from the experience of pain.

To Live Pain-Free, Take Care of Your Fascia: Here's How

Laurie Steelsmith, ND, LAc, medical director of Steelsmith Natural Health Center in Honolulu, where she has a busy private practice, and is an associate clinical professor at Bastyr University. She is coauthor of three books—*Natural Choices for Women's Health, Great Sex, Naturally* and *Growing Younger Every Day.* DrSteelsmith.com

Take a yoga class and chances are you'll hear your instructor mention the word fascia…in fact, you're likely hearing it everywhere, from "myofascial treatments" at your favorite spa to celebrities touting the benefits of cupping.

But what is fascia—and what role does it play in your physical health?

Fascia refers to your internal webbing. Located roughly two millimeters below the surface of your skin, it's made up of connective tissues such as elastic fibers, collagen, glycoproteins, and various other cells (including fibroblasts and fat cells). It stretches throughout your body, keeping your organs, bones, muscles, blood vessels, and nerves in their proper place, organizing your internal system and providing you with the capacity to both move and stay stable. It also plays a major role in your posture and determines where you are most likely to get injured, just as it influences your recovery time.

How Fascia Work

Your "second skin," as it's also called, is connected to your muscles, tendons, organs, and ligaments at thousands of contact points throughout your body. Fascia's fibrous connective tissues are tightly bound together, and can be slippery, wet, and like a robust rubber band inside of you, allowing your body to return to its original position after it's been elongated, and letting you elongate in the first place. It applies tension and compression to the body material it shields and surrounds (like joints and organs), absorbs shock, and reduces friction from everyday movement. It's also a superhighway of communication, sending information from your muscles to your organs to your bones, and balancing stressors and counter-stressors in the dance your body needs to be mobile, pliant, and strong.

What Can Go Wrong with Your Fascia—and How Does It Impact Pain?

Fascia is important for dozens of reasons, but one of the biggest of all is that it can be the source of chronic or acute soft-tissue pain.

When people have pain in their bodies, often the site of their pain is not the site of the problem. They may point to their lower back as the cause of their aches when it's really an issue with their hamstring.

How can this be? Remember: Every bit of you is encased in fascia. Sensitive to all movement, this highly innervated internal matrix bucks the notion of isolation exercises and "chest and biceps" days. All movement—and lack thereof—affects it. It runs in "trains," or lines, throughout the body, spanning from the bottom of your foot to the top of your head. Neck pain, then, could actually be due to a problem with your hip, or even your heel.

Trauma, disease, inactivity and more can impact the suppleness and "smooth glide" of your fascia, causing it to "thicken and become sticky," Harpreet Gujral, DNP and program director of integrative medicine at Sibley Memorial Hospital, told Johns Hopkins Medicine. When it "dries up" and constricts around muscles, it can decrease agility and cause painful adhesions, or knots, to develop.

What Can You Do to Keep Fascia Healthy?

Luckily, there's plenty you can do to keep your fascia healthy.

• **Fluid movement.** We tend to think we are supporting our muscles when we exercise, which in fact we are. But because each muscle is swathed in fascia—and because fascia hold the majority of your nerve fibers—fluid movements such as dance that engage multiple muscle groups or the majority of your body is one the savviest ways to keep your fascia well-oiled—and keep you able to perform effortless and painless movements. So pump it up at your aerobic dance lessons, Zumba classes, learn how to do the cha-cha or any other type of continuous movement, and enjoy knowing you are also supporting your fascial health.

• **Yoga and stretching.** Stretching is often overlooked for more vigorous forms of activity or due to a dearth of time. This is a shame. Safe stretching is central to the health of your fascia—not too little, but also not too much. You want to activate it physiologically without overactivating it, which may create scarring and reduce mobility.

That being said, bear in mind that, genetically, we have different fascial tendencies. People who are naturally superflexible tend to have structurally different fascia tissue than people who tend to be stiff. Naturally super-flexible people need more strength training, toning and ballistic stretching (bouncing on a trampoline or jogging) than stretching. Those who tend to be stiff, on the other hand, need more stretching, which is what they will find in a yoga class.

Indeed, during my training as an Iyengar yoga teacher, I discovered that yoga's ancient asanas (postures) tap into both the deep and superficial fascial lines of the body. By consistently doing asanas, the fascial lines are released, balanced, toned, and profoundly affected. Those who have chronic soft tissue pains, postural imbalances or stiffness would benefit tremendously by slowly and methodically starting a yoga or stretching practice that impacts on these fascial lines. When I immersed myself in the 5,000 year-old practice of Iyengar, hip pain that had haunted me on and off for years disappeared. The ache in my lower back—pain stuck in my left sacroiliac joint that I had tried to treat with a chiropractor—evaporated. I found myself sitting up straighter, smiling more, and thinking better. I even found myself standing erect and pinning my hips in, like in mountain pose, while pumping gas instead of unconsciously thrusting my hip out to the side. Yoga was re-aligning my entire being.

•**Sleeping—and Rising the "Right" Way.** Not just any sleep, but sleeping on a hard bed. Yes, hard. A soft bed may appear welcoming, but it makes it harder to get going in the morning because you've been "gelled up" in its cocoon. Also, your fascia become stiff when you don't move all night long. When you sleep on a hard bed, you have a greater tendency to move during the night, and shifting positions hydrates your fascia. This isn't for everyone! Make sure you have a mattress you sleep well on. A good night's sleep allows your connective tissue cells to do their job of knitting your fascial tissues back together.

When you rise, consider doing what's known as "pandiculating." You know when your cat or dog gets up from a long nap and does a big stretch? This is "pandiculation," and humans can do it too. It stretches your body's fascia and all the nerves that travel in it, literally waking up your sensory-motor system, while minimizing strain.

Techniques to Release Fascial Adhesions

Learning about fascia, how it works, and its makeup has helped me to understand more clearly how some of the therapies I offer patients work to treat their chronic pain.

•**Acupuncture** involves the use of fine needles, which are inserted into acupuncture points along meridians (highways of energy, or Qi) in the body. It is not scientifically known how acupuncture works, but I believe part of its efficacy in decreasing pain is due to stimulating blood and fluid to the area where the needle has been inserted. Interestingly enough, in Traditional Chinese Medicine, pain is always associated with what is called "Stuck Qi," and putting a needle into a painful area releases the Qi and allows for the free-flowing movement of Qi. My feeling is that this ancient technique "unkinks" fascia and allows it to return to its most optimal state.

•**Cupping,** also part of Traditional Chinese Medicine, is also used to break up stagnant Qi and decrease pain. The treatment utilizes sterile glass or ceramic cups that create a suction on the skin. The cups adhere to the skin either by applying heat to the inside of the cup before placing the cup on the skin, or by suction. The skin and fascia lift up and fascial adhesions break up when the cups are moved along the skin. Note that cupping can sometimes cause bruising of the skin and should only be done by a trained professional.

•**Perineural injection treatment** is a treatment that utilizes 5 percent dextrose (medical grade sugar) plus sodium bicarbonate in sterile water to treat stiffness and pain. Developed by New Zealand family physician Dr. John Lyftogt, the treatment is performed through small injections that are made along the peripheral nerves. (Your peripheral nervous system is a web of 43 motor and sensory nerves that link the brain and spinal cord to the body.) The dextrose in the solution is believed to block a particular receptor, known as Trpv-1, that releases proteins—or neuropeptides—that generate stiffness and pain. What remains under investigation is if the injected water also promotes the coveted "smooth glide" of fascia. I have seen patients who, within seconds of receiving perineural injections, felt "lighter, looser, and freer," and the taut, painful, restricted movements in their neck had suddenly diminished.

•**Prolozone therapy** utilizes a prolotherapy solution of dextrose, sodium bicarbonate and procaine (an anesthetic) that is injected into trigger points, where there are fascial adhesions, or joints followed by ozone (a gas that carries extra oxygen). When the ozone gas is injected, it immediately converts to oxygen and water. The oxygen then stimulates the cells to produce more energy, or ATP, and increases growth factors. The water, originally thought to just be an inert by-product, may also contribute to the smooth glide of fascia. I have witnessed countless patients—as well as myself—experience terrific fascial changes post-Prolozone injections that rolfing and other deep tissue therapies couldn't touch.

●**Foam rolling** is a self-treatment in which you use a foam roller to apply pressure to your fascia, thereby urging it to release tension, re-establish the integrity of the tissue and encourage flexibility.

If movement seems to be a recurrent theme here, that's because it's essential to keeping your fascia healthy and gliding. Ultimately, tending to your fascia can change your chronic body-pain patterns, improve your posture, and give you freedom of movement—keeping you healthy and gliding. Through life, that is.

3D Technology Makes Knee Replacement Better Than Ever

Daniel Wiznia, MD, orthopedic surgeon specializing in reconstructive surgery of the knee and hip, director of technology and innovation in the department of orthopaedics at Yale University School of Medicine, New Haven, Connecticut, and assistant professor of orthopaedics and rehabilitation and of mechanical engineering and materials science.

For decades, knee-replacement surgery has been allowing people with extreme pain and joint deterioration to return to an active life. Recently, the procedure itself has undergone an evolution, leading to even greater benefits. What's making the difference? Three-dimensional (3D) technology that personalizes the surgery for each individual's anatomy.

This is key because your gait (how you walk or run) is unique like a fingerprint. How your knee bends is different from how someone else's knee bends. This means that the shape of your bones also will be different from another person's.

With the use of 3D technology, surgeons now can "see" the precise uniqueness of your anatomy—and adjust the replacement accordingly—long before the first incision. *What you need to know about this high-tech breakthrough…*

How It Works

The first step of 3D knee replacement, as with the traditional approach, is to get high-resolution images of your knee, usually with a CT scan or an MRI. With the new technique, a computerized 3D replica of your joint then is created from the scan using specialized software. Your surgeon reviews this replica to evaluate your bone structure, surrounding tissues, joint alignment and the extent of joint damage, noting the subtleties of your anatomy.

Because the 3D images are so precise, your surgeon can generate a computerized model of exactly how the bones glide against one another as the joint connects with other bones, which helps in selecting the best size and shape of implant for you…and in determining the best placement and alignment of that implant. The 3D replica also shows whether modifications are needed, such as compensating for loose or injured ligaments with an implant that provides a tighter fit.

Many different versions of personalized knee replacement rely on the 3D model. For example, some surgeons who perform knee replacements have received specialized training in the use of robotic surgery. In other cases, the surgeon will use the computerized 3D model to formulate navigation guides for making incisions and choosing the optimal placement of the joint, sometimes using specially created 3D-printed instruments that will help align implant components during the surgery.

The 3D Advantages

Compared with traditional knee replacement, 3D-based knee replacement offers a variety of benefits for patients such as…

●**More precise positioning for a better fit.** Research shows that a customized pre-op plan means fewer errors in positioning the implant and reduces your chance of needing a revision, which involves replacing some parts of the original implant. Without 3D imaging, even the best surgeons have to do a bit of educated guessing to try to place the replacement knee as perfectly as possible. If the placement is even a little bit off, you could have extra pain and stiffness, and your recovery could take longer.

●**Smaller incision, less pain.** Because the surgeon uses 3D technology to model where the replacement joint will be positioned, clinical practice has shown that the incisions used for 3D-based knee replacement can be up to 20 percent smaller than with the traditional approach. There also is less stretching of ligaments and soft tissue, so there is less pain—and less need for narcotic medication, which can be addictive.

●**Safer procedure.** With 3D-based knee replacement, there is less blood loss and a far lower likelihood of needing a blood transfusion, which carries potential side effects, ranging from fever and chills to suppression of your immune system.

With better pre-op planning, the surgery also takes about 15 minutes less to perform than traditional knee replacement. Less time spent in the operating room means less time under anesthesia, which, in turn, reduces its associated risks, such as heart attack, stroke and infection.

●**Less need for hospital re-admission.** You're less likely to be readmitted to the hospital after getting a 3D-based knee replacement because there are fewer postsurgery problems, such as blood clots, infection and loose components.

●**Better recovery.** 3D technology leads to better biomechanics, too. By replicating your own anatomy as much as possible, the better-fitting implant you'll receive feels more natural, allowing you to resume normal activities sooner—usually in about six weeks versus roughly three months for traditional knee replacement. This is because 3D-based knee replacement causes less inflammation.

Bonus: There is less need for pain medication.

While participation in a rehab program is still essential, you should be able to bend your knee properly soon after surgery, and that will make it easier for you to build up strength and overcome the weaknesses caused by years of arthritis.

●**Longer-lasting implant.** When the implant fits better, there's less daily friction, so its life span may extend beyond the 20-year average for traditional implants (right now, 3D hasn't been used long enough to know for sure). A better fit means less loading and stressing being placed on the joint, which lengthens the life span of the implant.

Availability of 3D

3D-based knee replacement is increasingly available at most major academic centers but is conducted by only a few surgeons because it requires specialized training. Before scheduling a 3D-based knee replacement, make sure your surgeon has proper training and experience.

Best approach: Ask the surgeon whether he/she has completed an orthopedic total-joint-replacement fellowship, a one-year program that now routinely includes training in the use of 3D technology.

Nearly all insurance companies cover 3D-based knee replacement. Some may not cover the pre-op CT or MRI imaging (about $150), but that could be a small price to pay for the advantages of this type of knee replacement. All of the increased cost of 3D-based knee replacement is covered by insurance (including the costs of the robotic technology, computer navigation technology,

3D-printed cutting guides and 3D-printed implants).

Note: 3D technology also is available for hip replacements, using a 3D model of the femoral head (the ball at the top of the thighbone) and socket joint.

3D Boosts Implant Durability

With the use of 3D technology, manufacturing practices have become more advanced, improving the durability of knee implants. Most knee implants are made of metal (such as cobalt chromium or titanium) or ceramic, often in combination with polyethylene (a plastic). Ceramic is becoming the leader for longest-lasting material, with an average life span of 25 to 30 years.

One material-based innovation is oxidized zirconium (a proprietary material called Oxinium and developed by medical-device-maker Smith & Nephew), which starts as a metal but is processed in a way that turns it into a ceramic. Instead of polished cobalt chrome connecting with the polyethylene liner, the oxidized zirconium, which is a very smooth, wear-resistant surface, connects with the polyethylene, resulting in less wear and a longer life span.

Important: With so many implant options available, be sure to discuss your lifestyle and goals with your doctor so the best one for you can be chosen.

Fight the Rise of Autoimmune Disease

Susan Blum, MD, MPH, the founder and director of the Blum Center for Health in Rye Brook, New York. She is the author of *The Immune System Recovery Plan* and *Healing Arthritis*. BlumHealthMD.com and BlumCenterFor Health.com

---

The immune system is constantly working to fend off viruses, bacteria, and other invaders, but when it becomes overzealous, it can attack the very body it's defending. As a result, runaway inflammation wreaks havoc throughout the body. From rheumatoid arthritis to multiple sclerosis, there are more than 100 conditions attributed to what's called autoimmune disease.

And the problem appears to be growing: According to researchers from the National Institutes of Health, nearly 16 percent of Americans have a biomarker of autoimmunity called antinuclear antibodies, a significant rise from 11 percent a few decades ago.

Research suggests that this increase could be attributed to a handful of factors that are common in the 21st century: a diet loaded with processed foods, chronic stress, an imbalance in the gut microbiota, and a deluge of environmental toxins. Addressing those factors can lower your risk of developing an autoimmune disease or, if you already have one, to get it under control.

Eat a Mediterranean Diet

In a recent review paper in the journal *Bio sciences,* Greek researchers reported that the Mediterranean diet is linked to a lower incidence of multiple sclerosis, less severe psoriasis, and better quality of life in patients with rheumatoid arthritis and lupus. This anti-inflammatory diet calms rather than overstimulates your immune system. This diet emphasizes nutrient-rich vegetables and fruits, beans, nuts and seeds, fatty fish, and olive oil, and eliminates white sugar, white flour, and processed foods.

Some people may also want to eliminate foods that contain gluten, a combination of two proteins found in wheat, barley, and rye. In people with celiac disease, gluten triggers an immune response that damages the lining of the small intestine, interfering with the absorption of nutrients from food.

Relax

Studies show that stress is a risk factor for autoimmune disease. In October 2020, researchers reported that people who were diagnosed with a stress-related disorder, such as post-traumatic stress disorder, were more likely to be diagnosed with an autoimmune disease and were more likely to develop multiple autoimmune diseases.

To turn off stress, practice a relaxation technique every day. I teach many of my patients this simple, stress-relieving exercise, and use it myself: Sit up in a chair or bed, as erect as possible. Get comfortable and close your eyes. Loosen any clothing that feels restrictive. Breathe deeply, in through your nose and out through your mouth. Now, imagine your belly is soft. This will deepen the breath and improve the exchange of oxygen, even as it relaxes your muscles. Say to yourself in your mind "soft" as you breathe in and "belly" as you breathe out.

As you breathe in, imagine your belly puffing out. As you breathe out, imagine your belly flattening in. Sit quietly and practice "soft belly" breathing for five to 10 minutes. If you notice your mind wandering away, just come back to "soft belly."

Heal Your Gut

About 70 percent of your immune system resides in your gut. The two most important ways to keep your gut healthy are to eat a Mediterranean diet and to take a daily probiotic supplement, which supplies friendly, gut-balancing bacteria. Look for a gluten-free and dairy-free probiotic supplement with 25 to 50 billion colony-forming units of six or more strains of probiotics, with an emphasis on lactobacillus and bifidus strains. Also try to eat more fermented foods and beverages, such as sugar-free yogurt with live cultures, miso (fermented soy paste), kimchee (Korean sauerkraut), and kombucha (fermented green and black tea).

Detox Your Environment

From personal care products to cleaning supplies, our world is filled with toxins. To reduce your exposure, always use natural cleaning supplies and household products. Use a HEPA air filter to remove toxins from indoor air.

Don't spray pesticides around or in your home. Look for cosmetics and skincare products that don't contain synthetic fragrances, parabens, or phthalates. Go organic when it comes to fruits and vegetables, and opt for free-range, organic meats and eggs. Filter your tap water. Avoid using plastic bottles and containers with the numbers 3, 6, and 7 on them as they may leach chemicals into their contents. Support your liver, your most powerful detoxifying organ with 600 to 1,200 milligrams of N-acetyl-cysteine each day.

My Story

When I was diagnosed with Hashimoto's thyroiditis, I began using the principles of functional medicine to heal myself. My lifestyle was already very healthy—I was a vegetarian, exercised regularly, and practiced yoga and meditation. But I discovered from interviewing my family that I have a genetic predisposition to autoimmune disease. Genetic testing showed that I also had an issue with clearing out mercury, resulting in high levels in my body. To take my unique biological patterns into account, I went on a gluten-free diet, stopped eating fish that was high in mercury, had my mercury dental fillings removed and replaced, drank an inflammation-reducing protein shake every day, and took small amounts of thyroid hormone. Two years into my new regimen, my level of thyroid-attacking antibodies had returned to normal.

Autoimmune Disease Throughout the Body

Autoimmune diseases seem different from each other, but that's because antibodies are targeting and attacking tissues in different parts of the body…

• **Thyroid.** When the immune system attacks the thyroid gland, it can cause either Graves' disease (overactive thyroid) or Hashimoto's disease (underactive thyroid).

• **Nerve cells.** When it attacks the myelin sheathing around nerve cells, a process called demyelination, patients can develop multiple sclerosis.

• **Joints.** The immune system can attack the joints, causing the tissue damage and inflammation known as rheumatoid arthritis.

• **Intestines.** If the immune system attacks the microscopic, finger-like protrusions called villi that line the small intestine, it can cause celiac disease.

• **Mucus-secreting glands.** In Sjogren's syndrome, the immune system attacks mucus-secreting glands, leading to symptoms such as dry eyes and dry mouth.

• **Multiple systems.** In systemic lupus erythematosus, the immune system attacks the skin, joints, kidneys and nervous system.

Bee Venom Injections Relieve Knee Osteoarthritis

Study titled "Efficacy and Safety of Honey Bee Venom (Apis mellifera) Dermal Injections to Treat Osteoarthritis Knee Pain and Physical Disability: A Randomized Controlled Trial," by researchers at CHA University, Seongnam, The Republic of Korea, published in *The Journal of Alternative and Complementary Medicine*.

You might think of bees as pain inflictors more than healers, but researchers have recently shown that injections of European honeybee venom (HBV) can reduce pain and improve function for people with knee osteoarthritis.

Using bee venom as medicine is part of a discipline known as apitherapy (*api* is Latin for bee). Apitherapy has been used for hundreds of years and is practiced today as a complementary and alternative therapy. Some studies show that HBV has strong anti-inflammatory properties.

Recent research finding: The new study, published in *The Journal of Alternative and Complementary Medicine*, combined HBV injections with acupuncture, since the injections were given in the knees as well as in traditional acupuncture sites, including around the eyes and the spine. Injections were given just below the skin (called a dermal injection). This study was double blind, placebo-controlled, which means the researchers compared HBV to placebo injections, and neither the subjects nor the researchers knew which participants were given the HBV.

The researchers recruited 538 patients with X-ray-documented osteoarthritis of the knee and significant knee pain scores recorded before treatment. Patients were randomly assigned to receive injections of either histamine (the placebo) or HBV. All patients received 12 weekly sessions of 15 injections. Injections included five in each knee and other injections in various acupuncture points.

At the end of the 12 weekly injections the placebo group was compared with the HBV group for pain scores, physical function ratings, doctor evaluation and patient assessment. Compared with the placebo patients, the HBV patients had highly significant improvement in pain, which lasted four weeks after finishing treatment. The HBV patients had significant improvement in both doctor and patient assessment of their overall osteoarthritis condition.

The HBV patients had more injection-site reactions, but overall HBV safety was comparable to the placebo injections. The researchers conclude that HBV therapy can significantly improve knee osteoarthritis pain and function.

Tryptophan Shows Potential to Relieve Celiac Disease

Study titled "Aryl Hydrocarbon Receptor Ligand Production by the Gut Microbiota Is Decreased in Celiac Disease Leading to Intestinal Inflammation," by researchers at McMaster University, Ontario, Canada, published in *Science Translational Medicine*.

For people with celiac disease, maintaining a strict gluten-free diet can be extremely challenging. And even when making vigilant food choices, there's no guarantee that the symptoms (such as painful abdominal bloating) will subside.

Good news: New research shows that a common amino acid, combined with probiotics, may help celiac sufferers improve their response to a gluten-free diet while also helping intestinal healing.

Bonus: The amino acid, tryptophan, can be found in your favorite turkey meal.

Celiac disease develops when the small intestine triggers an exaggerated immune response to the presence of gluten, a protein found in the grains wheat, barley and rye. Eventually, the lining of the small intestine becomes damaged, making it harder for the body to absorb critical nutrients from food.

Gut damage from celiac disease is also usually accompanied by an impaired ability to stimulate protective receptors in the gut lining, such as AhR, the aryl hydrocarbon receptor. AhR is important in controlling inflammation in the gut.

When the AhR receptor does not function properly, celiac patients can struggle with intestinal healing even after all gluten is removed from the diet. Tryptophan can potentially combat this by helping to produce metabolites that signal to receptors like AhR to start controlling inflammation and better protect the gut barrier.

The study: A team of international researchers at McMaster University in Ontario, Canada, looked at how effectively tryptophan could help with celiac through stimulation of AhR. Their study was published in *Science Translational Medicine*. To test tryptophan's efficacy in managing celiac disease, the researchers observed the metabolism of tryptophan across three groups of people—those with active celiac disease, celiac patients two years into a gluten-free diet and healthy people with no celiac symptoms.

Results: The patients with active celiac had trouble breaking down the tryptophan necessary to activate AhR, although those who had been on a gluten-free diet had a somewhat improved response. However, according to additional testing on mice with genes predisposed to celiac disease,

researchers were able to jumpstart the metabolism of tryptophan by introducing the probiotic lactobacilli, successfully triggering the AhR pathway response.

While further research is needed to confirm study results, the researchers believe these findings offer hope for a potential therapy combining tryptophan and probiotics to manage celiac disease.

Thriving When There Is No Cure

Craig K. Svensson, PharmD, PhD, dean emeritus and professor of medicinal chemistry & molecular pharmacology in the Purdue University College of Pharmacy, as well as adjunct professor of pharmacology & toxicology in the Indiana University School of Medicine. Dr. Svensson is the author of *When There Is No Cure*. CraigSvensson.com

---

I am just one of the millions of people who live with chronic medical conditions. I have lived through the uncertainty of not knowing what was causing my symptoms, the frustration of not being able to find relief, and the fear of losing mobility and independence. Diseases such as systemic lupus erythematosus, fibromyalgia, multiple sclerosis, rheumatoid arthritis, ulcerative colitis, and chronic pain have no cure (yet), but those of us who have them can still thrive and experience fulfillment and joy.

Learn About Yourself

When you live with a chronic condition, you need to arm yourself with information. Keep a health diary to become familiar with how the ailment affects your body. What worsens your symptoms? What lessens them? What patterns can you discern?

Next, think about what behaviors you can change to be more comfortable. Do you need to limit the time you sit to avoid aggravating underlying pain? Do you need to limit the number of evening activities in a given week to avoid cumulative fatigue? Do vacation plans need to account for your heightened sensitivity to heat or cold?

Consider how your illness affects others. Studies have found that the quality of life for spouses and partners is sometimes poorer than the quality of life for a patient with chronic illness. Family and friends want to ease our burden, but don't always know how. Careful reflection and open communication can ease the way.

Learn About the Disease

Once you have a diagnosis for your symptoms, the second educational focus is about the disease. How does it manifest in most people? What does normal progression look like? Should you expect a decline in your functioning? What options exist for treatment or symptom relief?

While your primary care physician is a valuable source of information, you may need to dig deeper. A single physician may not have ample experience with your specific condition and may not have all of the answers you need. In many cases, chronic illnesses are misdiagnosed by busy doctors. Furthermore, studies show that patients who understand diseases such as diabetes, high blood pressure, and asthma have better health outcomes. We have every reason to believe the same to be true for other ailments as well.

While researching, be aware that websites often post bad health information. The Access to Credible Genetics Resource Network has created a helpful tool patients can use to assess the credibility of posted health information. You can find it at TrustOrTrash.org.

Disease-specific patient advocacy groups are often valuable for both information and support. The best groups include an expert advisory panel to assess the accuracy of the information provided.

Learn About Disease Progression

People living with a chronic disease often make two opposing errors. The first is seeing any change in health as a sign of disease progression. The second is ignoring signs that merit attention. It is imperative to learn how to strike the right balance between these two extremes.

Many chronic ailments, even those associated with a progressive decline, wax and wane over time. You need to identify benchmarks to pinpoint when it's time to self-manage and when it's time to seek a medical expert.

Speak frankly with your health-care providers about how they will assess progression over the years to come. Are there symptoms that suggest a more rapid progression? How will the disease affect functional and cognitive abilities? How might these impact your professional or personal plans?

If You Expect a Decline in Function

While some chronic conditions lead to unrelenting symptoms, others inevitably lead to functional decline. In that latter case, it is wise to consider ways you might change things in your life to accommodate future disability.

You may be able to make home modifications to accommodate future mobility challenges.

If you are very active, it's wise to consider less strenuous activities or hobbies that will still provide fulfillment in your leisure time.

It may make sense to consider alternative careers and even seek out essential education to prepare for them, if future decline will impair your ability to fulfill your current duties.

Evaluate your insurance policies and talk with a financial planner about what-if scenarios.

Discuss with loved ones how to address housing changes, if they become necessary.

If you find yourself in a perpetual cycle of worry, sadness, anger, or fear, consider seeking spiritual or professional counsel. Support groups can also help you find others who have traveled down the same road and found ways to overcome the challenges that you face.

Live Your Life

The foolish but oft-repeated mantra, "If you don't have your health, you don't have anything," represents a depressing and narrow view of life. The truth is, many who suffer from chronic illness have found their life journey to be fulfilling and marked by abundant joy. I am convinced this path is open to all who live with an incurable ailment that leads to chronic suffering. Yes, life is different from before chronic illness. Nevertheless, different can be fulfilling.

How to Live with Pain

For many people with chronic pain, there comes a point when you must recognize that eradicating pain is an unrealistic near-term goal. That doesn't mean giving in to suffering, but it does mean that you need to establish new goals to enable you to live life to the fullest extent possible.

- **Identify the most important areas of your life that are disrupted by pain and look for adaptation strategies.** For example, I suffer extreme back pain when driving, but I'm not willing to accept drowsiness or dulled cognitive ability to obtain this goal through medication. Ultimately, I purchased an SUV of substantial height that did not re-quire lowering myself into the seat of a car. That purchase did more to improve my pain while driving than any form of physical therapy or medication.

- **See a pain-management specialist.** Unlike a general physician, pain-management specialists have focused their training on the effective management of chronic pain. The growing trend toward telemedicine can make the limited number of pain-management specialists available to people no matter where they live.

- **Avoid idleness and isolation.** When the mind is idle, pain is more noticeable, and we are more prone to brood on thoughts of despair about our plight. Keeping your mind busy with activities and social interaction provides distraction, which actually alters sensory pain signals in the spinal cord, and it gives life more meaning and joy.

- **Manage stress.** People living with chronic pain will often experience increased pain during times of stress. Learning how to reduce stress or to better cope with its presence in our lives can reduce pain. Similarly, anxiety can provoke pain in patients with ailments like trigeminal neuralgia (painful attacks arising from a misfiring of the trigeminal nerve in the jaw). Addressing the underlying causes of anxiety can reduce the episodes of painful attacks in such patients.

Chapter 12

PHYSICAL INJURY AND BONE HEALTH

Physical and Emotional Trauma Linger in Your Body: How to Free Yourself

Trauma—whether emotional or physical—is a painful, horrifying experience that overwhelms your capacity to cope, and its effects often last for decades. Victims are more likely to be irritable, anxious and depressed...have difficulty focusing...miss work...have financial problems...sleep poorly...abuse alcohol or drugs...suffer from a major health problem...and/or feel suicidal.

There are many ways to be traumatized. Experts estimate that an astounding 75 percent of us have experienced one or more traumatic events of varying degrees.

Examples: You suffered through a childhood of abuse. Your parents had a bad divorce, or one or both were mentally ill, alcoholic or addicted to drugs. You were raped or sexually assaulted. You were mugged. You killed people in combat and watched friends die. You lived through a natural disaster. You were in a serious accident. You're a cancer survivor. More recently, losing a loved one

because of COVID-19 could have the potential to leave traumatic scarring on some.

What often gets overlooked: Beyond physical injury caused by the event, trauma leaves an imprint on your body, not just your brain, in the form of heartbreaking and gut-wrenching physical sensations.

For real healing to take place, your body needs to learn that the danger has passed and that it's possible to live in the safety of the present. *Here's what you need to know to lay the residues of trauma to rest—and recover...*

Goals of Recovery

The challenge of recovering from trauma is to know what you know and feel what you feel without becoming overwhelmed, enraged, ashamed or collapsed. *For most, this involves four goals...*

GOAL #1: **Finding a way to become calm and focused.**

GOAL #2: **Learning to maintain that calm in response to images, thoughts,**

Bessel van der Kolk, MD, founder and medical director of the Trauma Research Foundation in Brookline, Massachusetts. He is professor of psychiatry at Boston University School of Medicine and author of the #1 *New York Times* best-selling book *The Body Keeps the Score: Brain, Mind and Body in the Healing of Trauma.* BesselvanderKolk.com sounds and physical sensations that remind you of the past.

GOAL #3: Finding a way to be fully alive in the present and engaged with the people around you.

GOAL #4: Not keeping secrets from yourself, including secrets about the ways you have managed to survive (for example, by abusing alcohol or drugs).

There are several body-based methods that I have used extensively to help my patients, and I've also experienced their effectiveness personally. *In addition to those body-based techniques, there are several other approaches that research shows can be very helpful...*

• **Eye movement desensitization and reprocessing (EMDR).** In this well-researched technique, you recall a traumatic event while a therapist moves his/her fingers back and forth in front of you, and you follow them with your eyes. EMDR rebalances brain circuits, allowing you to experience the "true" present without interferences from trauma-related perceptions. It is most effective for trauma caused by a single event in adulthood, such as a car accident, but it can be useful as an adjunctive treatment for people struggling with the legacy of childhood trauma.

Scientific evidence: In a National Institute of Mental Health–funded study conducted by myself and my colleagues, 88 people with post-traumatic stress disorder (PTSD) were treated for eight weeks with EMDR...an antidepressant drug...or a placebo. At a six-month follow-up, 75 percent of those with adult-onset trauma who received EMDR had complete relief of symptoms, compared with zero percent in the antidepressant group. (We did not keep people on a placebo for the entire study.)

Resource: To find an EMDR practitioner, check the EMDR International Association (EMDRIA.org).

• **Yoga.** Traumatized individuals tend to become overwhelmed by their physical sensations and spend a lot of energy trying to block out what is going on in their bodies.

Some do this naturally...others turn to drugs, alcohol or eating disorders. The memory of helplessness during trauma tends to be stored as muscle tension in the affected areas—for example, head, back and limbs in accident victims...vagina and rectum in victims of sexual abuse. Also, trauma victims often are chronically angry or scared, which leads to muscle tension that produces back pain, migraine headaches, fibromyalgia and other forms of chronic pain. Yoga, which typically combines breath practices, stretches and meditation, can help people develop a harmonious relationship with their physical sensations, relax those muscles and normalize rage- and fear-causing circuits between the body and the brain.

Scientific evidence: We studied women with chronic, treatment-resistant PTSD, enrolling them in 20 weeks of trauma-sensitive yoga sessions. Participants experienced significant reductions in PTSD, which was amplified in two subsequent long-term follow-up studies.

Resource: Find a teacher certified in trauma-sensitive yoga at TraumaSensitive Yoga.com.

• **Neurofeedback.** When neurons (brain cells) communicate with each other, they generate electrical pulses—brain waves—that can be detected with sensors on the scalp. One study showed that people with PTSD can have brain waves that lack coherent patterns and don't generate brain wave patterns that filter out irrelevant information and help you pay attention to the task at hand, which is why lack of focus is a hallmark of PTSD. Neurofeedback helps correct these dysfunctional brain wave patterns.

The method "harvests" a person's brain waves and projects them onto a computer screen, allowing him/her to play therapeutic computer games with his own brain waves— reducing the brain waves that create fearfulness, shame and rage...and increasing the brain waves that create calm and focus.

Scientific evidence: My colleagues and I first studied 52 people with chronic PTSD from multiple events, dividing them into two groups. One group received neurofeedback, and one didn't. By the end of the 40-session study, only 27 percent of those receiving neurofeedback still met the criteria for a diagnosis of PTSD, compared with 68 percent of those who didn't get neurofeedback. Most dramatic was the improvement in executive functioning—being able to plan, be mentally flexible, being able to look at a problem from a variety of points of view and inhibiting their impulses. Another neurofeedback study of foster children with histories of abuse and neglect had similar positive results.

Resources: To find a neurofeedback provider trained in overcoming trauma near you, visit the website of the International Society for Neuroregulation & Research (ISNR.org).

•**Talk therapy.** As you use body-based methods to relieve the physical burdens generated by trauma, you can make better use of talk therapy. You need to acknowledge and name what happened to restore feelings of control. Feeling listened to and understood also changes your body—being able to articulate a complex feeling and having your feeling recognized creates an "aha moment." Modern-day therapy for PTSD has focused on treatment through prescription drugs such as antidepressants. These aren't a solution. They dampen the physical systems that create symptoms of trauma but don't resolve them. The only way to resolve the trauma is to understand and release it at your deepest emotional levels.

Another effective way to access your inner world of feelings is through writing. When you write to yourself, you don't have to worry about other people's judgment—you just listen to your own thoughts and let their flow take over.

Scientific evidence: In a study published in *British Journal of Clinical Psychology,* 88 trauma survivors received trauma-focused psychotherapy. After four months, the participants had better verbal memory, information processing and executive functioning (the ability to plan and make decisions). And in a six-month study on Afghanistan and Iraq war veterans, those who wrote expressively

about their feelings had greater reductions in PTSD, physical complaints, anger and distress compared with veterans who didn't write at all.

Look for a therapist who has mastered a variety of techniques—EMDR, psychodrama, expressive writing, neurofeedback and trauma-focused talk therapy. Feeling safe and comfortable with the therapist is necessary for you to confront your fears and anxieties. If you don't feel that connection or that he/she is curious enough to find out who you are and what you need, look for another therapist.

---

4 Common Moves That Lead to Injury...And How to Do Them the Right Way

Jonathan L. Chang, MD, orthopedic surgeon at Alhambra, California based Pacific Orthopaedic Associates (PACOrtho.org). He is a former clinical associate professor of orthopedic surgery at Keck School of Medicine of University of Southern California in Los Angeles and has served as spokesperson for the American College of Sports Medicine and the American Orthopaedic Society for Sports Medicine.

We tend to associate injuries with car accidents and major falls, but the truth is our days are filled with chances to make small mistakes during very common movements that can lead to painful injuries. But with a few strategic changes, you can minimize your risk for injury—and the painful recovery that would accompany it.

EVERYDAY RISKY MOVE #1: **Lifting Heavy Objects**

Nearly all adults will experience low-back pain at some point in their lifetime. One of the most common causes is lifting a heavy, unstable or unwieldy object. Most people know that they lift the wrong way, but they do it anyway thinking that they'll be fine.

How it happens: People overestimate how much they can lift or underestimate an object's weight, so they approach that bag of groceries or moving a box full of books with a false sense of confidence.

Next, they reach for the object by bending over, hinging from the waist, then attempt to lift it by simply straightening back up again. This leaves the lifting to the back muscles, which have evolved to hold the weight of your torso and head up when you are standing erect, not when bent over. Lifting in this position leaves the back vulnerable to injury.

If the object is unevenly weighted (such as a box stacked with books on just one side) or has moving parts (a wriggling child), your back muscles will automatically attempt to compensate for the instability, increasing injury risk.

Besides creating lower-back strain, improper lifting can exacerbate an existing herniated disk (also called a slipped disk) or create a new one.

Note: A strain results when muscles or tendons (the bands of tissue that connect muscles to bones) are overstretched or torn. A sprain occurs when the ligaments (the bands of tissue that connect two bones together in a joint) are torn or overstretched.

Do it safely: Preparation is key. Know the weight and weight distribution of what you're lifting. With your feet planted shoulder-width apart, squat halfway down until your thighs are approximately parallel with the ground, keeping your torso relatively upright, and then try lifting the object. Don't position your feet too narrowly, or you could lose your balance and topple over. And don't bend your knees more than 90 degrees or it will be difficult to stand back up.

Young children seeking to cuddle are a recipe for low-back strain. It may feel difficult to say no when they reach their arms up toward you, but if you're out of shape or have trouble lifting heavy objects, sit down and have them climb into your lap for that cuddle.

EVERYDAY RISKY MOVE #2: **Putting on a Jacket or Shirt**

We tend to take an everyday activity such as getting dressed for granted. But the motions required to put on a coat, jacket or a button-front shirt can trigger a rotator cuff injury.

How it happens: The rotator cuff is a collection of tendons and muscles surrounding and protecting each shoulder. It's what allows you to raise and rotate your arms. Dressing in the above items requires you to hold your arm up and out, often at a somewhat unnatural angle, which can strain a tendon in your rotator cuff. The tendon swells and becomes pinched by the shoulder joint, creating a sudden sharp, almost knifelike pain. Rotator-cuff injuries are more common with age.

Do it safely: Rotator cuff impingement pain intensifies when reaching behind your back or overhead—two positions involved in putting on a coat or a shirt. But there's no real need to put your arm into those positions. Instead, keep your arm below chest level and push your hand downward into the sleeve, using your other hand to pull the garment up.

EVERYDAY RISKY MOVE #3: **Overusing Your Neck**

If you have ever woken up with a "crick" or "kink" in your neck—pain accompanied by a limited ability to look from side to side or up and down—you likely attributed it to sleeping in an odd position. But a more likely culprit is neck muscle overuse the prior day.

How it happens: Gardening, housecleaning, too much time on your cell phone and even reading all are common activities that require you to do a lot of looking down, taxing your neck and shoulders. Poor form when working on a computer can cause it, too. Then, when you finally rest, those muscles tighten up, creating a strain.

Do it safely: The neck usually assumes a natural curved position at rest unless strained or overused. Chin tucks are a safe and effective move to strengthen the neck and help prevent strain from overuse. Sit in a comfortable chair looking straight ahead. Move your head backward, tucking your chin in toward your neck in a slow and easy manner. Keep your gaze forward, and do not tilt your head. Hold the tuck for five seconds, then return to the starting (rest) position. Repeat five times twice daily.

***EVERYDAY RISKY MOVE #4:* Navigating Stairs**

More than a million Americans hurt themselves on stairs every year. That's 3,000 injuries every day according to a study in *The American Journal of Emergency Medicine.* Injuries—usually sprains and strains, soft tissue injuries and fractures—typically are worse when descending rather than walking up. A common mistake? Missing the last stair or two.

How it happens: When you trip while climbing up, you may be able to catch yourself with the railing or the stairs in front of you. But should you miss a step or two while walking down, gravity conspires against you and it is difficult to catch yourself.

Do it safely: The advice here will sound obvious, but people still don't follow it. Paying attention is paramount. Hold the handrail when going up and down. Avoid carrying objects that can obscure your vision, such as laundry baskets or large packages. Enlist aid from others if needed… otherwise proceed with great caution. Wear nonslip shoes, and avoid overly long pants. If you have vision issues, wear appropriate glasses or contact lenses.

As a preventive measure, consider enrolling in a tai chi class. This traditional Chinese practice involves slowly moving your body through a series of poses, benefiting core strength and balance in the process. Tai chi has been shown to help prevent falls in older individuals. And because it cultivates mindfulness, it improves your awareness of your surroundings, which could reduce falls.

Important: Certain medications, such as sedatives, pain medication and antidepressants, can affect balance. Before taking any of these, talk to your doctor to make sure it is safe for you to navigate stairs.

3 Easy Ways to Relieve Your Pain from an Injury

Wanda Jean Swenson, PT, a retired physical therapist with more than 30 years of experience who currently leads workshops and lectures in Sonoma County, California. She is a former clinical instructor and outpatient physical therapist at Kaiser Permanente in Santa Rosa, California, and the author of *The How of Ow: Everyday Self-Care and the Art of Pain Relief.* TheHowOfOw.com

You strained your lower back after lifting a heavy box.

You reached for the top kitchen shelf and tweaked your shoulder.

Your neck is stiff after you overdid it at yoga.

You've got a muscle spasm in your hip after awkwardly getting out of bed.

How do most people cope with these muscle injuries? As soon as the pain hits, they may try to stretch it out on their own or pop a painkiller in the hopes of getting some relief—fast. What the majority of pain sufferers don't know is that they can avoid getting these common injuries in the first place if they practice some surprisingly easy movements while going about their daily activities. *Here's how…*

The Right Movement

Many people think they shouldn't move much after they've injured themselves…because it hurts. So they freeze up, equating pain with further injury.

These pain sufferers often stay in bed or park themselves on the couch, waiting for the pain to pass…sometimes for days. But avoiding movement doesn't help. In fact, it promotes joint stiffness and, if continued for days, lack of movement can lead to muscle weakness and continued discomfort.

The truth: The right type of movement, done in small amounts, is essential for healing and will promote a speedier recovery. To get relief, try using postural isometric lengthening (PIL) right after a muscle injury. This technique, which incorporates elements of yoga, lengthens the spine, which eases joint pressures while strengthening the deep muscles that are associated with these types of injuries. PIL also can be used for chronic arthritis pain that affects the neck and back. When you're not in pain, you can also do PIL movements throughout the day to help prevent muscle injuries and improve arthritis pain.

When to Use PIL

Whether you've hurt yourself lifting a heavy object, turning your neck while parallel parking, slipping and falling, exiting the car awkwardly…or whenever back, neck, hip or shoulder pain strikes, practice these moves right then and there to prevent and relieve pain.

If you're symptom-free, ideal times to practice PIL include before getting out of bed in the morning…before standing up after sitting for a while…and after spending time in awkward positions (such as gardening, plumbing or bending over cooking).

Got chronic pain? Doing PIL for flare-ups improves strength and muscle coordination, turning your mental focus away from the pain and relieving symptoms. *Three key moves…*

• **Seated PIL.**

What to do: Sit up as tall as possible, as if your height is being measured and the back of your head is being pulled up. Your pelvis (the area that connects the trunk to the hips) will naturally rock forward and your back moves away from the back of the chair. Gently lower your chin toward your throat while lengthening the back of your neck. Your shoulder blades should be pinched together and downward. Then pull in your belly as if you're trying to zip up a pair of pants that are too tight—this movement tightens your deep abdominal muscles.

Hold this position as you take three to five slow, deep breaths, inhaling for two counts, exhaling for three. Keep the belly pulled in toward the spine, and feel the breath expand the lower ribs without puffing up the chest.

Breathing this way initiates a natural pain-relieving relaxation response.

Important: If you do feel any pain, relax your body and slump over slightly. Slumping stretches any strained muscles that are in spasm. Take a few breaths and try again.

• **Standing PIL.**

What to do: Follow the steps above for seated PIL, but begin by standing tall, feet shoulder-width apart and knees slightly relaxed. Your arms should be at your sides, palms facing forward, shoulder blades pinched together and down.

• **PIL in bed.**

What to do: Lie on your side with a pillow beneath your head and a pillow between your knees, if needed for comfort. Start by rocking your pelvis back and forward a few times. As your pelvis rocks backward, you will naturally round your spine. Then straighten and lengthen the spine as your pelvis rocks forward. Pull the belly in toward the spine, and pinch the shoulder blades slightly together and down. Take a few breaths in the lengthened position, and then relax. Repeat three to five times.

Important: If a muscle injury is not improving or symptoms worsen after trying PIL for one or two days, consult your doctor or health-care provider.

Danger of Plant-Based Diets: Bone Fractures

Study of almost 55,000 adults in the UK by researchers at Nuffield Department of Population Health, Oxford University, published in *BMC Medicine.*

Vegetarians and vegans generally have lower bone mineral density than non-vegetarians, resulting in a higher risk for fractures in later life. Over a 10-year period, compared with meat eaters, there were 4.1 more fractures per 1,000 people in vegetarians…and 19.4 more cases in vegans. Part of the reason may be that calcium, important for bone strength, is more bioavailable when a diet includes meat.

Can the "Love Hormone" Prevent Osteoporosis?

The study titled "Oxytocin and Bone Quality in the Femoral Neck of Rats in Periestropause," led by researchers at São Paulo State University, Brazil, and published in *Scientific Reports*.

When it comes to reducing risk for osteoporosis, calcium, vitamin D and weight-bearing exercise are the standard recommendations—especially for menopausal women, whose bone health declines when their estrogen levels plummet.

Because osteoporosis also increases the odds of suffering a debilitating and sometimes deadly hip fracture, preventing significant bone loss can actually be a matter of life or death. Hip fracture is also a matter of urgent concern, as hip fractures are expected to increase by 50 percent in the U.S. by 2050, according to the World Health Organization.

Recent development: To help identify new ways of preventing osteoporosis-related hip fractures, researchers at São Paulo State University in Brazil conducted a laboratory study to investigate a novel approach—boosting levels of the so-called "love hormone" oxytocin.

Usually associated with social bonding, orgasm, childbirth and breast-feeding, oxytocin has recently been found to also play a role in bone health. Noting that oxytocin levels tend to decline along with estrogen levels as women enter perimenopause, researchers theorized that boosting levels of the hormone may help curb the development of osteoporosis and prevent future hip fractures.

Study details: To test their theory, the researchers gave 18-month-old female rats (the age of periestropause—the equivalent of perimenopause in women) two doses of oxytocin or two doses of salt water (placebo)

over 12 hours. The two groups were compared one month later by conducting blood tests and taking bone samples of femoral neck bone (the upper part of the thigh bone, where most hip fractures occur).

Results: The oxytocin-treated rats had higher levels of alkaline *phosphatase*—a protein that promotes bone formation—in their blood than the rats that had received the placebo. Unlike the control group, the rats that received oxytocin also had no evidence of osteopenia (a precursor to osteoporosis) and were found to have stronger and denser bones.

Takeaway: Oxytocin therapy is a promising strategy for preventing osteoporosis when given in the period just before menopause, according to the study, which was published in *Scientific Reports*. Based on these laboratory findings, the researchers now hope to move this inquiry into clinical trials in humans.

If oxytocin is found to help prevent osteoporosis, it could be a game changer, since it is a condition that many women cope with for up to one-third of their lives. The consequences are even more dire for those who suffer an osteoporosis-related hip fracture—less than half recover their previous level of mobility and 24 percent die within 12 months.

Steroids for Asthma Linked to Osteoporosis

Christos Chalitsios, MSc, is a PhD candidate at University of Nottingham, UK, and leader of a study published in *Thorax*.

Patients receiving the most oral steroids had 4.5 times higher odds...1.6 times higher from inhaled steroids. This steroid risk has been known in other health conditions but not for asthma.

Asthmatics: Use steroids sparingly. If you take steroids orally for two months or more, ask your doctor if a bone-protection treatment using bisphosphonates is for you, though there are reports of osteonecrosis of the jaw and atypical fractures with them. Vitamin D and calcium may protect bones, but data are scarce.

After an Accident: Healing Lasting Anxiety and Insomnia Naturally

Andrew Rubman, ND, is medical director of Southbury Clinic for Traditional Medicines in Southbury, Connecticut. SouthburyClinic.com. He is author of the "Nature Doc's Patient Diary" blog at Bottom LineInc.com.

The patient: "Denise" was a normal suburban housewife who had become horribly dysregulated after a car accident.

Why she came to see me: Referred by a friend, Denise had a virtual conference with me and told me of how she had suffered after the trauma of almost losing a sibling to a horrific car accident that had left them both in the intensive care unit for many weeks. She was waking repeatedly during the night profusely sweating and fearing that someone was breaking in. Not only was she afraid to drive but her anxiety was producing an angry disposition and short temper that she feared was threatening her marriage.

How I evaluated her: Denise had sent over consultation notes and laboratory test results from the many physicians that she had consulted, from her primary care doctor to a psychiatrist. There was little pertinent information revealed in any of it. We discussed the various ways in which her life had become dysregulated, from sleep disruption and irritable bowel to menstrual irregularity and emotional outbursts. She admitted to being extremely sensitive to pharmaceuticals and even found taking the vitamin B12 that her psychiatrist had prescribed disruptive.

How we addressed her problem: I explained to Denise that profound stress can not only deplete vitamin and nutrient re-serves but also degrade and disrupt communities of hormones and neurotransmitters. We agreed to put in place a regime of improved diet, more attention to regular sleep/wake cycles and supplements that would be introduced in stages.

I had her begin with a "broad spectrum" multi-B vitamin, twice daily, at a reasonable therapeutic level and a twice daily small dose of DHEA, a hormone precursor, in a form that would be absorbed directly from her mouth. These interventions would replenish the raw materials to allow Denise's body to create and balance her stress and reproductive hormones. This is often a better approach than providing direct hormone replacement therapy.

The patient's progress: My office received a call from Denise the next day. I was somewhat concerned to hear bad news that she had experienced some worsening of symptoms. Instead she was bubbling over with enthusiasm at how well she had slept and how improved her mood and temperament was after only 12 hours. We are waiting for a bit longer to allow the initial regime changes to "settle in," discussing areas of improvement and identifying any outliers. We'll design the second phase based on outcomes rather than supposition.

Beware of This Hidden Cause of Falls

The study "Auditory Input and Postural Control in Adults: A Narrative Review," conducted by researchers at the Ear Institute at Mount Sinai School of Medicine and New York University, both in New York City, and published in *JAMA Otolaryngology-Head & Neck Surgery*.

If your hearing isn't as good as it used to be, you already know that making a simple phone call can sometimes be difficult. Untreated hearing loss also has more serious dangers—increased risk for dementia, depression and even cardiovascular disease, to name a few.

Here's another risk you might not know about. The sounds that you hear (or don't hear) can strongly affect your risk of falling. Even mild hearing loss—the kind that can make conversations challenging—can nearly triple the risk.

Yet when doctors evaluate patients who have suffered falls—the leading cause of deadly injury for older Americans—they tend to focus on vision, neuropathy in the feet or bone problems, without giving a second thought to hearing, says Maura Cosetti, MD, director of the Ear Institute at Mount Sinai School of Medicine in New York City. That's a mistake.

People who can't hear normal background sounds (such as music, the clatter of dishes, etc.) are more likely to have balance problems than those with healthy hearing, according to recent research led by Dr. Cosetti and Anat Lubetzky, PhD, assistant professor of physical therapy at New York University in New York City. The research was published in *JAMA Otolaryngology-Head & Neck Surgery*.

We all use sound information to keep ourselves balanced, especially in cases where other senses—such as vision or proprioception (our awareness of the position and movement of the body)—are compromised, she explains.

Sadly, even though one in three older adults has some degree of hearing loss, about 85 percent don't use hearing aids or get other forms of treatment.

Important: People who notice symptom of hearing loss—muffled sounds, tinnitus or a sensation that one or both ears are blocked—should get a hearing test. Medicare and most private insurers pay for annual audiologic evaluations, along with some hearing-related tests.

And don't assume that you're too young to have hearing problems. Significant age-related hearing loss can begin as early as age 55…or even earlier if you've regularly been exposed to loud music or other loud environ-

ments, or take medications, such as certain antibiotics (including *gentamicin*) and chemotherapy drugs (including *cisplatin* and *carboplatin*), that are considered "ototoxic"—that is, known to cause hearing loss.

Researchers are planning additional studies to confirm whether hearing aids and other treatments for hearing loss can function as a "balance aid," similar to the way a cane can be used to improve balance and decrease fall risk.

In the meantime, if you're concerned about your risk of falling, get your hearing checked—especially if you're age 70 or older.

Balancing Act

Robert Cobbett, recently retired adjunct faculty member at Quincy College in Braintree, Massachusetts, and ACE certified personal trainer who teaches balance programs at several Councils on Aging.

Balance is often overlooked when it comes to putting together a workout plan, but it's an important part of achieving overall fitness, especially after age 50, when the risk of falls increases.

While balance issues can be caused by some medications and chronic health conditions, they can also result from simple age-related muscle loss. The remedy is to make balance exercises part of your daily routine.

The following targeted exercises involve shifting your weight from side to side to build lower body coordination and strength. Do them standing alongside a sturdy table or chair in case you need support at any point. And practice deep, steady breathing as you work out—don't hold your breath.

• **Toe taps.** Place a plastic cup on the floor two feet in front of you. Tap the top of the cup with the toes of your right foot; then switch feet and tap with the toes of your left foot. Keep alternating feet until you've tapped six to eight times on each side. As you gain strength, tap the cup twice before switching sides, building to six to eight double taps on each side. To progress, keep adding to the number of taps you do before you switch feet.

• **Soccer kicks.** Plant your right foot firmly on the floor and position your left foot behind you. Pretend there's a soccer ball in front of your right foot and "kick" the ball by bringing your left foot forward and crossing it in front of your right foot with some speed and control. Switch feet and repeat for a total of six to eight repetitions on each side. To progress, increase the number of repetitions and the speed of the movement

• **Tandem-stance heel raises.** Place your right foot directly in front of your left, with about three to four inches between your right heel and the toes of your left foot. Both feet should be pointed forward. With good posture and your eyes focused straight ahead, lift onto your toes and then lower back down with control. Repeat six to eight times and then switch the position of your feet and repeat. To progress, increase the number of repetitions.

• **Tandem-stance arms to sides.** Place your right foot in front of your left, heel to toe, with no space between. Both feet should be pointed straight forward. Balance in this position for 10 to 15 seconds, and then, with your fingers laced and your arms extended, move your arms to the left, back to the center, to the right, and back to the center. Repeat the arm extensions three to four times in each direction in a controlled manner. To progress, move your arms up and down as you extend them to the sides.

• **Knee raises to opposite elbow.** This exercise includes a cardiovascular component. Stand with your feet shoulder-width apart. Lift your left knee and cross your body to touch it to your right elbow just above your waist. Switch sides and repeat. Keep alternating your knees for a total of eight to 10 repetitions on each side. Use a vigorous yet controlled movement. To progress, pick up the pace and add repetitions.

• **Heel-to-toe walking with head turns.** Start with good posture, with your head up and shoulders back. Walk at least 8 to 10 feet in a straight line while turning your head from side to side. Pivot and return to the starting point. To progress, step over some soft objects placed along the way. You can also have fun by spelling words backwards or solving math problems as you walk.

• **Rounded routine.** There are many components to balance—you need strength, flexibility, and good posture. So in addition to these exercises, add twice-weekly strength training to improve muscle mass and frequent weight-bearing exercise, like walking, to maintain bone health.

Fall Prevention

Many falls occur because of tripping hazards, like loose area rugs or poor lighting, but some happen because of physical multitasking.

The ability to "walk and chew gum" can diminish with age. So when a neighbor waves while you're unloading the groceries, stop what you're doing and turn toward them, have your chat and then resume unloading the car.

Remember that it takes only a second to fall, but can take months to recover.

How to Do Computer Work With Thumb Pain

Leon S. Benson, MD, a hand surgeon at the Illinois Bone & Joint Institute, professor of clinical orthopaedic surgery at The University of Chicago Pritzker School of Medicine, and spokesperson for the American Academy of Orthopaedic Surgeons.

Doctors often blame hand and thumb pain in older individuals on arthritis... which means relief is elusive. Work often involves using a computer with a mouse all day. Is there anything you can do to prevent hand arthritis from making your computer work (and numerous other activities) next to impossible?

Yes, there are some steps you can take, but let's start with what it means to have arthritis. As you probably know, there are different types of arthritis. Hand pain while you work on your computer could be due to osteoarthritis. It is extremely common for this condition to develop at the base of the thumb—where the thumb and wrist join together.

Osteoarthritis develops when there's a wearing away of the cartilage that buffers and protects the area where two bones come together. It is similar to wearing the rubber off a tire after many miles of use. This "wear and tear" arthritis can result from the aging process, overuse or injury. Currently, there is no way to prevent cartilage damage from worsening, other than to not use the joint that's involved. Obviously, not using your hand is certainly an impractical—if not impossible—task.

There are, however, some simple ways to relieve your thumb arthritis pain. Using a splint to rest the thumb for a few hours a day can be very helpful. It is usually possible to use a mouse and keyboard even when wearing such a splint. To ensure that you get a splint that is customized for the shape of your hand, it's smart to see a certified hand therapist, an occupational therapist or physical therapist who specializes in treating the hand and upper extremity. Insurance often pays at least part of the cost of splint fabrication. To find a hand therapist in your area, check the online directory found on the website for the American Society of Hand Therapists (ASHT.org).

Sometimes heat or cold (like an ice pack) can help ease the pain. Hand exercises can also help relieve any pain and stiffness in your thumb. However, they should be pursued carefully, because too much exercise can worsen the pain from arthritis.

Anti-inflammatory medication, such *ibuprofen* (Motrin), can significantly help ease arthritis pain. If the pain persists, a steroid injection into the thumb joint space may be even more effective. An injection can often give relief for six to 12 months, and as long as it is not administered too frequently (more than twice per year), is a very safe treatment. Topical medications are also available, such as anti-inflammatory creams, but they typically are less effective than oral medications or injections.

Although there are different devices that can be used in place of a computer mouse (like a trackball) or instead of the keyboard (like voice-recognition software), computer use itself is actually not the main cause of arthritis symptoms. People use their hands constantly for activities of daily living outside of the workplace, so computer use is neither a particularly bad activity for your hands nor is it done for a long enough duration to be a major cause or aggravation of arthritis pain.

If none of the above treatments are effective or last long enough, joint replacement is an option. Surgery for the most common type of thumb arthritis has been around for decades. It is performed in an outpatient setting, usually under twilight-type anesthesia, and allows most patients to resume normal use of their hand without pain. Post-operative immobilization in a splint or brace is often required for about four weeks, after which time many patients can use their affected hand with minimal limitations.

Why Does Dizziness Linger After a Bad Fall?

Timothy C. Hain, MD, neurologist, Chicago Dizziness and Hearing. Dizzy-Doc.com

After a head injury, dizziness (feeling lightheaded, woozy or disoriented) and vertigo (feeling like you or the room is spinning) often are due to a condition called benign paroxysmal positional vertigo (BPPV). A head injury can cause BPPV, which develops when calcium carbonate crystals (known as otoconia) detach from their normal location in the inner ear. The otoconia, now free to tumble within the labyrinth of the inner ear, create currents that press on tiny hairlike sensors that transmit balance signals to the brain.

The classic sign of BPPV is dizziness or vertigo that appears when the person's head position changes—for example, when rolling over in bed, bending the head forward to look down or tipping the head back. Usually, this begins immediately after the fall, but there can be a delay of up to a week. In most cases, vertigo resolves itself when the loose otoconia dissolve after about six weeks.

Your physician can diagnose BPPV by evaluating you after these head movements. This condition is diagnosed by seeing the characteristic eye-jumping (nystagmus) when the patient is lying down with the head to one side. If this is not quickly confirmed, you should seek further medical evaluation. (See also pages 10–12 in chapter 1, "Aging Well," for more information on BPPV.)

BPPV can be treated with a procedure called particle repositioning, which involves a series of head movements to help shift the otoconia back into place. A physical therapist can guide you through these head movements. It's best to look for a physical therapist who specializes in vestibular PT. To find one near you, consult the Vestibular Disorders Association (VeDA). Vestibular.org

Is Whiplash More Dangerous If It Happens Again?

Robert Zembroski, DC, DACNB, MS, chiropractic neurologist, director, Darien Center for Functional Medicine, Darien, Connecticut.

Usually, whiplash symptoms resolve on their own within a few weeks or months. But for about one-third of people who get whiplash, it can be a long-term—even debilitating—disorder that never completely goes away. This is more likely to happen with repeated whiplash, especially when whiplash happens again before full recovery from the previous injury.

Whiplash is the term for neck injury caused by quick, forceful back-and-forth snapping of the neck—typically from being in an auto accident, but you can also get whiplash from any kind of accident, physical abuse or trauma. Symptoms can include neck pain, neck and shoulder stiffness, headache and tingling and numbness in the arms. It's also common to feel dizzy and to have trouble sleeping.

Getting whiplash multiple times can cause changes in your autonomic nervous system that can make you more sensitive to pain anywhere in your body and cause changes to blood pressure and abnormal sweating. Trauma to the nervous system can also cause postural muscle weakness and weakness to the limbs, usually on one side of the body. Repeated whiplash can also cause benign paroxysmal positional vertigo, a condition in which sudden movement causes a sensation of spinning or that the world around you is spinning. And the stress of chronic pain can lead to anxiety and depression.

How to Recover from Whiplash

Generally, it's best to start treatment as soon after injury as possible. *There is no one-size-fits-all therapy, but whether you're treating your first episode of whiplash or your second (or third or fourth), these therapies can help…*

• **Ice within the first 72 hours of initial injury to reduce pain and swelling…**after 72 hours, heat to improve circulation, improve motion and reduce pain.

• **Over-the-counter pain medications** such as *ibuprofen* (Motrin) or *acetaminophen* (Tylenol).

• **Gentle, assisted spinal manipulation from a chiropractor.**

• **Physical therapy.**

All of these potential treatments should be managed by a physician who examines you and tracks your progress—don't treat whiplash yourself.

What about those soft neck collars that are what many people think of when they imagine whiplash treatment? Your doctor may recommend that you wear one if an MRI shows ligament damage and/or there is significant pain both with movement and at rest. It's generally best to wear a neck collar immediately after the injury for up to seven days to prevent excessive movement while the muscles and soft tissues heal enough to receive therapy. Wearing a neck collar longer immobilizes neck muscles, which can cause them to become stiff and weak. In fact, moving your neck and staying active is important for full recovery. But do avoid activities that have a greater-than-average chance of leading to another neck injury.

If dizziness persists, the cause needs to be determined. Neck trauma can cause orthostatic hypotension, a drop in blood pressure when rising from lying down or sitting that causes dizziness. Pain or other symptoms that last longer than a day or two should be checked by a medical or chiropractic neurologist to see if there is nerve damage.

Since inflammation is a big part of neck pain and other whiplash symptoms, an anti-inflammatory diet including lots of vegetables and fruit and omega-3 fatty acids from such foods as nuts, seeds and cold-water fatty fish can be very helpful.

Is Shoulder Pain a Rotator Cuff Tear? Don't Trust Your MRI

Dr. Mitchell Yass, DPT, is the creator of The Yass Method, which uniquely diagnoses and treats the cause of chronic pain through the interpretation of the body's presentation of symptoms. Dr. Yass is the author of two books, Overpower Pain: The Strength Training Program That Stops Pain Without Drugs or Surgery, and The Pain Cure Rx: The Yass Method for Resolving The Cause of Chronic Pain.

I have been treating people with shoulder pain for what feels like forever. In most cases, they can't remember a specific incident that caused their pain or when the pain even began. But as time passed, the pain grew worse and eventually it ended up limiting their ability to perform many to most of their functional activities—like driving, hair

care (combing, blow drying), securing a bra, tucking in a shirt at the back of their pants, reaching behind them in the car and lifting objects over shoulder height. Lots of things that most people take for granted.

Then they sought medical attention. The proverbial MRI (magnetic resonance imaging) was taken and a rotator cuff tear was found. For the lucky ones who saw me before making an appointment for surgery, I worked with them to resolve their symptoms and their function fully returned. Those who had surgery for that rotator cuff tear that was supposedly the cause of their symptoms did not fare so well.

MRIs are not a reliable way to determine the root cause of most pain. If the rotator cuff tear only occurred at the time the pain began, say two weeks ago, and you can't remember a specific traumatic incident that occurred two weeks ago, isn't it possible that the rotator cuff tear that was found actually occurred more than two weeks ago? If an MRI were taken a few months prior to your pain beginning, the very same rotator cuff tear—the one being called the cause of your pain—would be present. And if it has existed for months or years prior to when your pain began, how can anybody assert that is what is causing your pain now?

Here is a little study that clearly illustrates this point. As reported in *The New York Times*, sports orthopedist Dr. James Andrews conducted MRI scans of the shoulders of 31 professional baseball pitchers with absolutely no shoulder pain or injury. He found that 87 percent had rotator cuff tears and 90 percent had labral (cartilage) tears.

Now let's talk about the rotator cuff tear itself. *Tears are classified as acute or degenerative…*

•**An acute tear is due to a trauma**—like falling off a ladder and trying to stop yourself by stretching your arm behind you.

•**A degenerative tear is due to wear and tear and progresses very slowly.** This occurs because the mechanics of the shoulder joint are not preserved as you lose strength

293

and balance of the muscles associated with shoulder function.

If you are troubled by shoulder pain, ask yourself which of these scenarios is more like yours...

• **Can you identify a specific trauma associated with your pain?** It would have to be something pretty dramatic. Prior to the event, you had no pain and you now have severe pain. Prior to the event you had full range of motion and now you have almost none. In this case, surgery to repair the tear is often advisable.

• **Is yours a case where nothing dramatic happened?** Degenerative tears create no immediate symptoms because they develop over years. And they also can be treated without surgery.

Let's talk about how the shoulder works and what part of the rotator cuff does what. The two primary aspects of the rotator cuff are the supraspinatus and infraspinatus. You will feel a bony portion running from the inside to the outside of the shoulder blade. This is called the spine of the shoulder blade. Above it (and above the shoulder joint) sits the supraspinatus. Its purpose is to support the weight of the arm bone when the arm is hanging at your side. It cannot help to keep the head of the upper arm bone in the right position when the arm is raised. That is pri-marily the job of the infraspinatus, which sits below the spine of the shoulder blade.

With this understanding, you can determine which muscle is eliciting your pain. If you have no real problem holding your arm at your side but you can't raise it even to shoulder height, the infraspinatus is involved. If you can raise your arm without much difficulty but just letting your arm hang at your side elicits the pain, then the pain involves the supraspinatus.

In pretty much every case I have treated where the rotator cuff was leading to shoulder-region pain, the person could not raise his or her arm; hanging it down was not a problem. Hence, the pain was from the infraspinatus. Yet in every case I have seen where an MRI indicated a tear of the rotator cuff, it was in the supraspinatus. This means that the tear had nothing to do with the pain.

The rotator cuff works with several other muscles to achieve normal function. If these other muscles are strained, it can cause the rotator cuff to overwork and strain. The key to resolving pain at the shoulder in most cases is physical therapy to teach you how to strengthen all the appropriate muscles associated with shoulder function, such as the exercise in the following article to strengthen the posterior deltoid: search "A Surprising Cure for Joint and Muscle Aches" at Bottom LineInc.com.

Chapter 13

PREGNANCY AND REPRODUCTION ISSUES

IVF Offers Clues to Future Health Problems

I f a woman struggling with infertility undergoes in vitro fertilization (IVF), she has a single goal—to conceive a healthy baby. Now, new research has shown that the IVF process can serve an additional purpose by offering important clues about the woman's future health.

With IVF, a woman takes fertility medication to stimulate her ovaries' release of mature eggs so that one or more can be fertilized with sperm in a lab ("in vitro" is the Latin term for "within the glass") and implanted in the uterus to create a pregnancy.

Because the process involves the retrieval of a woman's eggs, researchers at Aarhus University in Denmark wanted to investigate the link between varying levels of egg collection in women and later-life health risks—especially for cardiovascular disease (CVD) and osteoporosis. Risk for both conditions has been shown to increase during menopause—the point at which the ovaries stop releasing eggs.

New research findings: To begin their investigation, the researchers reviewed the medical records of almost 20,000 women under age 37 who had a first cycle of IVF.

(Women often undergo multiple cycles of IVF to achieve a successful pregnancy.)

During IVF, the more eggs a woman releases, the better her chances of creating a viable fertilized egg (embryo) in the lab to transfer to the uterus. A normal response to the hormonal stimulation that occurs during IVF is eight or more eggs, while five or fewer eggs is low and considered to be a sign of "early ovarian aging." Unlike men, who can produce sperm well into their older age, women have a set number of follicles in their ovaries that can release eggs during ovulation.

In the study, which was presented at the 2020 meeting of the European Society of Human Reproduction and Embryology, the researchers reviewed about six years of health records for the women who had undergone IVF to determine their rates of death or disease from any cause, along with reports of CVD, osteoporosis, type 2 diabetes and cancer. Of the women studied, 1,234 produced five or fewer eggs (the "early ovarian aging" group), while 18,614 produced eight or more eggs (the "normal ovarian response" group). *Among the key findings…*

Study titled "Response to Stimulation in IVF May Predict Longer-Term Health Risk" by researchers at Aarhus University in Denmark and presented at the 2020 meeting of the European Society of Human Reproduction and Embryology.

•**Women with early ovarian aging had a 26 percent greater risk of developing a chronic,** age-related disease compared with the normal ovarian response group.

•**The most significant risks for women with early ovarian aging** were a 39 percent higher risk for CVD and more than double the risk for osteoporosis.

•**The risk for cancer, other age-related diseases and death from any cause** was not significantly different between the two groups.

Bottom line: A low response to ovarian stimulation should be a warning sign for doctors to provide counseling for such women, especially for CVD and osteoporosis, according to the researchers. This counseling would include lifestyle changes, such as diet and exercise, and perhaps hormone replacement therapy. If your response to ovarian stimulation was limited and your doctor hasn't talked to you about this, speak up so you can begin taking steps to reduce your risk for future age-related health problems.

New Microbiome Therapy Fights Recurrent Vaginal Infections

The study "Randomization Trial of Lactin-V to Prevent Recurrence of Bacterial Vaginosis" led by researchers at the University of California, San Francisco and published in *The New England Journal of Medicine.*

Bacterial vaginosis (BV) is a bothersome bacterial infection of the vagina that affects close to 30 percent of women of reproductive age in the US. Even though BV can be treated with an antibiotic, it comes back within 12 weeks in up to three-quarters of women.

In addition to causing vaginal discharge and other troubling symptoms (see below), the infection has been linked to increased risk for preterm birth in pregnant women and low-birth weight babies. Having BV,

which upsets the healthy balance of "good" and "harmful" bacteria (known as the microbiome) in the vagina, also can increase a woman's chances on contracting a sexually transmitted disease, such as chlamydia or gonorrhea. In Africa, BV is associated with the spread of HIV, where the disease affects more women than men.

Risk for BV, which typically causes pain, itching or burning of the vagina and a strong, fish-like odor, especially after sex, is increased in women who douche and/or have a new sex partner or multiple sex partners—all of which can upset the balance of bacteria in the vagina. Using a latex condom during sex may help reduce the risk of developing BV.

Because this infection is so common and carries such serious potential harms, researchers from the University of California, San Francisco (UCSF) and other universities joined forces to investigate a so-called "live biotherapeutic"—a therapy that involves inserting healthy vaginal bacteria directly into the vagina.

Research findings: In the study, reported in *The New England Journal of Medicine,* 228 women with BV were treated with an antibiotic vaginal gel called *metronidazole.* After treatment some women were treated with a microbiome therapy called Lactin-V, a powder formulation derived from the healthy vaginal bacterium species Lactobacillus crispatus. Lactin-V is self-administered into the vagina with an applicator. The other women served as a control group and were not given the Lactin-V.

The women in the treatment group applied the powder every day for five days and then twice per week for 10 weeks. The other group used a placebo. After 12 weeks, the researchers found a significant reduction in BV recurrence—30 percent of the women treated with Lactin-V after the antibiotic treatment experienced a recurrence compared with 45 percent of those who received a placebo after the antibiotic. No safety risks were found from the bacteria used in the Lactin-V formulation.

"The initial indication for Lactin-V is for the prevention of BV, which millions of women in the US have each year," explained Craig R. Cohen, MD, first author of the study and professor of obstetrics, gynecology and reproductive sciences at UCSF. "But this product also has the potential to be an effective intervention to prevent HIV infection and preterm birth."

Before granting FDA approval for Lactin-V, which is produced by Osel, Inc. of Mountain View, California, the FDA will likely require a larger (phase III) trial. Funding for the study was provided by the National Institute of Allergy and Infectious Diseases (NIAID).

Drinking and Miscarriages

Study on week-by-week alcohol consumption in early pregnancy and miscarriage risk by researchers at Vanderbilt University Medical Center, Nashville, published in *American Journal of Obstetrics and Gynecology.*

Anything more than one drink per week during early pregnancy can increase the risk for miscarriage. In fact, for each week that alcohol is consumed in the first five to 10 weeks of pregnancy, the risk for miscarriage goes up by 8 percent Women who continued to drink before their first missed period or a positive pregnancy test also were at increased risk for miscarriage.

Best: If you are actively trying to get pregnant, stop drinking before you start trying.

If You're Having Trouble Getting Pregnant, Check Your Thyroid

Rima Dhillon-Smith, PhD, is a clinical lecturer at Birmingham Women's and Children's Hospital, UK. Her research was published in *Journal of Clinical Endocrinology & Metabolism.*

A study of more than 19,000 women with a history of miscarriage or difficulty becoming pregnant shows that one in five had mild thyroid dysfunction (not overt thyroid disease). Checking levels and treating dysfunction could improve your chances of a successful outcome.

Typical Drug Doses May Be Harmful for Some Pregnancies

Study titled "The Impact of Intrauterine Growth Restriction on Cytochrome P450 Enzyme Expression and Activity," led by researchers at University of South Australia, published in *Placenta.*

Nearly all pregnant women take prescription and/or over-the-counter (OTC) medication to treat a condition that may affect the health of the mother or the baby. Medications taken by the mother commonly include those used to treat pain, depression, diabetes, asthma and morning sickness. Drugs used to treat conditions such as abnormal heartbeats (arrhythmias) may be taken for the baby.

However, when the unborn child is not growing as quickly as expected—a condition known as intrauterine growth restriction (IUGR)—a typical medication dose taken by the mother may be too much for the fetus to break down (metabolize).

Because there are no professional guidelines for safe medication dosing in pregnant women with IUGR, researchers at the University of South Australia set out to investigate how drugs are metabolized during these pregnancies.

The review, which was published in *Placenta,* found that hormonal changes that occur during pregnancy may affect drug-metabolizing enzymes (DMEs), which play a key role in the baby's ability to break down medication. These enzymes are less effective in IUGR babies, which can lead to drug toxicity at normal doses.

"If the fetus is smaller and a mother takes 20 mg of a drug, it may effectively be a higher dose than in a normal-sized baby," said study author Janna L. Morrison, PhD, head of the University of South Australia's Early Origins of Adult Health Research Group. "The actual drug doesn't make the fetus smaller, but if it is already smaller, the fetus may be less able to metabolize the drug and get rid of it."

Worldwide, IUGR occurs in about one in seven pregnancies. During these pregnancies, the placenta fails to deliver the necessary nutrients and oxygen to the fetus. IUGR is more common in women with high blood pressure and in those who smoke, abuse drugs or drink alcohol during pregnancy.

While most babies weigh about six to eight pounds at birth, IUGR babies weigh less than 5.5 pounds. IUGR babies are at increased risk for diabetes, heart disease and impaired immunity throughout their lives.

Based on their findings, the researchers would like for additional studies to be conducted to better understand the effects of medication dosing during pregnancy. Depending on how the fetus metabolizes the drug, the optimal dose may need to be lower or higher.

"It doesn't automatically correlate that a lower dose would be better if the fetus metabolizes it faster," explained Dr. Morrison. "It may mean that with some complicated pregnancies, a higher dose is needed with some drugs. It's about making sure that the right dose is given to help the mother, without harming the baby."

Takeaway: Until more is known, pregnant women are advised to check with their health-care provider before taking any prescription or OTC medication. In IUGR pregnancies, the mother should also ask whether the baby could be at higher risk from any drugs she may take. Any pregnant woman also should consult her doctor before taking a dietary or herbal supplement.

Which Antidepressant Is Linked to the Most Birth Defects?

Study titled "Maternal Use of Specific Antidepressant Medications During Early Pregnancy and the Risk of Selected Birth Defects," by researchers at National Center on Birth Defects and Developmental Disabilities, Centers for Disease Control and Prevention, published in *JAMA Psychiatry*.

Even though antidepressant use in early pregnancy may increase the risk of some birth defects, many pregnant women are treated with these drugs, according to the Centers for Disease Control and Prevention (CDC). Doctors and pregnant women must weigh the risk of untreated depression against the risk of taking an antidepressant.

A new study from CDC researchers used data from the National Birth Defects Prevention Study to shed light on which antidepressants are linked to specific birth defects. They also looked at how much depression and anxiety may contribute to the risk of birth defects without medication. The findings were published in *JAMA Psychiatry*.

Study details: The researchers looked at antidepressant use in more than 30,000 mothers of babies born with birth defects and compared them to a control group of more than 11,000 mothers of babies without birth defects. Just over 5 percent of the birth-defect group reported taking an antidepressant compared with just over 4 percent of the control group. *These were the key findings…*

• ***Venlafaxine*** **(Effexor)** in early pregnancy was linked to several birth defects including heart, brain, spine and cleft palate defects.

• **Selective serotonin reuptake inhibitors (SSRIs),** including *sertraline* (Zoloft), *fluoxetine* (Prozac), *paroxetine* (Paxil) and *citalopram* (Celexa), were linked to a small number of birth defects, including heart defects.

To learn how much depression, anxiety or other mental health disorders contribute to birth defects, the researchers compared women exposed to antidepressants in the first three months of pregnancy to women with mental health disorders not exposed to antidepressants in early pregnancy. This comparison suggested that some of the risks linked to SSRI antidepressants may be caused by mental health conditions and not medication.

Overall, *venlafaxine* was associated with the highest number of birth defects, and this risk was not decreased by accounting for mental health conditions.

Takeaway: This study does not suggest that women who are pregnant and on antidepressants should stop taking their medication. Stopping an antidepressant during pregnancy may be more harmful than taking it. Women should talk to their doctor about the risks and benefits of managing depression during pregnancy with antidepressants. Psychotherapy without medication may be another option.

Postpartum Depression (PPD) Alert

Jean Guglielminotti, MD, PhD, assistant professor of anesthesiology, Columbia University, New York City.

When general anesthesia was given to women undergoing a cesarean delivery, they had a 54 percent greater likelihood of developing PPD and an increased risk of up to 91 percent for suicidal thoughts or self-inflicting injury versus those receiving regional anesthesia.

Possible explanations: A delay in mom-baby bonding and longer-lasting postpartum pain.

Self-defense: If possible, ask for regional anesthesia and, after delivery, get help for PPD warning signs such as extreme sadness and crying, and feelings of anxiety, guilt or hopelessness.

"Vascular Storm" Blamed for Severe Flu During Pregnancy

Study titled "Influenza A Virus Causes Maternal and Fetal Pathology Via Innate and Adaptive Vascular Inflammation in Mice," by researchers at Royal Melbourne Institute of Technology University, Australia, published in *PNAS*.

A new study led by researchers in Australia may change the way we understand the danger of flu during pregnancy. The prevalent theory has been that pregnancy decreases the woman's immune response, leading to more severe flu complications. The new study, published in *PNAS*, flips this theory, suggesting instead a drastic over response—what the researchers call a "vascular storm."

The finding is important because all pregnant women will be exposed to some part of flu season. Those who are infected with the flu virus are at higher risk for pneumonia and other lung and heart complications. Even though the flu virus itself does not cross into the placenta to affect the developing baby directly, the fetus is at higher risk from brain damage, low birth weight and preterm birth.

Study details: Using pregnant and nonpregnant mice, the researchers were able to show that the flu virus remained in the lungs of nonpregnant mice. In the pregnant mice, however, the virus passed from the lungs into the major blood vessels and spread through the circulatory system. This triggered a drastic immune response. The response caused inflammation in blood vessels that reduced their ability to dilate by about 70 percent to 80 percent.

This vascular storm is caused by immune-system proteins and white blood cells that flood blood vessels, causing the insides to swell and narrow. This reaction may explain why flu that does not cross into the womb still affects developing babies. It may drastically cut down their blood and oxygen supply. Vascular inflammation can also occur with preeclampsia (pregnancy hypertension) and with certain individuals suffering from COVID-19.

More studies are needed to understand why the vascular storm occurs. One theory is that the placenta releases proteins and fetal DNA into a mother's circulatory system...foreign elements that put the immune response on high alert. Adding the flu virus may somehow tip the immune system into a drastic response. Further research will also be needed to confirm this response in humans, but vascular inflammation is being targeted by new drugs currently being tested.

Takeaway: For now, the best defense against the flu and a vascular storm during pregnancy is for pregnant women to get their flu shots.

Natural Birth May Reduce Infants' Health Problems

Study of data from nearly 500,000 healthy, low-risk women who gave birth between 2000 and 2013, and of their children up to age five by researchers at Western Sydney University, Penrith, Australia, published in *Birth*.

Babies born with medical intervention, such as hormones used to induce labor, or surgical intervention, such as caesarean delivery, are more likely to have jaundice and feeding problems in their earliest weeks—and may be more likely to develop diabetes, respiratory infections and eczema later. The association does not prove cause and effect, but it adds to earlier research suggesting that intervention during childbirth should be done only when medically necessary.

Is Your Daughter or Daughter-in-Law Pregnant? For Family Harmony, Follow These Five Rules!

Kathy Hartke, MD, an obstetrician/gynecologist in Brookfield, Wisconsin. She is past chair of the Wisconsin section of the American College of Obstetricians and Gynecologists as well as its legislative cochair. She also serves on the board of the WI Association of Perinatal Care and the WI Perinatal Quality Collaborative. She has seven grandchildren.

There's a baby coming! It might be your daughter's, your daughter-in-law's, your niece's or even your grandchild's. You can hardly hold your enthusiasm—or your concerns. You want to share your own experience, give advice and be a part of the picture.

That's great—to a point. But what you say and do could actually help or hurt the situation, and the last thing you want to do is cause trouble...right? To help "expectant" grandparents understand what to say and do and what not to say and do, we spoke with Kathy Hartke, MD, an obstetrician/gynecologist in Brookfield, Wisconsin, who sees both sides of this equation all the time—expectant parents and the grandparents-to-be—and who happens to have seven grandchildren of her own. *Here are her five rules for expectant grandparents...*

RULE #1: Spare the gory details. Expectant women don't want to hear scary childbirth stories. They're upsetting. Even if you labored for 48 hours and tore from here to there, every labor is different—even among moms and their own daughters.

RULE #2: Be nonjudgmental and more thick-skinned. Ask, "Is this something new since I had children?" if you think your pregnant daughter (or daughter-in-law) is doing something amiss. And don't feel hurt if your child doesn't follow your advice. Pregnant women (and women with babies) tend to listen to their doctors and their friends with kids, not their moms.

RULE #3: Stay out of the birthing room. Childbirth is perhaps the most personal experience possible, which is why in most cases, a woman wants to share it just with her partner. So unless you're invited, hang out in the waiting room or at home. No hinting about going into the room, either—that just puts pressure on the parents.

RULE #4: Support the partnership between the new parents. Fathers these days want to be involved—and that's what their wives want too. So resist the urge to praise your son or son-in-law for simply doing his share, like diapering the baby or getting up for a nighttime feeding. And don't say he's babysitting when he's…parenting.

RULE #5: Retire the heirloom equipment. Once the baby arrives, you can provide invaluable grandparenting—not to mention, sorely needed babysitting. But safety standards for cribs, playpens, high chairs, swings, car seats and other infant equipment have changed dramatically and for the better even in the past few years—so the equipment you have in the attic should not be used. To know what's needed to equip your home safely for your new grandchild, either research "safe baby gear" online…or, yes, ask the expectant parents about it!

"Mommy Brain" Is Largely a Myth

Study by researchers at Purdue University, West Lafayette, Indiana, published in *Current Psychology*.

It's true that women are bombarded by hormones and exhaustion during and just after giving birth and those circumstances can result in memory lapses and lack of focus.

But: Mothers who were tested one year post-partum did better than nonmothers on attention-related tasks.

Important: Mothers' perceptions of their own levels of focus and attention were highly accurate, so the distractedness that many report is real but probably related to stress and poor social support, not lingering brain changes from childbirth.

Late Pregnancy and NSAIDs Alert

Center for Drug Evaluation and Research, US Food and Drug Administration, Silver Spring, Maryland.

Beware: Taking NSAIDs late in pregnancy can cause rare but serious kidney problems in an unborn baby. Nonsteroidal anti-inflammatory drugs include *ibuprofen, naproxen* and *celecoxib* (Celebrex). They have been used for decades to treat pain and fever. But new research shows that if women take NSAIDs about 20 weeks into pregnancy or later, fetal kidney problems can result—and in turn can lead to low levels of amniotic fluid and potential pregnancy-related complications.

Surgery for Benign Breast Disease Does Not Affect Breastfeeding

Study titled "Breastfeeding Capability After Benign Breast Surgery," by researchers at Boston Children's Hospital, Boston, presented as a clinical poster at the virtual American College of Surgeons Clinical Congress 2020.

Benign breast disease is very common in women of child-bearing age. In fact, about one million women are diagnosed with a benign breast condition, such as breast cysts or benign tumors, every year. As a result, many of these women will need breast surgery. Even though there has been concern whether this type of surgery would reduce a woman's ability to breastfeed successfully, few studies have researched this question.

Now: There is good news for women with benign breast conditions and their health care providers, according to a new study that was presented at the 2020 meeting of the American College of Surgeons Clinical Congress.

Study details: In a study of 85 women ages 18 to 45, researchers compared the breastfeeding experiences of those who had been diagnosed and treated for a benign breast condition with those who had not. Using a questionnaire, the subjects reported on their ability to breastfeed and their overall satisfaction with breastfeeding. The amount of time after giving birth ranged from six weeks to several years.

Of the 85 women, 15 reported benign breast disease before breastfeeding. Their symptoms included cysts, benign growths and enlarged breasts. Sixteen women reported surgery for a breast condition prior to breastfeeding. The surgeries included biopsies of cysts or removal of benign growths, breast-reduction surgery and breast-augmentation surgery.

Regardless of whether they had previous breast surgery, all women in the study reported about an 80 percent success rate for breastfeeding or pumping enough milk for bottle feeding. Overall satisfaction for breastfeeding was about the same in all women.

Conclusion: While the researchers are continuing to gather information on the effects of surgery for benign breast conditions prior to breastfeeding, their hope is that the results of this research and subsequent findings will reassure women and their doctors that breast surgery should not be withheld if it benefits a young woman of child-bearing age.

Chapter 14

RESPIRATORY CONDITIONS

Why You Can't Catch Your Breath...

I f you have difficulty catching your breath or feel a sudden chest tightening that makes it feel as if you can't take in enough air, you're experiencing dyspnea. Nowadays, that feeling may immediately bring the novel coronavirus to mind, but there are many other possible culprits—and they are often treatable.

Deconditioning

Your heart is a muscle that grows stronger with exercise. Without sufficient physical activity, it weakens and can't efficiently pump blood throughout the body. That means less blood reaches the lungs, leading to shortness of breath. Deconditioning, also known as being out of shape, is responsible for about 60 percent of dyspnea cases.

The treatment is exercise. Dyspnea due to deconditioning may be felt more acutely during physical activity, which often turns people off from doing what they need to. "I'm gasping for breath. I must be straining my heart!" is a common refrain, but it's not true. The authors of a 2020 *European Heart*

Journal study deemed the risk of exercise triggering a heart attack extremely low.

You're harming your heart by not exercising. Lack of physical activity heightens your risk of heart disease, obesity and depression, and each of these conditions is linked with shortness of breath. (In the case of depression, individuals with this serious mental health condition may be less likely to exercise, leading to weight gain and heart disease, which then causes the dyspnea.)

Your goal is to build up to 30 minutes of exercise per day on most days of the week. It needn't be fancy. Try fast walking, dancing or playing a favorite sport. If time is short, your workout can be broken into smaller chunks of time throughout the day. You want your heart rate up, but you should still be able to talk. The heart grows stronger remarkably quickly: Expect to feel less dyspnea after two weeks of your new routine.

If your dyspnea is so intense that you fear you'll pass out, if it is accompanied by chest pain or pressure, or if you have a family his-

John J. Ryan, MD, director of the University of Utah Health Dyspnea Clinic and the University of Utah Pulmonary Hypertension Comprehensive Care Center. Dr. Ryan is an associate editor of several American Heart Association journals and a cardiology consultant for the National Basketball Association and the U.S. Olympic Committee.

tory of heart disease, consult your doctor before starting to exercise.

Cardiovascular Disease

When sticky plaque accumulates in the arteries, it can impede blood flow. When blood can't move freely through the arteries and other blood vessels to the heart, the heart can't properly perform its primary job. As previously noted, that means the lungs can't efficiently perform their job—breathing—leading to shortness of breath.

The leading cause of death among U.S. women and men, cardiovascular disease is preventable and treatable, typically with lifestyle modifications that include exercise, diet, moving towards a healthy weight, and quitting smoking. Some people may also be prescribed medication to lower blood pressure or cholesterol.

Chronic Obstructive Pulmonary Disease (COPD)

Your lungs contain elastic airways and air sacs that inflate and deflate as you breathe. COPD is an umbrella term for a group of diseases that make it harder for them to fill with air. In emphysema, for instance, the air sacs stiffen. In chronic bronchitis, the airway lining becomes inflamed and clogged with mucus. These issues can cause shortness of breath, wheezing, chest tightness, and frequent coughing.

About 75 percent of COPD sufferers are current or former smokers. If you smoke, stopping is your first step. Your doctor may prescribe a medication called a bronchodilator, which relaxes the airways, easing airflow. Other options include steroids, oxygen therapy, endurance-building exercises, or, in extreme cases, surgery.

In some cases, COPD can cause pulmonary hypertension or increased pressure in the arteries inside your lungs. (Heart failure, obesity, blood clots, and other factors can cause pulmonary hypertension, too.) Tell your doctor if your shortness of breath is accompanied by fatigue and leg swelling. You may be referred to a pulmonologist or cardiologist.

Asthma

In asthma, the airways in the lungs become hypersensitive to stimuli such as mold, smoke and air pollution, pollen, and other allergens. These irritants trigger the airway muscles, causing them to constrict and become inflamed in what's called bronchospasm, while increased mucus takes up valuable space. As the airways narrow, you can experience shortness of breath, wheezing, dry cough, and chest tightness. In some individuals, exercise can also trigger asthma.

While many asthma sufferers are first diagnosed in childhood, it is possible to develop the breathing condition in your 50s, 60s, or beyond. Asthma tends to be more severe in women, who may experience their first asthma symptoms during menopause.

A combination of short- and long-acting inhalers are the go-to treatment for many people with asthma. In more severe cases, steroids may be prescribed.

Obstructive Sleep Apnea (OSA)

For 30 million Americans, breathing stops and starts during sleep—sometimes hundreds of times a night. (Apnea means "without breath" in Greek.) The resulting snoring and gasping strains more than a marriage: It also weakens the heart and lungs. Those overnight hours of stressful breathing exhaust your heart, leading to the same chain of events seen in heart disease: The heart can't do its job, so the lungs can't either. In addition to daytime dyspnea, OSA symptoms include drowsiness, high blood pressure, depression, and increased risk of heart attack and stroke. If your collar size is greater than 17 inches (men) or 16 inches (women), and you snore or have fragmented sleep, tell your doctor, who may prescribe a sleep study to diagnose apnea.

Weight loss is often encouraged, as about 70 percent of OSA patients also have obesity, and fat stored in the neck and tongue can impede breathing. Obesity can also cause dyspnea when fat presses on the diaphragm, making it difficult for the lungs to expand. Another key treatment is a continuous positive airway pressure machine, which uses pressurized air to keep the airway open.

If your shortness of breath comes on suddenly and affects activities you can normally do easily, let your doctor know so you can learn the cause. It's often treatable—if you catch it early enough.

Know the Symptoms of a Lung Emergency

Kevin McQueen, MHA, RRT, director of respiratory care, sleep diagnostics, hyperbarics and wound care at University of Colorado Health, Colorado Springs.

Most respiratory illnesses share the same set of symptoms, making it difficult to determine if you have pneumonia, flu, vaping-related illness or coronavirus (COVID-19).

Many people recover with a little rest at home, fever reducers and fluids. But others progress to a dangerous point before they seek medical care. In fact, five of the 30 most common causes of death are related to lung diseases, according to the World Health Organization.

Individuals who notice a slow progression in their shortness of breath should contact their primary care provider or go to an urgent-care facility. It may be best (and more convenient) to utilize telehealth if available.

If symptoms come on rapidly or are severe, seek care at a hospital emergency department. *Key symptoms…*

•**Respiratory distress.** You may climb a flight of stairs and feel "winded," or wheeze or grunt as you inhale and exhale. You might breathe better if you change positions, such as leaning forward. You may sweat but feel cool and clammy. Sometimes, air becomes trapped inside the lungs so you can't take in a normal breath.

•**Significant shortness of breath.** This usually is the key sign that a respiratory illness may be worsening to the dangerous level. Shortness of breath may worsen quickly—sometimes within hours. Stay aware of significant changes in your ability to complete normal daily activities. If you can usually walk several blocks or climb a flight of stairs without becoming winded but your illness makes you short of breath just walking across the room or if you can say only one or two words between breaths, you need medical care.

•**Signs of decreased oxygen levels.** Rapid, shallow breathing or sharp pain when you breathe, especially associated with a bluish tinge in your fingertips or lips, could indicate low oxygen in your blood—seek medical attention.

Having an underlying medical condition, such as cardiovascular disease or lung disease or undergoing treatment for cancer, puts you at greater risk. It's better to err on the side of caution and seek medical attention should you start developing symptoms.

Danger of Using Petroleum Jelly in the Nose to Moisturize Nostrils

Breathing in tiny particles of products such as Vaseline or Vicks VapoRub can cause a pneumonia-like reaction called lipoid pneumonia that can cause significant shortness of breath. The condition is rare but in extreme cases can cause significant lung inflammation. Using edible oils—such as vegetable oil—as nasal lubricants also can cause lung problems.

Safer alternative: Saline nasal spray or water-based gel.

Terry Graedon, PhD, medical anthropologist and cofounder of PeoplesPharmacy.com.

Breathe Better: Four Easy Exercises to Strengthen Your Lungs and Restore Good Health

Belisa Vranich, PhD, a clinical psychologist, founder of The Breathing Class, and former director of Breathing Science at the Ash Center for Comprehensive Medicine in New York City. Her books on breathing are *Breathe: The Simple, Revolutionary 14-Day Program to Improve Your Mental and Physical Health,* and *Breathing for Warriors: Master Your Breath to Unlock More Strength, Greater Endurance, Sharper Precision, Faster Recovery, and an Unshakeable Inner Game.* TheBreathingClass.com.

V*iruses, pollution, chemicals, dust:* Our lungs are constantly under attack. For people with chronic lung disease, such as chronic obstructive pulmonary disease and asthma, strong breathing muscles are crucial to keeping the blood oxygenated, but that's not the only thing that benefits from better breathing. Deep breathing reduces anxiety. Even the CDC urged the populace to "take deep breaths" to reduce stress due to COVID.

That advice can even strengthen your immune system during stressful times: Researchers from the University of Texas-Houston taught deep breathing and other relaxation techniques to 49 women with newly diagnosed breast cancer and saw a significant increase in the activity of natural killer cells, a type of white blood cell that is part of the immune system, and other virus-killing immune components.

Stronger breathing muscles and deeper breaths are fundamental to good health. Studies show that they can help to lower blood pressure, ease back pain, banish insomnia, sharpen memory and focus, and resolve digestive problems like heartburn, constipation and irritable bowel syndrome.

Poor Breathing Technique

Most of us are under-breathers: We don't have the strong breathing muscles that allow us to take consistently deep, oxygenating breaths. It's likely that your breathing muscles are weak and constricted if you're under chronic stress or anxiety; spend a lot of time in front of a computer or texting; sit for many hours a day; or routinely carry a heavy purse, bag or knapsack. Former smokers, people who live with smokers or those who live in polluted cities are at risk, as are people who snore, carry extra abdominal weight, or have a history of nose or lung issues, allergies, sinus problems or even neck, shoulder or back injuries.

Breathing Basics

The main muscle that controls breathing is the diaphragm, a pizza-sized, parachute-shaped muscle at the bottom of your rib cage that flattens and spreads when you breathe properly. The intercostals—the muscles between the ribs—are also vital to breathing. Other muscles used during breathing include those on either side of your spine (erector spinae), the muscles that flank your abdomen (transverse abdominis), and your pelvic floor muscles, which form a kind of sling or hammock at the base of your torso.

When those muscles are weak, other muscles must step in to help: Shoulder muscles move up when you inhale and down when you exhale, and neck muscles tense during inhalation. But those muscles aren't built for the job, and they don't allow you to take full, deep breaths.

The Four-Exercise Fix

While cardio exercises like brisk walking, biking and jogging make you breathe more heavily, they don't actually help your breathing muscles (though they are wonderful for your heart). You can strengthen the breathing muscles only when your body is relatively motionless.

The following exercises, done for less than 20 minutes each day, will strengthen all of your breathing muscles so that you can take deeper, deeply oxygenated breaths.

• **Rock and roll.** Sit in a chair or cross-legged on the floor. If you're sitting on a chair, don't lean back. If you're on the floor, make sure you're seated on a blanket or pillow.

On the inhale, expand your belly as you lean forward. If you're very thin, you may have to push your belly out to get the right posture in the beginning. If you're heavier around the middle, think of releasing your belly or putting it in your lap.

On the exhale, lean back as if you were slumping on a couch. Contract your belly, narrowing your waist, and exhale until your lungs are completely empty. Every time you move your belly, you're actually teaching your diaphragm to activate when you breathe. Do 20 repetitions.

• **Diaphragm extensions.** Lie down on your back. Place a large book (or a small stack of small books) on your abdomen, right on top of your belly button.

Gaze toward the books: You should be able to see them at the very bottom of your field of vision. As you inhale, try to make the books rise. On the exhale, watch them lower. Do 20 repetitions.

• **Cat and cow.** Get on your hands and knees. Exhale audibly and round your back up. You should resemble a hissing cat at Halloween, with its back arched. Hollow out your belly and blow air out toward your belly button. Drop your head completely and stretch the back of your neck. Your tailbone should be tipped under.

On the inhale—the cow portion of the exercise—drop your body, relaxing your belly, and letting it expand downward toward the floor. Let gravity help. Your tailbone should now be tipped out. Swivel your head upward as if you're looking toward the sky. When doing cow, your belly should be relaxed and hanging low, and your head positioned up as if you're mooing.

Alternate the cat and cow 10 times, synchronizing the movement until it flows and you can easily rotate back and forth.

• **The perfect standing breath.** Change to a standing position and continue to inhale and exhale as you were doing in cat and cow.

As you inhale, let your belly expand forward. Arch your back a bit and let your bottom pop back slightly. On the exhale, contract your belly, feel your lower abs tighten, and tuck in your bottom.

Your neck, chest and shoulders shouldn't move: Only your belly and pelvis should be moving back and forth.

Do 20 repetitions.

Daily Routine

Practice the four exercises in a sequence twice per day. It should take three to 10 minutes. If you feel lightheaded, start with fewer repetitions and work your way up over time.

• **Do rock and roll 20 times.**

• **Roll over onto your back and do diaphragm extensions 20 times.**

• **Roll over and push up on all fours.** Do cat and cow 20 times.

• **Sit back on your feet momentarily (or come back onto a chair) and do 20 rock and roll breaths again.**

• **Stand up and do the perfect standing breath 20 times.**

For the first two weeks, breathe through your mouth while doing the exercises. This will help keep your attention on your breath so you don't default to your old way of breathing. After two weeks, start breathing through your nose, which is the best way to take full, deep breaths.

Pulmonary Rehabilitation for COPD Saves Lives

The study "Association Between Initiation of Pulmonary Rehabilitation After Hospitalization for COPD and 1-Year Survival Among Medicare Beneficiaries" published in *JAMA*.

Medical guidelines say that any patient admitted to the hospital for chronic obstructive pulmonary disease (COPD) should enroll in a pulmonary rehabilitation program after discharge. Not surprisingly, a new study from researchers at the University of Massachusetts found that pulmonary rehabilitation starting within 90 days of hospital discharge reduced death at one year significantly. What was surprising was that less than two percent of patients took advantage of a pulmonary rehabilitation program.

COPD includes the diseases emphysema and chronic bronchitis. It affects about 16 million Americans. Causes include smoking and air pollution. COPD is a progressive disease. One way to slow down the progression is implementing the lessons learned in a pulmonary rehabilitation program, which includes instructions in exercise, diet and taking medications. Pulmonary rehabilitation has been shown to improve exercise tolerance, reduce flare ups, reduce hospital admissions and improve quality of life for COPD patients. In fact, pulmonary rehab is one of the most effective treatments for COPD.

The recent study is published in *JAMA*. Using Medicare records, the researchers went back and looked at pulmonary rehab use following hospital admissions for COPD in 2014. There were close to 200,000 admissions at more than 4,000 US hospitals reviewed. The average age of the patients was 77. They found that only 1.5 percent of the patients actually entered a pulmonary rehab program in the three months after discharge from the hospital.

The researchers compared the rate of death at one year after discharge between patients who had pulmonary rehab within three months to patients who did not have rehab in those first three months. Although only about 7 percent of the rehab patients had died at one year, the death rate for the other patients was about 20 percent—a significant increased rate of death.

This study answered the main question the researchers were looking at—does pulmonary rehab after hospitalization for COPD improve survival? It does. But the study raised another serious question. Why do so few patients take advantage of pulmonary rehabilitation?

Editorial comment accompanying the study suggests that both doctors and patients need to be more aware of the importance of pulmonary rehab and its effect on survival. Another problem may be lack of funding for and availability of these programs. If you or someone you care about has been discharged from the hospital with COPD, this study suggests that you really need to find a pulmonary rehabilitation program within 90 days. The study found that people who started rehab earliest and had more sessions had the best chance of being alive after one year.

Why We Sigh: The Biology and Psychology of Those Deep, Audible Breaths

Jack L. Feldman, PhD, distinguished professor of neurobiology, David Geffen School of Medicine at UCLA and a member of the UCLA Brain Research Institute.

Ramani Durvasula, PhD, professor of psychology at California State University, Los Angeles, and author of *"Don't You Know Who I Am?": How to Stay Sane in an Era of Narcissism, Entitlement, and Incivility.* She is former vice chair of the American Psychological Association's Committee on Women in Psychology. Doctor-Ramani.com

Often associated with feelings of exasperation, annoyance or relief, sighing is a ubiquitous act. Every mammal does it, from humans to rodents. But what's the point of these sudden, deep breaths? And if you live with a heavy "sigh-er," should you ignore it? Or is there a deeper message you need to listen to? *We asked a neurobiologist and a psychologist to explain…*

The Neurobiologist Jack L. Feldman, PhD

Ask average people how often they sigh, and they'll say two, maybe three, times a day. But the truth is, humans tend to sigh every five minutes…or 12 times per hour. We sigh a lot! Since most people say that we sigh only a few times a day, I think it is clear that we don't notice our sighs. I am sure if you listen closely to someone you're chatting with, you may not notice any sound, but you may notice (if you are looking for it) the deep breath.

Human lungs contain a branching system of airways, at the end of which are tiny, spherical air sacs called alveoli...400 to 500 million of them. These alveoli are in charge of gas exchange, passing oxygen from inhaled air into the blood and then helping to remove carbon dioxide from the blood via exhalation.

Alveoli are lined with a liquid substance called pulmonary surfactant that lubricates the inhalation-exhalation process. During normal breathing, some alveoli collapse, sticking together like a wet balloon. Sighing involves a sort of double inhale—a normal inhale followed by a second, deeper one before exhaling—and it happens unconsciously. It brings in about twice the volume of an average breath and is nature's way of reinflating those collapsed alveoli. Going too long without sighing actually can cause the lungs to fail. In fact, ventilators (machines that help people with respiratory failure breathe) include mechanical sighs every few minutes to ensure optimal lung functioning. Sighs often are referred to as "augmented breaths" for their ability to expand the lungs.

But there may be more to sighing than just sustaining life. Research suggests that sighing also may relieve stress. When my colleagues and I injected *bombesin*, akin to a peptide normally produced by the brain during times of stress, into the brain stems of rats, the rodents went from sighing 25 times per hour to 500 times per hour. We know that humans sigh more when we are stressed, so it may be that neurons in those brain regions responsible for processing stress-related emotions trigger the act of sighing as a way of providing a sort of psychological reset. More research is needed, but it would make sense, considering that other types of slow, paced breathing can have a profound, calming effect on one's emotional state. For example, deep breathing slows the fight-or-flight response and can increase activity in your parasympathetic nervous system (the one responsible for breathing and heart rate) to reduce stress.

Harness the "sighing effect": In healthy individuals, the body and brain do an excellent job of maintaining regularly scheduled sighs. But you can replicate their stress-easing effects by proactively taking a few slow, deep breaths whenever you're feeling nervous or anxious...or before a high-pressure moment such as delivering a speech or trying to sink a putt. Yes, you will feel calmer even though these aren't actual sighs. Even better, start a meditative practice such as meditation or yoga that features slow, paced breathing. There's also box breathing, which involves inhaling for four counts...holding your breath for four counts...exhaling for four counts...and holding your breath for another four counts. The type of practice you choose isn't as important as whether you enjoy it and will stick with it. Work your way up to 15 minutes a day, and you'll likely notice meaningful improvements in your stress level.

The Psychologist Ramani Durvasula, PhD

When done purposefully and audibly, sighs are a potent form of communication. They're considered nonverbal vocalizations, like laughter and crying out, and their power lies in their ability to convey a range of emotions, from satisfaction to contentedness to exasperation to annoyance to irritated acceptance. Interestingly, sighing seems to mean the same thing regardless of culture or language. Even deaf individuals use sighs to express relief, per a 2017 *Current Biology* article on this breathtaking topic.

Often impulsive, emotional sighs can show up during arguments, where they send the message, *Here we go again,* to the other person. If your spouse is being toxic, for instance, going on yet another rant, you might sigh out of frustration, resignation or just as a form of internal acknowledgment that this person isn't going to change. For the sigher, it feels less taxing than conjuring up the actual words needed to convey those thoughts.

Keep your sighs on a leash: Nonverbal communication of all kinds, such as sighs, raised eyebrows and glares, needs to be monitored as carefully as verbal communication. We often use the sigh as a means of communicating sentiments that feel frustrating or scary. But taking that same moment to recognize that you can communicate respectfully, with mindfully chosen words, can mean the difference between escalating a tense situation or defusing it. Use the seconds before the sigh to realize that you have something that deserves to be said and make the decision to either say it...or say nothing at all and walk away...or ask for a moment to process things, instead.

When you're close with a frequent sigher: It's easy to make assumptions about another person's motivations or intentions when you're on the receiving end of a sigh. Calmly check in with him/her by asking whether everything is OK. Keep a soft tone when making this inquiry so it doesn't feel accusatory. It might turn out that the sigh wasn't directed at you at all but just the other person's own cleansing breath. On the other hand, if the sighs seem to be his way of expressing negative emotion, take a moment before responding. This may help prevent a blowup by serving as a much needed pause to regroup.

Ready for some positive news? Sighs also are used to express a feeling of satisfaction, such as during the first few minutes of a massage...or relief, perhaps when your doctor tells you the lump is benign. In the latter example, sighing also represents a moment of processing—you're waiting for, or receiving, an important piece of information, and once you've received it, you experience a letting go of those emotions with a big, cathartic sigh.

Air Pollution Damages Gut Bacteria

Air pollution damages gut bacteria, reducing microbial diversity and encouraging growth of species associated with obesity, diabetes and other chronic diseases. The relationship between air pollutants such as ozone and diseases such as type 2 diabetes and inflammatory bowel disease has been known for some time—but now a study suggests that these and other diseases actually occur because pollutants damage the diversity of microorganisms in the gut. The study suggests that parks, playgrounds and housing should be moved away from high-pollution areas and more money should be spent to improve air quality.

Tanya Alderete, PhD, assistant professor of integrative physiology, University of Colorado, Boulder, and senior author of a study published in *Environment International*.

A Healthier Home

Tasha Stoiber, PhD, a senior scientist at The Environmental Working Group. EWG.org

As people have spent more time at home than ever before and undertaken a variety of home-improvement projects, many have unwittingly increased their exposure to a host of toxic chemicals that have been linked to both acute and long-term health risks.

We reached out to Tasha Stoiber, PhD, at the Environmental Working Group to get some tips on staying safe.

What toxins are people commonly exposed to at home?

Indoor air can be two to five times as polluted as the outdoors because of a variety of chemicals in everything from building materials to cleaning and personal care products. *Here are a few to be aware of...*

• **Per- or polyfluoroalkyl substances (PFAS)** are notoriously persistent in the environment and the human body. Exposure to high levels of PFAS may reduce the antibody response to vaccines and lower resistance to infectious diseases. You may be exposed through drinking water, nonstick cookware, stain-resistant carpeting and upholstery, and cleaning and personal care products.

• **Flame retardants,** found in foam furniture, insulation, carpet padding and electronics, have been linked to cancer and hormone disruption.

• **Phthalates** are used in soft plastics, vinyl flooring and wall coverings, personal care products, and cleaning agents. Exposure is linked to male reproductive problems, asthma, and allergies.

When making small home improvements, what are sources of toxins people should know about?

Pay attention to the volatile organic compound (VOC) content in paint. VOCs have been linked to respiratory irritation, nervous system damage and cancer. Choose paint that is free of VOCs, and skip those that are marketed as anti-microbial or anti-fungal, as they may contain harmful chemicals. Some options include Benjamin Moore Aura, Sherwin-Williams Harmony, Valspar Simplicity, Old Fashioned Milk Paint Company and Behr Premium Plus. Also look for paints that are certified by Green Seal-11.

Installing a new floor can expose you to toxins as well. I recommend avoiding carpet as much as possible since it can contain PFAS or flame retardants. Carpets also tend to trap dust, which contains allergens and chemicals shed from products. It's also wise to avoid laminate and vinyl flooring.

Instead, choose natural linoleum, tile that was made in the United States, or solid wood with a water-based, Green Seal 11-certified finish. Look for nail-down or click-lock options so you can avoid glue that can contain formaldehyde.

Is it necessary to replace floors, repaint walls and buy new furniture to lower risk?

Dangers in Dust

The chemicals in our homes wind up in dust that we can inhale or get into our mouths. Our exposure to dust is a lot like exposure to soil, so my colleagues and I applied the standards that the U.S. Environmental Protection Agency (EPA) uses to assess contaminated ground to samples of dust we'd gathered. We found that the levels of some phthalates and flame retardants exceeded the EPA's screening numbers for both cancerous and non-cancer effects.

To reduce your exposure to these chemicals, keep household dust to a minimum by dusting with a damp cloth, washing floors with a wet mop, and using a vacuum with a high-efficiency particulate air filter. Wash your hands with soap and water frequently and always before eating.

Tasha Stoiber

No, you don't have to revamp your whole house, but it's important to avoid bringing any new sources of these chemicals into your home as you do renovations or even when spring cleaning. To reduce the health effects of chemicals that are already there, it's imperative to remove household dust (see box above) and ensure adequate ventilation.

Secondhand e-Cigarette Exposure Is Dangerous

Meghan E. Rebuli, PhD, is assistant professor at Center for Environmental Medicine, Asthma and Lung Biology at University of North Carolina at Chapel Hill.

It contains toxic chemicals that are linked with lung and cardiovascular diseases and eye, nose and throat irritation. Exposure can potentially harm still developing brains of infants, children and teens, but there has been little research done on it. Vaping aerosols are particularly dangerous for babies and young children who touch contaminated objects then put their hands in their mouths.

Cleaning Products Linked to Childhood Asthma

Tim Takaro, MD, professor of health sciences, Simon Fraser University, Burnaby, British Columbia, Canada, and leader of a study published in *Canadian Medical Association Journal*.

Infants from birth to age three months living in homes where household cleaners were used with high frequency were more likely than other children to develop asthma by the time they were three years old. The relationship between product exposure and respiratory problems was much stronger in girls than boys—for unknown reasons. The households studied used 26 different types of cleaners, including dusting sprays, antimicrobial hand sanitizer, disinfectants, polishes and air fresheners.

Teas That Relieve Asthma

Ginger—its compounds reduce airway inflammation. Green—the antioxidants lower inflammation and improve lung function. Black—contains caffeine, which relaxes the airway. Eucalyptus—reduces mucus production and expands the passageways inside the lungs. Licorice—one of its compounds relieves asthma symptoms, but don't exceed one cup per day. Mullein—relaxes the muscles in the respiratory tract. Breathe Easy Tea—a branded herbal formulation from Traditional Medicinals that contains ginger, licorice and eucalyptus.

Note: Don't replace your asthma meds with tea—instead, use both.

Roundup of studies on tea and asthma, reported on Healthline.com.

Milk Allergy in Babies May Be Overdiagnosed

Robert Boyle, PhD, consultant allergy specialist, Imperial College London, England, and lead author of a study published in *JAMA Pediatrics*.

Up to 14 percent of parents believe they have a child who is allergic to cow's milk—but only about one percent of children actually have a milk allergy. Overdiagnosis may be caused by official medical guidelines that mention symptoms including excessive crying, regurgitating milk and loose stools. Those symptoms are very common in normal, healthy babies who don't have a milk allergy. Seven of nine guidelines studied advised breast-feeding women to avoid all dairy products if their child was suspected of being allergic—but less than one-one-millionth of the protein from cow's milk travels through to breast milk, and that is far too little to cause an allergic reaction.

A Simple Pill Could Block Severe Allergic Reactions

Study titled "Bruton's Tyrosine Kinase Inhibition Effectively Protects Against Human IgE-Mediated Anaphylaxis," by researchers at Northwestern University Feinberg School of Medicine in Chicago, published in *The Journal of Clinical Investigation*.

For people with drug or food allergies, anaphylaxis is a danger that's always lying in wait. This sudden and severe reaction can occur within seconds or minutes of exposure to an allergen, leading to life-threatening anaphylactic shock that causes blood pressure to drop severely and/or the airway to close up. These severe reactions affect one in 50 Americans, according to research, though many experts believe that number is actually closer to one in 20.

Until recently, an injection of epinephrine, using an EpiPen, has been the only treatment for anaphylaxis. In 2020, the FDA approved a drug called Palforzia to help reduce the risk of allergic reactions in children with peanut allergies.

Now: A new study suggests that an oral medication being used to treat some cancer patients may become the first pill to prevent anaphylactic reactions that result from any drug or food allergy.

Study details: In the new research, published in *The Journal of Clinical Investigation,* researchers from Northwestern University found that medications known as Bruton's tyrosine kinase (BTK) inhibitors successfully blocked anaphylaxis in human test-tube mast cells, which release allergy-causing substances in response to an allergen.

When an allergy exposure occurs, BTK (an enzyme) activates the release of histamine and additional substances in mast cells and other cells. BTK inhibitor drugs block this trigger. A BTK inhibitor was also shown in the study to block anaphylaxis in mice that had transplanted human mast cells in a so-called "humanized" mouse model.

"This pill could quite literally be life-changing and life-saving," explained Bruce Bochner, MD, the study's senior author and Samuel M. Feinberg Professor of Medicine at Northwestern University Feinberg School of Medicine in Chicago. "Imagine being able to take medication proactively to prevent a serious allergic reaction."

Previous research involving humans uncovered similar responses. For example, cancer patients who were allergic to airborne allergens, such as cat dander or ragweed pollen, and took the BTK inhibitor *ibrutinib* (Imbruvica) had allergy skin test reactions that were reduced by 80 percent to 90 percent within one week. Adults without cancer who took the drug for a few days also had reduced food allergy skin test reactions.

What's ahead: Human clinical trials will be needed to confirm that BTK inhibitors can be used to prevent allergic reactions. To do this, the researchers plan to give study participants who are allergic to a medication or food a BTK inhibitor then do skin testing to see if allergic reactions are reduced or eliminated.

Caveats: BTK inhibitors, which are FDA-approved to treat blood cancer, are not currently approved for use in children, who are often affected by food allergies (including milk, eggs and tree nuts) and drug allergies (such as antibiotics and antiseizure medication). Cost is also an issue. At $500 a day, using the drug preventively on an ongoing basis would be prohibitively expensive at its current cost.

Still, if these issues can be resolved and the drug proves effective in further research, people who have lived in fear of having a serious allergic reaction may have their worries removed by simply taking a daily pill.

Your Heartburn Could Be Caused by an Allergy

George Kroker, MD, retired allergist, formerly of Allergy Associates of La Crosse, Onalaska, Wisconsin, quoted on AllergyChoices.com.

If you experience heartburn symptoms that don't respond to antacids, it's possible you're suffering from a condition called eosinophilic esophagitis (EoE), a buildup of disease-fighting white blood cells in the esophagus reacting to a food allergy (often milk, wheat or eggs) or even seasonal allergies. People who have the condition experience pain and difficulty when swallowing, chronic cough and, for some, heartburn.

A gastroenterologist can diagnose EoE through an endoscopy and a biopsy. Once the culprit allergens have been identified, diet changes and/or allergy medication can be effective treatments.

Surprising Solution to Recurrent Nasal Infections

Andrew Rubman, ND, is medical director of Southbury Clinic for Traditional Medicines in Southbury, Connecticut. SouthburyClinic.com. He is author of the blog "Nature Doc's Patient Diary" at Bottom LineInc.com

The patient: "Anabel," a woman in her mid-60s who loves to spend her free time "exploring deep woods and trails."

Why she came to see me: Anabel simply could not escape her frequent nasal infections. She was referred to me by her friend whom I treated for ear infections.

How I evaluated her: I first sat and simply talked with Anabel about her ongoing problem. She shared that no matter what drugs and procedures had been tried, her nasal infections returned—sometime diagnosed as "viral," occasionally "bacterial," and often "allergic." She had tried dehumidifiers, HEPA filters, wheat- and dairy-avoidance diets, multiple antihistamines, allergy medications and many, many antibiotics. I did a physical examination of her nose and took a swab of the tissue relatively deep within the nasal passage. I then applied the swab to a microscope slide and stained it with a small amount of tincture of iodine. I placed it under my microscope that had output into a laptop computer in my exam room. This stain would reveal if there were yeast organisms present in her nose.

Indeed, there were yeast organisms in the mucus sample. I explained that often these organisms can disrupt the physical and immunological strength of the underlying membrane and allow bacteria or viruses to take hold, and that common allergens found in the environment can further aggravate inflammation in the nose.

How we addressed his problem: While it is virtually impossible to eliminate yeast in the nose, it can be held at bay by simply deeply rinsing both nasal passages with a salt solution containing some aromatic alcohols like eucalyptol (from the eucalyptus tree bark), menthol (from a number of plants in the mint family), or thymol (from the cooking herb thyme). I made up a solution in my pharmacy and dispensed it to her. She performs the rinse at least twice a day and often when she returns from her woodland outings.

The patient's progress: Anabel reported feeling that her nose had "opened up" substantially and that she was breathing more freely. As of one month, she's had no reoccurrences of any of the past infections that had plagued her. Did we find a "cure"? Only time will tell, but I believe that we found and limited a substantive trigger.

Thirdhand Smoke Can Affect People Even in Nonsmoking Environments

Study by researchers at Yale University, New Haven, Connecticut, published in *Science Advances*.

Residue that contains measurable amounts of harmful substances found in cigarette smoke adheres to walls and other surfaces where smoking has occurred. The residue can cling to the bodies and clothing of people who enter those places—and be transported to other locations.

Chapter 15

VERY PERSONAL

Demystifying Incontinence

I t's an alarming moment: You sneeze, cough, laugh or pick up a heavy package, and a bit of urine leaks out.

Urinary incontinence is incredibly common—affecting about 25 million American adults, three-quarters of them women—but it isn't inevitable. No one needs to endure the distress and disruption of what is often a closeted problem, since 80 percent of those with incontinence can now be helped or cured using a tailored treatment menu that may combine several leading-edge therapies.

Unwanted Intruder

Always unwelcome, incontinence comes in two main forms. By far, the most prevalent is stress incontinence: urine leakage when the bladder feels pressure from a sudden movement. Urge incontinence, dubbed overactive bladder, occurs when the bladder squeezes down without "warning" the urethra—allowing even larger amounts of urine to escape. Some people can even be dealt a double whammy, suffering from a combination of stress and urge incontinence. But why does incontinence happen?

Stress incontinence stems from weakness in the muscles and connective tissue supporting the bladder, uterus and rectum. Age is a predisposing factor, with the loss of estrogen from menopause thinning these vital structures. More famously, pregnancy and childbirth take a toll, as do smoking, obesity and chronic coughing.

The incidence of urge incontinence ticks up with age, but it can also coexist with a variety of other conditions, such as spinal cord injury or irritable bowel syndrome. Simply put, overactive bladder happens when there's a disconnect between the nerves that relax and contract the bladder. Notably, 300 different medications, from sleep aids to high blood pressure pills, can contribute to this disconnect.

Men are more often spared from incontinence not only because they can skip childbirth and menopause, but because their urethras are much longer than women's, making it easier for this "gatekeeper" against urine loss to close off against bladder pressure.

Jill Maura Rabin, MD, a professor of obstetrics and gynecology at Zucker School of Medicine at Hofstra Northwell in Hempstead, New York. Dr. Rabin is the coauthor of *Mind Over Bladder: A Step-By-Step Guide to Achieving Continence.*

Thorough Diagnostic Process

As with many medical problems, accurately diagnosing incontinence and its causes begins with your doctor asking a bevy of questions about your symptoms, medical and surgical history, and number of pregnancies and births. He or she should also review a full list of your medications and supplements.

Next is a thorough physical exam to understand the size, shape, consistency, and placement of the pelvic organs. This crucial exam can reveal if organs have prolapsed, slipping from their normal positions and placing pressure on the bladder or other organs. The answers will help point to type of incontinence—whether stress, urge, or another form. *A variety of tests may also be done, including…*

- **Urine sample** to detect infection
- **Ultrasound** to reveal any fluid remaining in the bladder after urination
- **Urodynamic testing,** which fills the bladder with sterile water through a catheter placed into the urethra. This tube and another placed in the rectum monitor pressure in both organs. Then you're asked to cough, showing stress incontinence if fluid leaks from the bladder. You're also asked to urinate to check for any blockages and ensure the bladder muscle works properly.

Tailored Treatment Menu

While there's no one-size-fits-all approach to treating incontinence, several tactics tend to provide at least some relief. Losing five to 10 pounds lowers pressure on the bladder by 10 to 15 percent, for example, while changing medications can zap urine leakage for a surprising number of those affected. Even avoiding food triggers such as alcohol, chocolate, spicy foods, or aspartame, which can prompt bladder contractions, spells drier days for some with overactive bladder.

After zeroing in on the type of incontinence and learning about your day-to-day lifestyle, your doctor should be able to offer a menu of treatment options tailored to your individual situation and severity. And just like any menu, you get to pick and choose—in this case, typically two or three approaches to try simultaneously or sequentially.

New Options

The latest treatment options include techniques to quiet an overactive bladder—in many cases without medication. *Nonsurgical interventions include…*

- **Behavioral therapy** that "retrains" the brain to suppress unwanted bladder contractions
- **Keeping a diary** of fluid intake and trips to the bathroom
- **Bladder training** that gradually increases the amount of urine you can hold in your bladder
- **Kegel exercises** and physical therapy to strengthen pelvic floor muscles
- **Mechanical devices** such as a pessary, inserted to support prolapsed pelvic organs
- **Tibial nerve stimulation,** wherein a small electrode sends pulsating signals to calm bladder muscles.

Surgical Treatments

There are also several minimally invasive surgeries that boast a quick recovery…

- **Bladder neck injection,** which injects synthetic "bulking agents" into the urethra wall to hamper urine leakage
- **Sling procedure,** which places a sling under the urethra that's attached to the abdominal wall to support the bladder and block leakage
- **InterStim,** a "pacemaker" for the bladder that implants a device sending mild electrical signals to the sacral nerve at the bottom of the spine, calming overactive bladder.

If you're hesitant to get help, ask yourself: "How important is my quality of life?" Ultimately, it takes getting out of your emotional comfort zone to achieve physical comfort.

Be Your Own Advocate

Astoundingly, more than two-thirds of women don't consider urine leakage while coughing or sneezing a health problem, and one-third think a loss of bladder control is a natural part of aging. Yet the typical incontinence sufferer spends between $1,000 and $3,000 each year on absorbent products whose chirpy names are the polar opposite of how these women feel while buying them. Serene and poised on the checkout line? Probably not. So it's somewhat perplexing that only one of 12 people affected by incontinence seeks medical help, waiting an average of nearly seven years after first experiencing bladder control issues.

Less Sex Linked to Earlier Menopause

Analysis of data on 2,936 women by researchers at University College London, UK, published in *Royal Society Open Science*.

Women who reported some form of sexual activity at least weekly were 28 percent less likely to have experienced menopause at any given age during the study period than women who reported sexual activity less than monthly. Sexual activity was defined to include intercourse, oral sex, sexual touching and caressing, or self-stimulation. It is possible that the bodies of women who do not often have sex stop using energy for ovulation and direct it elsewhere, which may lead to earlier menopause.

Talking Testosterone

Gary Donovitz, MD, FACOG, founder of BioTE Medical. His latest book is *Testosterone Matters More: The Secret to Healthy Aging in Women*. Donovitz.com

With so many supplements on the market being touted for "low T" to restore men's virility, it's easy to forget that testosterone plays a wide variety of roles, even with women. To learn more, we spoke with Gary Donovitz, MD, author

of *Testosterone Matters More: The Secret to Healthy Aging in Women*.

Low T Consequences

Many of the signs and symptoms of low testosterone are the same in men and women: lower libido, mood swings, weight gain, problems with sleep, muscle loss and brain fog. *Without adequate levels of testosterone, both women and men are at increased risk of serious conditions…*

• **Cognitive decline.** You might experience memory, focus and concentration issues and, in women in particular, Alzheimer's disease.

• **Cardiovascular disease.** As testosterone levels decline, systemic inflammation increases, including in coronary arteries. It can also precipitate more plaque deposits in arteries.

• **Osteoporosis-related fractures.** Low testosterone and the resulting loss of bone and muscle mass can lead to frailty, which increases the risk for falls and breaking a bone.

• **Diabetes.** Diabetes, obesity and low testosterone are dangerously linked, especially in men. A man with diabetes has a 50 percent chance of having low testosterone. A man with diabetes who is also obese has a greater than 80 percent risk of having low testosterone.

Testosterone and Age

Testosterone levels in women start to decline as early as age 25. By age 40, they're half of what they once were. Menopause can simultaneously trigger low testosterone, uncontrolled inflammation and increased LDL (bad) cholesterol. For men, testosterone loss starts in the 30s, with levels declining 1 to 1.5 percent every year. Low testosterone likely affects more than one-third of men over age 45.

Restoring Testosterone Levels

The optimal range of testosterone levels in women has still not been established. Other than in the area of sexual dysfunction, testosterone's importance to women isn't appreciated enough. Restoring testosterone with hormone replacement therapy can mean better energy, sleep, and mood, less depression, and greater sexual satisfaction. Some studies show that it can be protective against cancer, specifically breast and prostate cancers. It can boost brain function, decrease inflammation and limit plaque buildup, improving blood flow and cardiac function, and increase bone mineral density to a greater degree than bone drugs.

Low testosterone in men is diagnosed when total testosterone is less than 300 nanograms/deciliter, but many men have signs of testosterone deficiency even above this level.

Testosterone Therapy

There are various testosterone formulations available, but they aren't equally effective. The testosterone replacement should be bioidentical, not synthetic. Synthetic testosterones have a different molecular structure and don't chemically match the hormone as naturally made by the body, so the benefits are never as good and the risks are higher.

Testosterone comes in topicals, such as patches, gels, and creams, but their absorption rates vary, and they can deliver too much or too little testosterone. Pills seem to increase inflammation markers. Pellets provide a more consistent blood level over time as the testosterone is released slowly over a period of weeks or months. This eliminates the rollercoaster effect of symptom relief and resurgence, and reduces the risk of side effects, such as hair thinning in women. Contrary to myth, in the right dose, it does not cause masculine traits like a deep voice.

Hormone Optimization

The best results for women come from hormone optimization, which is more than just hormone replacement. It means finding the right hormones—which might include thyroid and/or estrogen for some women—at the right dose for the right person. This is an example of precision medicine. Because

testosterone is not commercially available in doses made for women and is used off-label, hormones should be made at a compounding pharmacy so the dose can be individualized.

Pornography Doesn't Affect Relationship Satisfaction—at Least Not in the Short Term

Study of 77 same-sex and 140 mixed-sex couples by researchers at Université du Québec à Trois-Rivières, published in *Journal of Social and Personal Relationships*.

Researchers tracked porn use among partnered individuals for a 35-day period. Seventy-six percent of men with female partners and 40 percent of women with male partners used explicit material during the study. Their use had no bearing on relationship satisfaction. When women used pornography, they were more likely to have partnered sexual activity the same day. However, while male porn use was associated with reduced desire on the part of their female partners—possibly because men were turning to pornography when their partners weren't in the mood—that lowered desire was not expressed as dissatisfaction with the relationship.

Clean Your Bottom Better

James Lin, president of BidetKing, Monterey Park, California, which sells major bidet brands and provides bidet comparisons and information.

Bidets have been more of a European thing than an American thing—but the temporary shortage of toilet paper in 2020 created a surge in sales.

The bidet's stream of water not only reduces the amount of toilet paper you need to use, it's also more comfortable than wiping for people who have hemorrhoids or irritable bowel syndrome. Some research even suggests that bidet use can reduce the risk for bacterial infections, especially among older people.

Although you might think of a bidet as the stand-alone fixture common in countries such as France, there's an easier, less expensive option—a version that consists of a water-squirting seat or an attachment for the traditional toilet. It isn't even necessary to call a plumber to install one—many models can be added to existing toilets by a homeowner in less than a half-hour. However, all but the entry-level bidet attachments require an electrical outlet near the toilet.

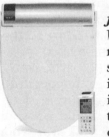

Best overall bidet seat for elongated bowls: Bio-Bidet Bliss BB-2000, which replaces a toilet's existing seat, delivers warm water instantly when activated via its remote or built-in controls, followed by warm-air drying. Unlike with some bidets, there's no initial cold spray before the water is properly heated…and the temperature can be adjusted ranging from room temp up to 105°F. It also has a seat-heating system, nightlights, a remote control that can be used to activate the unit and adjust settings, and a self-cleaning system for the unit's stainless-steel nozzle. At its highest setting, the water pressure is superior to most other bidets, which even can be useful for those who are constipated—it can act as an enema. It's available only in white and only in "elongated" shape, which fits toilet bowls measuring 18 inches to 20 inches from the seat mounting bolts to the front edge. $699. BioBidet.com

Best overall bidet seat for round bowls: Brondell Swash 1400 offers many of the same features as the BioBidet above, including adjustable warm water temperature (from 85°F to 104°F)…adjustable air drying…heated

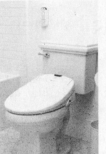

seat…remote control…and a self-cleaning function. But it's available for round toilet bowls (16 to 17¾ inches from the mounting hardware to the front edge of the seat) in addition to elongated bowls…and in beige and white. The Swash 1400 falls short in a few details— it can't match the BioBidet's top water pressure setting, although it's enough pressure for the average user…and its tankless water-heating system doesn't deliver warm water quite as quickly. $649. Brondell.com

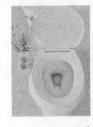

Best budget bidet "attachment": Tushy Classic is a simple plastic spray device that attaches to the seat bolts of most toilets in minutes. It's the only one in this article that doesn't require access to an electrical outlet.

Downside: The water it sprays is as cold as the water from the bathroom sink's cold-water tap. Most bidet users prefer warmer water. Tushy also sells a warm-water unit called Tushy Spa that requires attachment of an additional nine-foot hose to the hot-water supply under your sink. $99/Tushy Classic… $119/Tushy Spa. HelloTushy.com

Best bidet if price is no object: Toto Neorest NX2 Dual Flush Toilet is the Rolls-Royce of bidet toilet bowls. This bidet/toilet combo offers virtually everything the bidet seats above do—plus sensor-operated automatic toilet seat open/close…"tornado flushing" that's extremely effective at clearing waste despite using only 1.28 gallons per flush…germ-killing UV lighting…and an advanced ceramic glaze that remains cleaner than other toilet bowls.

Downside: It costs as much as a small car. $17,800. TotoUSA.com

Beware This Smell When You Pass Gas

Jacob Teitelbaum, MD, is a world-renowned fibromyalgia specialist and author of *Real Cause, Real Cure*. Vitality101.com

A strong rotten egg smell when you pass gas, particularly if accompanied by bloating and diarrhea, suggests small intestinal bacterial overgrowth (SIBO). It's commonly treated with the antibiotic *rifaximin* (about $1,400 for 14 days). Instead, the herbal supplement Ultra MFP Forte (about $56 for one month) often is as effective. It contains olive leaf, berberine and burdock. Gassiness without much sulfur smell suggests Candida overgrowth.

Helpful: Take a good probiotic and an antifungal, and avoid sugar. See an integrative doctor for comprehensive treatment.

How to Sweat Less and Stop the Stink

Ahmad Shatil Amin, MD, medical practice director at Northwestern Medicine Dermatology in Chicago and assistant professor of dermatology at Feinberg School of Medicine at Northwestern University.

You know that perspiration is the sign that your body's internal thermostat is working. But what happens if it works too well…and you're faced with constant telltale sweat marks on clothes, not to mention the odor? Here are strategies you can use, depending on how bad the problem is.

Sweat Glands 101

You have two main types of sweat glands. The eccrine glands are over most of your body. This type of sweat is what gives your skin that moist glow when you exercise, but most people don't notice the loss of moisture during low-exertion times. As your temperature goes up, these glands release fluid, mostly water, that cools you off as it evaporates. The sweat from the eccrine glands has no odor.

The apocrine glands are more problematic. They're found mostly in areas where hair grows—underarms, scalp, groin. When you're stressed, they release a milky fluid that's odorless on its own, but once it mixes with the bacteria on your skin, that's when the stink starts.

Why Am I Sweating So Much?

You expect to sweat when you work out, start feeling nervous in social and business situations or have a fever that breaks. But there are health conditions—and it's not just menopause—that ramp up the level of sweating.

Heavy sweating can be traced to infections…the nervous system, heart, lung and thyroid diseases…and diabetes (often from low blood sugar), among others. Hyperthyroidism and other hormone-related problems that stem from the hypothalamus, the part of the brain that regulates temperature, can cause excessive sweating during sleep. Managing those conditions should get your sweating under control, so check with your doctor to rule out these causes.

Some medications, such as antidepressants and heart and blood pressure medications, also can cause night sweats. Ask if a change in prescription is possible.

Being overweight can make you sweat more—you might notice it even with just a few pounds of weight fluctuation. Losing weight can help.

Important: Because changes in your perspiration pattern can be a warning of an undiagnosed medical condition, such as diabetes, leukemia or non-Hodgkin's lymphoma, see your doctor if…

•**You suddenly begin to sweat much more or less than usual.**

•**You experience night sweats for no apparent reason.**

•**You notice a change in your body odor.**

There also are millions of people who experience excessive sweating with no underlying cause. Called primary hyperhidrosis, there's no rhyme or reason to when the sweating happens. *But there are ways to resolve it…*

Simple At-Home Solutions to Sweat Less

Slight changes to your daily routine can have a big impact…

• **Double up on deodorant/antiperspirant.** Most people apply a combination deodorant/antiperspirant each morning to their underarms to block sweat and fight odor.

Better: Also apply it each night before bed. This gives your sweat glands the time needed to absorb the aluminum, which is the active ingredient in antiperspirants. Choose a higher strength product, which often will say "clinical grade" on the label.

Note: Many people have switched to deodorant-only underarm products, because of skin irritation or because they believe that the aluminum in antiperspirants can increase the risk for breast cancer, dementia, kidney disease and other health problems. There is no substantial scientific evidence to support these fears. And deodorant-only products do nothing to stop the sweat.

• **Dry off.** Before getting dressed or putting on your pajamas, carefully dry yourself—especially between your toes and under your arms—to reduce bacteria growth on skin, which is the foundation for odor. Skin also must be thoroughly dry before you apply antiperspirant for optimal absorption.

• **Relax.** If your emotions bring on perspiration, practice relaxation techniques such as yoga, meditation and biofeedback. These can help you learn to control the stress that triggers sweating.

• **Change your pajamas and your bedding.** If you sweat in your sleep, whether or not it's related to hot flashes, try cooling, moisture-wicking sleepwear, underwear and sheets—it is easy to find these using an Internet search. Certain fabrics, such as cotton flannel, can make sweating worse. As comfy as they are, down blankets can trap heat, causing you to sweat more, too.

Serious Remedies for Hyperhidrosis

If you're sweating through your clothes during the day and the amount is bothering you, see a dermatologist to discuss treatment options, starting with prescription-strength antiperspirants. *If that's not enough, here are other medical options to try…*

Topical: Glycopyrronium (Qbrexza) is available as an underarm wipe. In clinical trials, participants who used it for one month reported that it decreased sweating severity by up to 30 percent and sweat production by 50 percent, with some improvement seen after the first week. While glycopyrronium can be used in other areas of the body, it is approved only for underarms and may not be as effective elsewhere.

Glycopyrronium is an anticholinergic, meaning that it blocks the neurotransmitter acetylcholine, responsible for activating the sweat process. As with other anticholinergics, it's not for anyone with glaucoma, severe ulcerative colitis, myasthenia gravis or Sjögren's syndrome because it can make those conditions worse.

Injection: Botulinum toxin (Botox) is the most effective treatment we have for excessive underarm sweating. It also can be used on the palms of the hands and soles of the feet. For most people, it reduces sweating by 75 percent to 90 percent, bringing it down to a normal level. The treatment needs to be repeated every six months. Some health insurers will cover the injections because they're for a medical reason although Botox is not covered for cosmetic purposes. Check with your dermatologist's billing office—some may need repeated requests to do the paperwork and follow-up phone calls required for insurance approval.

Oral: Glycopyrrolate. For people who aren't helped by Botox, off-label use of glycopyrrolate may help. This is another form of the active ingredient in Qbrexza but is given in pill form. It was developed to reduce other types of body secretions and a decrease in sweating is one of its side effects. It works for some people, but not everyone finds its other side effects—dizziness, drowsiness, nervousness, loss of taste and headache—worth the benefit.

Noninvasive procedure: miraDry. This noninvasive, FDA-approved procedure uses a handheld device to target thermal (heat) energy at sweat glands in the underarms while keeping skin at the surface cool. One to two treatments are all that's needed to destroy underarm sweat glands. You will continue to sweat normally in other parts of the body.

How to Stop the Stink

Sweat by itself doesn't cause body odor. That happens when it meets bacteria on your skin. Washing off sweat after a workout will help. So will washing workout clothes every time you wear them—something that a surprising number of people don't do. But if you've ever felt that these clothes weren't becoming truly stink-free, your nose isn't deceiving you. High-performance fabrics tend to hold on to odors. Try specialty detergents developed for these fibers.

You can wash your hands or dab on sanitizer when your palms get sweaty, but it's harder to keep your feet odor-free when they're in shoes and unable to breathe all day. One of the best things you can do is not wear the same pair of shoes two days in a row. This gives the shoes a chance to completely dry out. *Try any or all of these additional tips to conquer foot odor…*

• **Wash feet nightly with an antibacterial soap, and dry them completely.**

• **Use a spray underarm deodorant or antiperspirant on your feet.**

• **Place deodorizing insoles in every pair of shoes, and change them as needed.**

• **Buy socks and hosiery made from breathable,** moisture-wicking fabrics and shoes made from natural materials such as canvas, especially important for closed-toe shoes that limit air circulation around your feet.

Bad Breath Despite Good Dental Hygiene?

Isabel Suastegui-Mursuli, DDS, Winston Dental, Palatine, Illinois; Chris Lewandowski, DDS, president, Princess Center Dentistry, Scottsdale, Arizona; Elizabeth Kampschnieder, DDS, Kennedy Dental, Bellevue, Nebraska; Eugene Gamble, BDS, MFD RCSI, MClinDent, MPerio RCSEd, FFD RCSI, Rosedale Dental Centre, St. Michaels, Barbados; and Leann Poston, MD, BeWell Medical Clinic, North Vancouver, British Columbia, Canada.

Patients often believe that bad breath is only related to the care and maintenance of their teeth, but halitosis can have numerous causes.

1. Gingivitis. Brushing and flossing regularly are indeed important, but you need to be sure you are brushing and flossing properly. Don't just pass your toothbrush and or floss over your teeth: You really need to clean them. If not, biofilm settles on your teeth and creates plaque, which builds up along the gum line, causing gingivitis.

2. Tonsil stones. Food and mucus can become trapped in the crevices of your tonsils and emit a foul odor. A dentist may be able to manually remove the stones. In some cases, lasers or surgery may be necessary.

3. The ketogenic diet. The popular "keto" diet, is notorious for causing bad breath, as are foods like garlic and onions. Unexpected culprits include citrus, dairy, cheese, and peanut butter.

4. Old broken fillings and crowns. If you have a broken filling or crown, you may not be able to clean the areas sufficiently. This will allow odor-creating bacteria to fester unhindered.

5. Health conditions. Gastric reflux conditions, sinus infection, tonsilitis, diabetes, and throat and other cancers can cause bad breath.

6. Medications such as antihistamines can decrease saliva production, while others have halitosis as a side effect.

7. Your tongue. One of the biggest reservoirs of bacteria in the mouth is the tongue. Clean it with the roughened back of your toothbtush (this is designed precisely to clean the tongue) or a specialized tongue scraper.

Visit your dentist at least twice a year for thorough cleanings and check-ups. If your problem persists, make an appointment with your primary care provider to check for any underlying health conditions.

Treat and Prevent "Maskne"

If your skin is irritated from wearing a mask, you may be a victim of "maskne," or mask acne, which can be either actual acne (in which case you'll see blackheads or whiteheads) or just irritation.

To prevent either condition: Don't wear makeup under your mask. Use a gentle cleanser in the morning, and apply sunscreen to put a barrier between the mask and your skin. After removing the mask, cleanse your face and apply moisturizer. Wash your mask daily using fragrance-free detergent.

To treat: Use an over-the-counter hydrocortisone cream for itching or an acne cleanser for pimples. See a dermatologist if your problem persists.

Allison Truong, MD, dermatologist, Cedars-Sinai Medical Group, Los Angeles, quoted at Cedars-Sinai. org.

Drug-free Constipation Cure: A Vibrating Pill

Satish S.C. Rao, MD, PhD, professor of medicine, director of neurogastroenterology, Medical College of Georgia, Augusta University, and coauthor of study titled "Brain Fogginess, Gas and Bloating: A Link between SIBO, Probiotics and Metabolic Acidosis," published in *Clinical and Translational Gastroenterology.*

Constipation is often the butt (sorry!) of crude humor, but for sufferers it's no joking matter. And when the condition is chronic, the desire for relief is chronic, too. Now, a new high-tech cure may change that. It doesn't use drugs, has virtually no side effects, is amazingly effective—and works by literally shaking the you-know-what out of you. Here are the details.

About 16 percent of Americans, including one-third of adults older than age 60, suffer chronic constipation. Eating more fiber, drinking more water and exercising are all well and good. But that's often not enough for people with chronic constipation—their constipation can be caused by problems with peristalsis, the natural contractions of the bowel that help move things through.

Laxative drugs are the common go-to solution for chronic constipation. These laxatives work chemically by stimulating or irritating the colon, or by attracting fluid to flush out stool. But they may become less effective if used regularly and may lead to dependency.

An Israeli company called Vibrant came up with a remedy that works mechanically. The remedy is a small capsule that is swallowed and programed to vibrate when it reaches the large intestine. The vibrations both relieve the constipation practically immediately...and also induce natural peristaltic activity, stimulating additional spontaneous bowel movements. The capsule is then excreted with bowel movements.

In early clinical trials, the Vibrant capsule almost doubled the number of bowel movements and achieved effective relief of constipation in close to 90 percent of patients with chronic constipation within eight weeks.

Researchers at Augusta University in Georgia and other institutions also recently tested the new device. They conducted two studies with a total of 245 patients with chronic constipation. For eight weeks, some of the patients took five Vibrant capsules (programmed to vibrate either one or two times a day) for five days per week…while others (the control group) took the same number of sham capsules.

Results: Compared to the control group, the patients who took vibrating capsules had twice as many spontaneous complete bowel movements. (The study did not track what happened to the patients after they stopped taking the vibrating capsule, so they don't know if the beneficial effect persisted.)

The capsule is about the size of a fish oil pill, and the mechanism inside the pill that vibrates uses novel technology similar to the vibrating device you get at a restaurant when you wait for a table. The device is activated (the pill starts flashing) using a small magnet just before swallowing and is preprogrammed to start vibrating in eight to 12 hours.

The vibrations are not felt by most people. (One out of 10 patients did sense some vibration but did not find the sensation unpleasant—and none dropped out of the study.) There were no other side effects—including no diarrhea or stool leakage, as can be the case with drug laxatives—and the device was found to be safe, according to the researchers.

Note: The researchers don't know whether the magnetic component within the pill will cause problems for people with implantable electronic medical devices, such as pacemakers. Safety studies are currently ongoing. In the meantime, it is not recommended that people with such devices use the vibrating pill.

The Vibrant company are testing their vibrating pill in 10 to 12 research centers using larger numbers of patients. If the pill continues to perform well and gets FDA approval,

Floating Poop Could Be a Sign of Trouble

An occasional bowel movement that floats is not cause for alarm—it probably just means that you ate something that made you extra gassy, and some of that gas got lodged in the waste. But if you get floaters more than a few times a week over the course of a month, you may be suffering from malabsorption, an inability to absorb nutrients during digestion. Malabsorption can be caused by celiac disease, lactose intolerance and pancreatitis. All three conditions come with other symptoms such as diarrhea, nausea and abdominal pain. If you experience such symptoms along with frequent buoyant bowel movements, see your doctor.

Roundup of gastroenterologists reported at Health.com.

they hope to have it available in about three years. While cost has not yet been determined, most likely it will be competitive with other prescription medications for chronic constipation. The researchers also are planning long-term studies to determine whether constipation relief persists without continuing to take the pill…and if so, for how long. If you are interested in getting onto a clinical trial, check Vibrant's website and/or ClinicalTrials.gov for upcoming trials and when they start recruiting.

New Treatment for Heavy Bleeding from Fibroids

James A. Simon, MD, is clinical professor of obstetrics and gynecology at George Washington University, Washington, DC, and leader of a study published in *Obstetrics & Gynecology*.

These noncancerous tumors have long been treated by surgery. In a trial of the twice-daily combination hormone pill Oriahnn (*elagolix*), blood loss dropped by at least half for 90 percent of the 433 participants—64 percent had no period—and subjects reported fewer hot flashes and better quality of life. The ideal patient is in her 40s, not interested in pregnancy and wanting symptom relief until reaching natural menopause.

Swelling in the Legs? Consider May-Thurner Syndrome

Kurtis Kim, MD, director of the vascular laboratory at the vascular center at Mercy Medical Center, Baltimore.

May-Thurner syndrome (MTS), also called iliac vein compression syndrome, is a potentially debilitating condition that isn't even on the radar of most vascular medicine specialists and surgeons. It primarily affects women between the ages 20 and 45, but can last into years beyond. Until about five years ago, medical schools taught doctors that MTS is so rare that they'd likely never see it and, if they did, the best course of action would be to ignore it.

It turns out that neither of those things is true.

What Is MTS?

MTS is essentially a pinched vein in the pelvic area. A quick anatomy lesson can best explain the cause. We have two types of blood vessels: Arteries carry oxygenated blood from the heart throughout the body, and veins work in the opposite direction to carry the oxygen-depleted blood back to the heart. We have more arteries on the left side of the body, which must cross over the veins that originate on the right side. In the pelvic area, the right iliac artery crosses over the left iliac vein, which rests against the spine. The artery has higher blood pressure and thicker walls than the vein, so when the two are competing for space, the artery wins, and the vein, trapped against the spine, starts to flatten.

Most people have some compression—about 10 to 20 percent—without any symptoms. But when that compression increases, the vein can flatten into a pancake-like shape. If the diameter is reduced by 60 percent or more, blood can't readily pass through the tight spot. Without a way to get back to the heart, blood can pool in the leg, causing sometimes intense swelling, skin cracking, pain, leg varicosities, throbbing, burning, numbness and discoloration.

Bodywide Symptoms

MTS can affect other bodily symptoms too. It's a bit like a car accident. When an accident first occurs, traffic builds up on the road immediately behind it, but as the backup increases, drivers start to pull off onto side roads to find alternate routes. Soon, those roads are congested as well. In the body, when blood can't pass through the narrowed iliac vein, blood first backs up in the leg, but then quickly overwhelms other veins in the pelvic area, leading to constipation, pelvic inflammation, urinary symptoms, varicose veins in the vulva, and hemorrhoids. It can also cause postural orthostatic tachycardia syndrome (POTS), a condition that causes lightheadedness, fainting, and a rapid increase in heartbeat when standing up from a reclining position. One of the most dangerous complications of MTS is that the swollen leg can be filled with a large number of clots. If a clot breaks off, it can move to the lungs and cause a pulmonary embolism.

Missed Diagnoses

Because of the constellation of symptoms, patients often see a multitude of doctors and receive a variety of incorrect diagnoses and incorrect treatments in their search for relief. One of my patients suffered from MTS symptoms for 40 years before she was referred to me. As noted above, even vascular specialists may not be thinking about MTS. In fact, most people don't learn they have MTS until they experience a deep venous thrombosis (DVT), a blood clot that partially or completely blocks blood flow through the vein. The standard treatment for DVT is to administer medication that dissolves the clot, but if there's a significant compression in the vein, thrombolysis won't solve the patient's problem, and further investigation reveals the presence of MTS. We now know that about 40 percent of cases of DVT in the left leg have underlying MTS. While MTS can occur in the right leg, it is very rare.

Treatment Options

Here's where things take one of two diverging roads. The vast majority of vascular specialists and surgeons were trained to leave veins alone as much as possible. Vein problems don't cause the same level of risk to life and limb that arterial issues do, and they're notoriously difficult to operate on. As a result, most vascular physicians will treat MTS with blood thinners, compression socks, elevation and weight loss.

And then there are vascular specialists and surgeons like me, who find great value in using a stent inside that vein to keep it open. In my practice, I work with patients who have symptomatic MTS without DVT. When I suspect MTS, I insert a small ultrasound device mounted on a wire into the vein to find and measure the narrowed point. If it is 60 percent or more narrowed, I diagnose MTS and place a stent at the same time.

Because not many vascular surgeons do this procedure yet, many of my patients have traveled long distances to find relief from their MTS symptoms. As a result, many have experienced an extraordinary improvement in their quality of life—and research suggests that those improvements will endure. There is convincing data that shows these stents are durable and effective for at least 15 years.

Drooping Eyelids: Aging Isn't Always the Cause

Michael S. Lee, MD, director of neuro-ophthalmology at University of Minnesota Medical School in Minneapolis and a professor in the departments of ophthalmology, visual neurosciences, neurology and neurosurgery.

If your eyelids droop, chances are you simply chalk it up to aging. But that could be a mistake.

What most people don't realize: Even though drooping upper eyelids are most often caused by excess skin and fat that accumulate and sag with age, an underlying medical condition—sometimes serious—can be to blame.

Finding the Real Cause

An open upper eyelid edge normally sits 4 mm to 5 mm above the center of the pupil. When the eyelid sags below that level, it is known as ptosis (pronounced "toe-sis" and derived from the Greek word for "falling").

Besides drooping, ptosis can blur or impair sight by physically obscuring your field of vision. Women and men of all races and ethnicities are affected equally. *Among the most common causes of eyelid ptosis…*

•**Muscle slippage.** The levator, a muscle in the upper eyelid that helps hold the lid open, often begins to slip from its original connection in one's 50s or 60s, resulting in a droopy appearance to one or both eyelids. But age alone isn't the only factor.

The contact lens link: Muscle slippage of the eyelid is up to 20 times more common in contact lens wearers…of any age. Inserting and removing contacts requires chronic eyelid manipulation that can cause levator detachment.

What helps contact wearers: Use of a DMV suction-cup device to reduce levator manipulation. This device gently adheres to the contact lens and can facilitate insertion and removal of the lens, reducing the amount of wear and tear on the eyelid. Wearing clean lenses with a thin, smooth edge may help, too.

Excessive eye rubbing also may contribute to this form of ptosis.

What to do: Visit an oculoplastic surgeon, an ophthalmologist specializing in eyelid repair. This physician will do a visual field test, in which you look through a special machine with one eye patched and the other eyelid carefully taped up so vision is unobscured.

If taping significantly improves vision, insurance often pays for corrective surgery. If the drooping doesn't disrupt your vision, expect to pay from $1,000 to $5,000 out of pocket (per eye) to correct it.

Note: The same test is used to determine whether vision is obscured by excess eyelid skin (mentioned earlier). If this condition obscures vision and vision improves with removal, insurance typically covers surgery for this, too.

Corrective surgery is performed under conscious sedation by an oculoplastic surgeon or sometimes a facial plastic surgeon. You can expect some bruising and swelling for up to two weeks. As with all surgery, there are risks. It is possible that the eyelids do not end up in the desired location—they can be higher (or lower) than you wanted. Other risks include infection, scarring or, in rare cases, vision loss.

•**Botox.** Drooping eyelids can be caused by Botulinum toxin type A (often sold under the brand name Botox), which is widely used to paralyze facial muscles to reduce and improve wrinkling and to treat migraine.

In 4 percent to 10 percent of patients who receive Botox for wrinkles, when the injection is given into the forehead, around the eyes or in the "frown lines" between the eyes, it migrates to the surrounding areas, including the upper eyelids. The drooping usually starts about three to seven days after the injection, occurring in one or both eyelids. This is also a risk when Botox is given for migraine.

Warning: Botox-induced drooping eyelid tends to occur when a less experienced practitioner is administering the injection. With an experienced practitioner, expect it to occur less than one percent of the time.

What to do: If you develop eyelid drooping in the week following facial Botox, tell your doctor. He/she may prescribe thrice-daily eyedrops containing 0.5 percent *apraclonidine* (Iopidine) until the drooping subsides. This medication, which is commonly used to treat glaucoma, stimulates the eyelid muscle to open. Even without treatment, most of these cases resolve within three to four weeks.

•**Horner syndrome.** With sudden drooping of just one eyelid, a neurologic condition called Horner syndrome (HS) may be suspected. It has three main symptoms—drooping of an upper eyelid…a small pupil only in the affected eye…and lack of sweating on the affected side of the face.

Other symptoms may include eye or neck pain…and "upside-down" ptosis in the affected eye, meaning that the lower lid rises up slightly.

Any sort of interruption in the nerve fibers that travel from the brain to the face and eyes can lead to HS—such as a tumor (in the brain or lung, for example)…or a spontaneous or trauma-induced tear of the carotid artery, one of the main arteries to the brain.

What to do: If you suddenly experience one-sided eyelid drooping and a small pupil in that eye, go to the emergency room…or to your ophthalmologist if you can be seen immediately. Your doctor will use apraclonidine eyedrops to test your pupils for reactivity—in healthy eyes, the pupil will not dilate when exposed to apraclonidine, but in HS, the affected pupil will dilate. The majority of HS patients with eyelid drooping will not improve on their own—surgery is needed to raise the eyelid.

A head-and-neck MRI also may be ordered to look for blood vessel tears. If a tear is identified, treatment may range from aspirin (to prevent blood clots) to surgery to fix the tear, depending on its severity. If no obvious cause is found but eyedrops confirm HS, it is considered idiopathic (no known cause).

Important: If you're experiencing sharp, one-sided head, face or neck pain in addition to eyelid drooping, call 911—that suggests a carotid artery tear, which can lead to a stroke if not treated immediately. Carotid tears, called carotid artery dissections, are rare. They can happen at any age but tend to occur in those under age 50.

• **Myasthenia gravis (MG).** This rare autoimmune disorder disrupts communication between nerves and muscles, resulting in muscle weakness that often affects chewing, swallowing and walking. Most people with MG also experience eyelid ptosis and double vision. In fact, more than half of all MG cases involve only ocular features.

Ptosis from MG tends to affect both eyes… can change moment to moment…and worsens as the day progresses. Men who are in their 60s and older are at highest risk…for women, MG usually occurs under age 40.

What to do: See your primary care physician for a physical and neurological examination to check for issues with eye movements, overall muscle strength, coordination and more. You may be referred to a neurologist who can order several tests, including a blood test used to help confirm MG.

The drug *pyridostigmine* (Mestinon) can improve MG symptoms by increasing communication between nerves and muscles. Oral prednisone may help by suppressing the immune response.

Women Fall Asleep Faster After Intercourse

Study by researchers at State University of New York at Albany, published in *Evolutionary Behavioral Sciences*.

A recent study found that sex had a greater sedative effect on women than men. The finding may indicate an evolutionary development—lying prone promotes sperm retention and increases the likelihood of pregnancy.

INDEX

A

ABC (air, brakes, and chain) check, 145
Abdominal fat. *See* Belly fat
Abdominal pain, 29, 48, 231, 249, 324
Ablation, 205, 208
Acamprosate, 30
Acceptance, 96
ACE inhibitors, 199
Acetaminophen (Tylenol), 167, 203, 218, 292
Acetyl-L-carnitine, 33
Acetylcholine, 33, 37, 321
Acetylcholinesterase inhibitors, 37
ACE2 (angiotensin converting enzyme 2), 63, 230, 232
Acidic drinks and cavities, 16
Acid reflux
    and cavities, 16
    and diabetes risk, 60
Acne, 8
    "maskne," 323
Acne rosacea, 244
Activated charcoal (AC), 241–42
Active listening, 93
Actos, 58–59
Acupressure massagers, 257
Acupuncture, 178, 237
    for chronic indigestion, 240
    for COVID-19, 231
    for fascia, 272
    for knee osteoarthritis, 277
    before surgery, 245
Acute myeloid leukemia (AML), 56
Adenosylcobalamin, 130
Adrenal glands, 199, 215, 231–32
Adrenaplex, 214
Adult child returning home, 83–86
    five key topics, 85–86
    setting stage for successful return, 84–85
    upside of, 86
Advance health-care directives, 13
Aerobic exercise. *See* Exercise
Affirmations, 22
A-Fib. *See* Atrial fibrillation
African Americans, colorectal cancer risk, 50
Ageism, 4, 5
Age-related macular degeneration (AMD), 18
Aging well, 1–20
    belly fat, 19–10
    cavities, 15–16
    dizziness, 10–11
    earwax, 16–17

erasing undereye dark circles and bags, 8–9
    eye floaters, 17–18
    five things better after 70, 3–5
    hearing and heart-healthy diet, 17
    independent living, 13–15
    intermittent fasting, 20
    menopause and man-made chemicals, 7–8
    menopause and resveratrol, 6–7
    menopause and vaginal estrogen, 5–6
    secret to successful, 1–3
    and sitting, 9–10
    and sugar, 15
    vertigo, 11–13
    vision and dementia, 17
Agreeableness, 25
Airbnb, 3
Air pollution, 33, 304, 308, 310
Alcohol
    and atrial fibrillation, 206
    before bedtime, 2
    and belly fat, 19
    and the brain, 28–30
    and chronic inflammation, 238–39
    content in drinks, 30
    and folate deficiency, 131
    and menopause brain, 24
    and miscarriages, 297
    and older women, 86
    and remembering names, 28
    and SIBO, 244
    and stroke, 210
    before surgery, 158–59
    and undereye dark circles and bags, 8
Alcohol-free hand sanitizers, 225
Alcohol-related deaths, 87
Alcohol use disorder (AUD), 28–30
    medications for, 29–30
Alignment and sitting, 9–10
Allay Lamp, 261
Allergies. *See also* Food allergies
    and anaphylaxis, 312–13
    and heartburn, 313
    and undereye dark circles and bags, 8
"All or nothing" approach to eating, 103
Aloe vera juice, 67
Alpha lipoic acid (ALA), 106
Alzheimer's disease, 3, 21, 48, 317
    blood test for, 38
    early detection of, 38–39
    natural prevention of, 33–34
Ambien, 2, 149

Amino acids, 112
Amitriptyline, 259, 261
Amygdala, 29
Amyloidosis, 188–89
Anaphylaxis, 312–13
Anaplastic lymphoma kinase (ALK), 47
Anemia, 198, 203–4
Angina. *See* Chest pain
Animal protein, myth about, 112
Ankylosing spondylitis, 255
Annoying people, 95–96
Antacids, 130, 169, 244, 313
Anthracycline, 51
Anti-anxiety medications, 26–27, 65–66, 255
Antibiotic resistance, 170, 211–12
Antibiotics
    and gut microbiome, 170–71
    side effects, 169, 170
    and tinnitus, 167
    in toxic foods, 66, 118
    for UTIs, 212
Anticholinergics, 37, 169, 321
Antidepressants, 199
    and birth defects, 298–99
    and menopause, 45
    for migraines, 259
    side effects, 169
Antihistamines, 169, 219, 314, 323
Antioxidant supplements, for dementia, 33–34
Antiperspirants, 321, 322
Anti-seizure drugs, 259
Anti-VEGF, 18
Antivirals, 217, 226
Anxiety
    chamomile tea for, 250
    and COVID-19, 230, 232
    gut's role, 65–68
    and increased gas, 265
    and memory, 73
    natural healing of, 67–68, 288
    prevention tips, 66–67
    and sleep disruptions, 2
    stress of caregiving, 72
    ways to keep from spiraling, 67
    worry and neuroticism, 24–27
Apitherapy
    for breast cancer, 46–47
    for knee osteoarthritis, 277
Apocrine glands, 320–21
Apps
    free workouts, 140–41
    heart-rate, 164
    indoor-cycling, 146–47

for vital signs, 163, 164–65
walking, 138
Arch Rocks, 267
Arm sweeps, 148
Arm wrestling, 22
Arrhythmia, 128, 200, 201, 206, 297
Arthritis. *See also* Osteoarthritis; Rheumatoid arthritis
and depression, 254–55
hands, 253–52, 290–91
and *hydroxychloroquine,* 172
and menopause, 251–53
resveratrol for, 6–7
Arthritis gloves, 253–54
Artichokes and Shell Beans Braised in White Wine, 114
Artificial sweeteners, 113, 244
Ashwagandha, 33–34
Asking for help, helping people, 92–94
Asking medical doctors right questions, 152–54, 161, 163
Aspirin
and cancer, 55
and heart disease, 55, 194–95
Association strategy for remembering names, 28
Asthma, 130, 238, 306
and cleaning products, 312
and dyspnea, 304
steroids and osteoporosis, 287–88
teas for, 312
Atherosclerosis, 7, 200
Atherosclerotic Cardiovascular Disease (ASCVD) Risk Score, 192–93
Athletic shoes, 141
Ativan, 26
Atopic eczema, 249
Atrial fibrillation (A-fib), 153, 187, 205–8
after surgery, 205–6
and blood clotting, 128
heart monitor, 201
prevention, 206–8
protein intake, 209
tracking app, 163
Attention deficit/hyperactivity disorder (ADHD) and car crashes, 72
Attire and mood, 70–712
Autoimmune diseases, 275–77. *See also* Arthritis
stopping inflammation, 238–39, 275
Avocados, 20, 33, 67, 108–9, 127, 229
Avocado Sweet Potato "Toast" with Hummus, 108–9
Azacitidine, 56

B

Back pain, 176, 177, 178, 266, 269–70, 285–86
Backward lunges, 148
Bacterial vaginosis (BV), 213, 296–97
Bacteriophage therapy, 212–13
Bactrim, 212
Bad breath, 322–23
Baker's cyst, 247
Balance, 289–90
and hearing loss, 289
Baldness, 3
Bamlanivimab, 217
Banded crunches, 140
Barre exercise, 148
Bathroom scales, 163, 165
Beans, 20, 62, 67, 117–18, 191
Bedtime routine, 2, 105, 206, 214
Bee venom
for breast cancer, 46–47
for rheumatoid arthritis, 46, 277

Belly fat, 19–10
and coffee, 110
risks, 61–62
Benadryl, 37
Benign breast disease, 301–2
Benign paroxysmal positional vertigo (BPPV), 10–11, 12, 291–92
Berberine, 244, 320
for colon polyps, 49–50
Bereavement, 76–78
Bergamot, 236
Beta-blockers, for migraines, 259, 261
Beta-carotene, 108, 248
Beta glucan, 229
Bicep curls, 142–43
Bidets, 318–19
Big change in small increments, 76
Biking, 144–48
affordable bikes, 145–46
"Peloton" experience, 146–48
safety tips, 145
types of, 144–45
for varicose veins, 246
Biking shoes, 141, 145
Binge eating, 106
Biologics, 242, 255
Birth defects, 297–99
Black olives, 117
Black tea, 201, 312
Bladder neck injections, 316
Bladder training, 316
Bladder wrack, 54–55
Blood clotting and calcium, 128
Blood donations, 158
Blood glucose monitors, 163
Blood oxygen, 163, 164, 165
right way to measure, 166
Blood pressure
high. *See* High blood pressure
low, 198–99, 259
testing mistakes, 196–97
Blood pressure medications, 172
taking at night, 198
Blood pressure monitors, 163, 165, 196–97
Blood sugar, 59, 61
and COVID-19, 63
Blue light therapy, 235
Body mass index (BMI), 61, 62, 186, 187, 201, 268
Bonding hormone, 25–26
Bone health, 286–90
Bone mineral density (BMD), 128, 286–87, 318
Botox
and drooping eyelids, 327
for hyperhidrosis, 321
for migraines, 259–60
Bowel movements, 48
floating poop, 324
Braces, 254
Bradycardia, 198, 200
Brain
aging and myths about, 2–3
gut's role, 65–68
Brain fog, 35, 44, 66, 214, 235, 317
Brain health, 21–40. *See also* Alzheimer's disease; Dementia; Headaches
and alcohol, 28–30
calcium for, 128
diet for, 33
exercise for, 21–22, 40
four brain hacks, 21–23
meditation for, 22–23, 31–32
and memory, 21–24, 32
and menopause, 23–24

mind makeover, 30–32
multiple sclerosis and meditation, 39
remembering names, 27–28
strength training for, 27
and TV watching, 40
worry and neuroticism, 24–27
Brain plasticity, 21, 22, 33–34
BRAT diet, 243
BRCA (BReast CAncer gene), 44
Breast cancer, 161, 172–73, 195, 253, 318
CT scans for, 50–51
earlier screening age for, 42–43
fasting diet for, 43
honeybee venom for, 46–47
and hormone therapy, 44
mammography for, 41–43
and menopause, 43–46
PPIs and cognitive issues, 53
Breast-feeding, 25
and for benign breast disease, 301–2
and berberine, 50
and coffee, 110
and ovarian cancer, 46
and PFOA, 123
Breathe Easy Tea, 312
Breathing
for anxiety, 67, 265
for autoimmune diseases, 276
basics of, 306
calming "monkey mind," 102
for chronic inflammation, 239
difficulty (dyspnea), 303–5
exercises to strengthen lungs, 306–7
and menopause, 45
poor techniques, 306
sighs (sighing), 304, 308
Breathing problems. *See* Respiratory conditions; Shortness of breath
Brine-cured olives, 117
Broccoli, 17, 33, 107, 129, 191, 229, 246, 265
Broken-heart syndrome, 195
Bruises (bruising), 256, 272, 327
Bruton's tyrosine kinase (BTK), 313
Bupivacaine, 158
Butterbur, 262
Buttocks (glutes), exercises for, 133, 138, 139, 147
Byetta, 58, 171

C

Cabbage, 119, 121, 129, 265
Lemon Dill Kraut, 120
Caffeine. *See* Coffee
Calcitonin gene-related peptide (CGRP), 260
Calcium, 49, 127–29
nutritional teamwork, 128–29
supplements, 129
testing for, 128
Calf Raises, 133
Calf toners, 143
Calorie restriction, 19, 43
Cancer, 41–56. *See also specific types of cancer*
and aspirin, 55
CAR therapy, 51–53
CBT for, 78–79
colon protection, 47–49
and gum disease, 50
hats for, 3
HPV-related, 53–54
and IVF, 296
mammograms for, 41–43
misdiagnosis of, 161
and PFAS, 7

psilocybin for, 53
seaweed for, 54–55
and sunburn, 50
treatment side effects, 56
Cannabidiol (CBD), 67, 167
Cannabis
in pain management, 264
before surgery, 167
Cantaloupe, 127, 248
Carbohydrates, 112, 116
in Mediterranean diet, 183
Car crashes and ADHD, 72
Cardiac amyloidosis, 188–89
Cardiovascular disease. *See* Heart disease
Caregiving, stress of, 72
Carpal tunnel syndrome, 188–89
Car safety, 80–81
Cast iron pans, 123
Cat and Cow, 307
Cataracts, 171
Cataract surgery, 19, 173
Catheter ablation, 205, 208
Cavities, 15–16, 173
prevention tips, 15–16
Celecoxib, 301
Celiac disease, 129, 131, 174, 265, 275, 277
tryptophan for, 277–78
vs. sourdough, 123–24
Cerumen, 16–17
Chair Pose, 10
Chair sitting, 9–10
Chamomile tea, 214, 248–50
Changing minds, 90–92
Charcoal, 241–42
"Cheesy" Popcorn with Nutritional Yeast, 109
Chemotherapy, 289
and dry mouth, 15
menopausal symptoms from, 44
side effects, 56
Chest pain, 181–82, 185
Chest presses, 133
Chicken Almond Satay Wraps, 124–25
Chilblains, 226
Child returning home. *See* Adult child returning home
Chimeric antigen receptor (CAR) therapy, 51–53
China
berberine, 49–50
and food safety, 118
Chin tucks, 284–85
Chiropractic care, 176–78, 292
types of, 176–77
what to look for, 177–78
Choco-Banana "Nice Cream," 108
Cholesterol
and heart disease, 186, 189–90
and insulin resistance, 190–91
Chronic bronchitis, 304, 308
Chronic indigestion, acupuncture for, 240
Chronic inflammation, 65, 116, 238–39, 249
Chronic obstructive pulmonary disease (COPD), 158, 304, 306
cordyceps sinensis for, 231
and low blood oxygen, 163, 166
medications and side effects, 169
pulmonary rehabilitation for, 307–8
Chronic tendonitis, 247–48
Chronic worry and neuroticism, 24–27
Cirrhosis of the liver, 110, 226
Cleaning products, 220, 276, 311, 312
Clonidine, 45

Closets, cleaning out, 70–71, 104
Clostridium difficile, 174, 221
Clothing
cleaning out closets, 70–71, 104
for exercising, 135
and mood, 70–712
for mosquitoes, 221
Coachable moments, 92–93
Coenzyme Q10 (CoQ10), 175, 191, 194, 215, 246
Coffee, 110–11
and body fat, 110
health benefits of, 22, 110
unfiltered, 111
Cognitive behavioral therapy (CBT), 167, 316
for inflammation, 78–79
for neuroticism, 26
Colds
beta glucan for, 229
Pelargonium for, 229
probiotics for, 227–28
vs. COVID-19, 218
Cold sores, 224–25
Collagen, 8, 17, 178, 270
Cologuard, 48
Colon, protection tips, 47–49
Colon cleanses, 48–49
Colonoscopies, 48, 49, 54, 221
Colon polyps, berberine for, 49–50
Colorectal cancer, 47–49
screening for, 48–49, 50, 54
Community involvement, 1, 14
Computer screens
doomscrolling, 75–76
and eye floaters, 18
Computer use
and sitting, 9–10
thumb pain from, 290–91
Concentration
frankincense for, 34
"menopause brain," 24
PPIs and breast cancer, 53
and saturated fats, 122
and testosterone, 317
transcendental meditation for, 31
Concussions, morning light for, 235
Congestive heart failure. *See* Heart failure
Conscientiousness, 25
Conscious eating, 106
Constipation, 323–24
as medication side effect, 169
Contact lenses, 17, 222, 285, 326–27
Cooling down, 134–35
COPD. *See* Chronic obstructive pulmonary disease
Cordyceps sinensis, 231
Core exercises, 20, 133, 140, 142, 148
Corlanor, 202
Corn syrup, 107, 238, 244
Coronary artery calcium (CAC), 51, 180, 193–94
Coronavirus. *See* COVID-19
Corticospinal tract (CST), 27
Cortisol, 87–88
and belly fat, 20
and chronic worry, 21
and memory, 21
Cortisone injections, 264
Couch exercises, 142–43
Coughing, 304, 315
as post-COVID-19 symptom, 215
Coumadin, 246, 250
Countertop pushups, 142
Countertop squats, 142

Counting down, 270
"Country of Origin Labeling" law, 118
COVID-19, 213–18
alcohol-free hand sanitizers for, 225
and blood oxygen, 166
and blood sugar spikes, 63
and broken-heart syndrome, 195
cleaning tips for, 220
clothing and mood, 70, 71
and diabetes, 63–64
and diet, 112
and divorce, 81
doomscrolling, 75–76
eyeglasses for, 222
glutathione for, 228–29, 231
and *hydroxychloroquine*, 172, 216, 217
and immune system, 216
long-haul symptoms, 213–15
losing your quarantine weight gain, 106
and MMR vaccine, 219
natural healing after, 229–32
and NSAIDs, 175
pulse oximeters, 163, 164, 165, 166
and sore feet, 226
supplements for, 214–15, 217–18
and surgery procedures, 158–60
telemedicine, 159, 162–64
treatment of, 216–18
vs. colds, 218
Coxsackie B (CVB), 64
Cranberry juice, 212
C-reactive protein, 59, 60, 238, 39
Creamy Curried Red Lentil Dip with Raw Veggies and Tortilla Chips, 109
Creative endeavors, 89
Creativity and brain health, 22
Crohn's disease, 171, 174, 244
Cross-training shoes, 141
Cruciferous vegetables, 191, 229, 246
CT (computed tomography) scans, 50–51
Cucumbers, tea-and-honey soaked, for puffy eyes, 8–9
Cuddling, 25–26
Cultured (lab-grown) meat, 115
Cupping, 270, 272
Curcumin
for amyloidosis, 188
for arthritis, 253
for COVID-19, 230
for dementia, 33
for inflammation, 239
for ulcerative colitis, 240–41
Curfews for adult child returning home, 85
Curiosity, and aging well, 1
Cycling. *See* Biking
Cytokine release syndrome, 52
Cytokine storm, 218, 229, 230

D

Dancing, for brain health, 22
Dantrolene, 162
Dark chocolate, 191
DASH (Dietary Approaches to Stop Hypertension) diet, 62
Dating behaviors, playing hard-to-get, 81
Death of loved one, finding meaning after, 76–78
Deconditioning, 303–4
Deep, audible breaths, 308–10
Deep brain stimulation (DBS), 35–36
Deep venous thrombosis (DVT), 326

Dehydration, 35, 134–35, 138, 198
Dementia, 3, 21, 33–38. *See also* Alzheimer's disease
    and alcohol, 28
    and calcium, 129
    coffee for, 110
    and DBS risk, 35–36
    and dehydration, 35
    and hearing loss, 16, 288–89
    and hypertension, 32
    and ineffective medications, 38
    natural prevention of, 33–34
    and openness, 25
    piracetam for, 32
    and poor vision, 17
    risk factors for, 36
    in younger people, 36
Dental care, 16, 80
Dental visits, 16
Deodorants, 321
Deodorizing insoles, 322
Depression
    after surgery, 76
    and arthritis, 254–55
    and cortisol, 87–88
    and COVID-19, 229, 230, 232
    and hearing loss, 288–89
    psilocybin for, 101–2
    and sleep disruptions, 2
Dexamethasone, 217
DHA (docosahexaenoic acid), 183–84
DHEA (dehydroepiandrosterone), 6, 45, 288
Diabetes, 57–64
    and acid reflux, 60
    and belly fat, 19
    and COVID-19, 63–64
    and dry mouth, 15
    flax and pumpkin seeds for, 62
    and glutathione, 228
    and gut microbiome, 59–60
    and heart disease, 186
    and heart failure, 202
    and hot flashes, 57–58
    and keto diet, 111
    medications for prevention, 58–59
    and normal-weight obesity, 61–62
    and pregnancy, 180
    probiotics for, 58
    resveratrol for, 6–7
    and sleep disruptions, 2
    and statins, 64
    stem-cell treatment for, 64
    and testosterone, 317
    vaccine, 64
    and weak grip strength, 64
Diagnostic medical errors, 160–61
Diaphragmatic breathing, 67
Diaphragm Extensions, 307
Diarrhea
    activated charcoal for, 242
    fecal transplant for, 221–22
    as medication side effect, 169
Diet, 103–27. *See also* Recipes
    for aging well, 1–2
    for anxiety, 66–67
    for arthritis, 253
    and atrial fibrillation, 207
    for autoimmune diseases, 275, 276
    for Baker's cyst, 247
    for belly fat, 19–10
    for chronic inflammation, 238
    for colon health, 49
    for COVID-19, 232
    craving bad food, 106–7
    for dementia, 33

and diabetes, 59–60
exercise and keeping cool, 134
for eye floaters, 18
fasting, for breast cancer, 43
5 ways to change your attitude and get healthy, 103–5
guilt-free snacks, 107–9
and gut microbiome, 171
for headaches, 262
for hearing, 17
for heart health, 62, 182–83, 191, 201, 203, 207
hidden dangers in food from China, 118
immune-boosting recipes, 124–26
intermittent fasting, 20
keto, 111, 112, 322
lab-grown meat, 115
Mediterranean, 49, 62, 182–83, 238, 275
and menopause, 24, 45
for normal-weight obesity, 62
pickled vegetables, 118–20
for post-COVID-19 symptoms, 215
prebiotics and sleep and stress, 121
probiotics, 227–28
removing temptation from home, 104
shared success stories, 105
and SIBO, 244–45
smaller portion sizes, 106
sourdough bread, 123–24
spices, 116
before surgery, 158–59
"taste bud rehab," 106–7
for tendonitis, 248
3 food myths, 111–13
for varicose veins, 246
vegetarian. *See* Vegetarian diet
Dietary supplements. *See* Supplements
Difficulty breathing (dyspnea), 303–5
Dificid, 221–22
Diflunisal, 188
Digestive enzymes, 242–43, 245, 249–50
Digital breast tomosynthesis (DBT), 41–42
Digoxin, 172, 202
Diosgenin, 253
Disease-modifying antirheumatic drug (DMARD), 255
Disease progression, 279
Disinfecting, 220
Diuretics, 12, 169, 199, 202
Dizziness, 10–11, 161, 181
    and BPPV, 10–11, 12, 291–92
    diagnosis of, 10–11
    and medications, 13
D-mannose, 212
Docetaxel, 46
Doctor-patient relationship, 152–54
Doctor phobias, 156–57
Dogs. *See* Pets
Donations, 78
Donepezil hydrochloride, 37
Doomscrolling, 75–76
Dopamine, 23, 28, 29, 30, 65, 236
Dried fruit, unsweetened, 126
Drinking water. *See also* Hydration
    PFAS in, 7
Driving and cataract surgery, 19
Drooping eyelids, 326–28
Dry, chapped hands, 225
Dry brining, 119
Dry eye and migraines, 263–64
Dry mouth, 15–16, 277
    as medication side effect, 169
Dust, 311

E
Ear candles, 16
Ear infections, 12, 165
Early-onset dementia, 36
Earplugs, 2
Ears, ringing. *See* Tinnitus
Earwax, 16–17
Ebola virus, 217
Eccrine glands, 320–21
E-cigarettes, 311–12
E-coaching, 156
Eczema, 249
EGFR (epidermal growth factor receptor), 47
Eldercare, 14–15
Electric-assist (e-bikes) bikes, 144–45
Electro-acupuncture, 269–70
Electronic health records (EHRs), 158, 159
Elimination diet, 66
Emergency care, 155, 175
    heart attacks, 181–82
Emergency contacts, 158
Emergency information, 13, 14
Emergency plan for responders, 14
Emotional rescue, 65–102. *See also* Negative emotions
    ADHD and car crashes, 72
    adult child returning home, 83–86
    annoying people, 95–96
    bereavement, 76–78
    best ways to "regulate" emotions, 94
    big change in small increments, 76
    calming "monkey mind," 102
    changing minds, 90–92
    clothing and mood, 70–72
    coping with life transitions, 88–90
    and COVID-19, 232
    detoxing relationships, 99–101
    doomscrolling, 75–76
    faux daily commute, 72–73
    forgiveness, 97
    gut's role, 65–68
    helping people asking for help, 92–94
    imposter syndrome, 97–99
    marriage killers, 81–83
    "micro-moments" of connection, 86
    narcissistic partners, 68–70
    playing hard-to-get, 81
    preventing problems before they erupt, 79–81
    procrastination, 79, 97
    small talk, 94–95
    social anxiety and memory, 73
    stress. *See* Stress
    time and money traps and happiness, 73–75
    toxic person in workplace, 96
    volunteering and happiness, 86
Emotional trauma, 281–83
    goals of recovery, 281–83
Emphysema, 304, 308
Encephalitis, 161
Endocarditis, 160, 161
Endometrial cancer, 43
Endometrial hyperplasia, 43
Endothelial progenitor cells (EPCs), 182–83
"Energy gels," 134
Entresto, 202
Eosinophilic esophagitis (EoE), 313
EPA (eicosapentaenoic acid), 183–84
Epilepsy, 29, 173
Epinephrine (EpiPen), 313
Epstein-Barr virus (EBV), 214

Erectile dysfunction (ED), 168, 199
Erenumab, 260
Escherichia coli (E. coli), 121, 170
Essential oils
    for dementia, 34
    for headaches, 262
    for Parkinson's disease, 236–37
Estring, 44, 45
Estrogen dominance, 230
Estrogen replacement therapy, 7, 252–53,
    288, 296
Eszopiclone, 2
Eucalyptus tea, 312
Evaporative humidifiers, 223–24
Excuses, making, 104
Exercise, 132–48
    for aging well, 1
    for anxiety, 67
    for arthritis, 253
    athletic shoes for, 141
    and atrial fibrillation, 206–7
    for balance, 289–90
    barre, 148
    for belly fat, 20
    for benign paroxysmal positional
        vertigo (BPPV), 11, 12
    and brain health, 40
    for brain power, 21–22
    for colon health, 49
    for diabetes, 60
    and dyspnea, 303–4
    "fidget-cisers," 142–44
    fitness capacity, 184–85
    for heart health, 184–85, 192, 203
    and independent living, 15
    keeping cool, 134–35
    for menopause brain, 24
    for neck pain, 258–59
    for normal-weight obesity, 62
    "Peloton" experience, 146–48
    for post-COVID-19 symptoms, 215
    postural isometric lengthening (PIL),
        285–86
    RHR for, 200
    "rubber band" workouts, 138–40
    to strengthen lungs, 306–7
    for varicose veins, 246
    for weight loss, 106
    winter hiking, 136–38
Exercise With Oxygen Training
    (EWOT), 231
Exparel, 158
Expired milk, 122
Exposure therapy, 157
Extroverts (extroversion), 25, 71–72
Eyes
    medications and problems, 171–73
    pupils and heart failure, 187
    undereye dark circles and bags, eras-
        ing, 8–9
Eye creams, 8
Eye exams, 171–72, 173
Eye floaters, 17–18
Eyeglasses and viral infections, 222
Eyelids, drooping, 326–28
Eye movement desensitization and re-
    processing (EMDR), 282, 283
Eye rubbing, 327
Eye strain, 10

F

Face masks
    honey-and-lemon, 8
    tea-and-honey-soaked raw
        cucumbers, 8–9
Face rash, 242–43

Fainting
    heart monitors for, 201
    from sight of blood, 199
Falls (falling), 288–90
    balance, 289–90
    and BPPV, 10–11, 12, 291–92
    fall-proofing your house, 14–15
    and hearing loss, 288–89
    medical-alert devices for, 13–14
    prevention tips, 290
    sleeping pills as cause of, 2
Family travel, 3–4
Fascia, 270–73
Fashion psychology, 70–71
Fatigue, as post-COVID-19 symptom,
    214–15
Faux daily commute, 72–73
Fecal immunochemical testing (FIT), 48
Fecal microbiota transplantation (FMT),
    221–22
Femring, 6, 44
Fermented foods, 66, 228, 276
    basics of fermentation, 119
    pickled vegetables, 118–20
Fertilizers, 80, 121
Fever, 218–19
    danger signs of, 219
    treatment of, 219
Fever blisters, 224–25
Fiber
    for anxiety, 67
    for colon health, 49
    and diabetes, 59–60
Fibroids, 324–25
Fidaxomicin, 221–22
"Fidget-cisers," 142–44
Finances after 70, 4–5
Fish oil. *See* Omega-3 fatty acids
Fitbit, 199
Fitbit Care, 156
Fitness. *See* Exercise
Fitness capacity, 184–85
"5-4-3-2-1" method for anxiety, 67
Flame retardants, 311
Flavanols, 191, 201
Flax, for diabetes, 62
Flomax, 173
Flonase, 172
Floors (flooring), 311
Flow-mediated dilation (FMD), 182–83
Flu. *See* Influenza
Fluvoxamine, 218
Foam rolling, 256, 273
Focus blocks, 75
FODMAP, 244–45
Fogginess, 35, 44, 66, 214, 235, 317
Folate, 49, 131
Food. *See* Diet; Recipes
Food allergies, 66, 115, 312–13
Food cravings, 106–7
Food diaries, 201
Food labels, 66
    "Country of Origin Labeling" law, 118
    unlisted ingredients, 115
Food poisoning, 121, 243, 244
"Forest bathing," 237
Forgiveness, 97
Fosamax, 172
Fractures. *See also* Hip fractures
    misdiagnosis of, 160
    and plant-based diet, 286–87
Fragrance-free products, 220
Frankincense, 34, 236
Fremanezumab, 260
Front planks, 133
Fruit flies, 15

Fruits. *See also specific fruits*
    dried, unsweetened, 126
    exercise and keeping cool, 134
    ice cubes, 127
    leather, homemade, 126–27
Fulvestrant, 43

G

GABA (gamma-aminobutyric acid),
    32, 65
Gabapentin, 45, 214
Gait, 39, 273
Gaiters, 137
Galantamine hydrobromide, 37
Galcanezumab, 260
Gardasil, 54
Garlic, 191
Garlic Lemon Yogurt Topping, 125
Gastric bypass surgery, 173–74
Gastroesophageal reflux disease
    (GERD), 169, 173–74
Gatorade, 135
Genitourinary syndrome of menopause
    (GSM), 5–6
Geriatric-care managers, 15
Gerotranscendence, 3
GI issues, 249
    as post-COVID-19 symptom, 215–16,
        231
Ginger tea, 312
Gingivitis, 322
Ginseng, 33–34, 232
GI Revive, 245
Glaucoma, 171–73
GLP-1 receptor agonists, 58–59, 171
Glucose. *See* Blood sugar
Glutamine, 215–16
Glutathione, 215, 228–29, 231
Glutes (buttocks), exercises for, 133,
    138, 139, 147
Glyburide, 171
Glycogen, 134
Glycopyrrolate, 322
Glycopyrronium, 321
Glyphosate, 66, 117–18
Goiter, 122
Golden rule, 82
Go Red for Women, 179
Gout, 15
Graft-versus-host disease (GVHD), 52
Grandchildren, loneliness and caring
    for, 97
Gratitude, 2, 23, 75
"Gratitude jars," 75
Greek olives, 117
Green light for migraines, 263
Green tea, 8, 9, 20, 201, 231, 312
Green-tea extract, 188
Grief, death of loved one, finding
    meaning after, 76–78
Grip strength and type 2 diabetes, 64
GU Energy Gels, 134
Guests of adult child returning home, 85
Guilt-free snacks, 107–9
Gum disease, 16, 50
Gut microbiome, 170–71, 221
    and air pollution, 310
    and anxiety, 65–68
    and autoimmune diseases, 276
    and colon health, 48–49
    and diabetes, 59–60
    and medications, 170–71
    and organic apples, 121
    and PPIs, 170, 171
    and SIBO, 243, 244, 245
    and stevia, 127

H

Hair loss
    hats for, 3
    and iodine, 122
Hand arthritis, 253–52, 290–91
Hand creams, 225
Hands
    dry, chapped, 225
    stretches for, 267
Hand sanitizers, 225, 312
Hand therapy, 254, 291
Happiness
    and aging well, 2
    and making changes in your life, 81
    time and money traps, 73–75
    and volunteering, 86
Hashimoto's thyroiditis, 276
Hats, 3
Headaches, 262–63. *See also* Migraines
    hydration for, 262
    and menopause, 23–24
Head/scalp massages, 257
Health-care design, 4
Health-care goals, 151–52
Health coaches, 154–56, 164
    asking questions, 154–55
    choosing, 156
    finding, 156
    sessions, 156
    stages of behavior change, 155–56
Health insurance and independent
    living, 13
Healthy home environment, 310–11
Hearing, heart-healthy diet for, 17
Hearing aids and earwax, 17
Hearing loss, 16, 17
    and falls, 288–89
    and Ménière's disease, 12
Hearing tests, 289
Heart attacks
    diet for, 182–83
    hot flashes and night sweats, 184
    and low blood pressure, 198–99
    silent, 185–86
    sudden cardiac arrest, 195
    and vitamin B12, 131
    vs. panic attacks, 181–82
Heartburn, 16, 170, 174, 313
Heart bypass surgery, 202–3
Heart disease, 61, 179–81
    and aspirin, 55, 194–95
    and belly fat, 19, 61
    CBT for, 78–79
    and cholesterol myth, 189–92
    CT scans and breast cancer, 50–51
    and diabetes medications, 59
    and dyspnea, 304
    gender differences in, 149
    and hearing loss, 288–89
    and insulin resistance, 190–91
    and IVF, 295
    misdiagnosis of, 161
    new paradigm for, 179–81
    and normal-weight obesity, 61–62
    omega-3 supplements for, 183–84
    preventive care, 180–81
    resveratrol for, 7
    risk factors, 116, 180, 181
    screening for, 180–81
    and sleep disruptions, 2
    and spices, 116
    statins for. *See* Statins
    and testosterone, 317
    and unhealthy relationships, 99
Heart failure, 155, 181, 184, 201–5
    and carpal tunnel syndrome, 188–89

causes of, 202
    lifestyle changes, 203–4
    and low blood pressure, 198–99
    LVADs for, 203, 204–5
    new treatments, 202–3
    predicting prognosis, 187
Heart health, 179–210
    blood pressure mistakes, 196–97
    diet for, 62, 182–83, 191, 201, 203,
        207
    exercise for, 184–85, 192, 203
    and mealtime, 201
    omega-3 supplements for, 183–84
    supplements for, 191
    thyroid hormone T3 for, 184
Heart monitors, 201
Heart rate, 187
    and calcium, 128
    resting (RHR), 199–200
Heart-rate apps, 164
Heat and cooling down, 134–35
Heat stroke, 135, 219
Hemorrhoids, 319, 325
Hemp oil, 67–68
Hepatitis C, 217, 226
HER2 gene, 46
High blood pressure (hypertension)
    and coffee, 110
    and dementia, 32
    and heart disease, 181, 186
    and heart failure, 202
    and long work hours, 198
    misdiagnosis of, 160, 196
    and obesity, 61
    and PFAS, 7
    and pregnancy, 180
    and sleep disruptions, 2
High-fructose corn syrup, 107, 238, 244
Hiking boots, 136
Hiking in winter, 136–38
Hip flexor, 143, 266
Hip fractures, 2, 6, 287
Hippocampus, 22, 25, 29, 34, 87, 88
HIV/AIDS, 193, 213, 296, 297
Home care agencies, 14
Home environment, 310–11
Homemade fruit leather, 126–27
Honey-and-lemon face masks, 8
Honey-and-tea-soaked raw cucumbers,
    for eye bags, 8–9
Honeybee venom
    for breast cancer, 46–47
    for knee osteoarthritis, 46, 277
Hormone optimization, 318
Hormone tests, 252
Hormone therapy, 7, 252–53, 288, 296,
    318
    and breast cancer, 44
    and menopause, 5–6, 44
Horner syndrome, 327–28
Hot flashes
    alternative therapies for, 45
    and breast cancer, 44
    and diabetes, 57–58
    and heart attacks, 184
    medications for, 45–46
    and vaginal estrogen, 5, 6
Hot peppers, 45
Household dust, 311
Householder cleaners, 220, 276, 311,
    312
House rules and adult child returning
    home, 84–85
Housework, 84
HPV (human papillomavirus), 53–54
HPV vaccines, 54

Humidifiers, 223–24
Hummus, 117–18
    Avocado Sweet Potato "Toast" with
        Hummus, 108–9
    Super Spinach Hummus, 126
Hydration
    exercise and keeping cool, 134
    for fever, 219
    for headaches, 262
    for tendonitis, 248
    for UTIs, 212
Hydroxychloroquine, 172, 216, 217
Hyperbaric oxygen therapy, 231
Hyperhidrosis, 321–22
Hypertension. *See* High blood pressure
Hyperthyroidism, 320
Hypotension. *See* Low blood pressure

I

Ibuprofen, 24, 130, 167, 203, 218, 248,
    269, 291, 292, 301
Idleness aversion, 74–75
Iliac vein compression syndrome,
    325–26
Imitrex, 260, 261
Immune system
    and breathing, 306
    and COVID-19, 216
    and PFAS, 7
    and sleep disruptions, 2
Immunity boosters
    chamomile tea, 250
    natural healing for, 227–29
    recipes, 124–26
    ourdough bread, 123–24
Imposter syndrome, 97–99
Incontinence. *See* Urinary incontinence
Independent living, 13–15
Indian ginseng, 33–34
Indigestion, 60, 113, 186
    acupuncture for, 240
Infections, misdiagnosis of, 161
Infectious diseases, 211–26. *See also*
    COVID-19
    cleaning tips for, 220
    and fever, 218–19
    humidifiers, 223–24
Infertility and IVF, 295–96
Inflammation
    CBT for, 78–79
    and "mind over matter," 78–79
    and undereye dark circles and
        bags, 8
Inflammatory bowel disease, 129, 170,
    171, 238, 310
Influenza (flu), 238
    NAC for, 227
    "vascular storm" and pregnancy,
        299–300
Insect bites, activated charcoal for, 242
Insecticides, 239
Insomnia, 58, 251
    natural healing of, 288
    as post-COVID-19 symptom, 214–15,
        230
Instagram, 76
Insular cortex, 29
Insulin-like growth factor 1 (ILGF1), 43
Insulin resistance, 190–91
Intentional exercise, 22
Intergenerational family travel, 3–4
Interior design
    after 70, 4
    for eye floaters, 18
Intermittent fasting, 20
InterStim, 316

Intestinal bloat, 243, 265
Intestinal gas, activated charcoal for, 242
Intralipid, 162
Intrarosa, 6, 45
Intrauterine growth restriction (IUGR),
  297–98
Intravenous (IV) nutrient therapies, 231
Introverts (introversion), 71–72
Invisible balance beam, 143–44
Invisible hula-hoops, 143
In vitro fertilization (IVF), 295–96
Iodine, 119, 122, 214, 314
Iodized table salt, 119, 122
IRA contributions, 5
Iron deficiency, 203–4
Iron supplements, 203–4
Irritable bowel syndrome (IBS), 48, 49,
  171, 174, 306, 315, 319
    walking for, 238
ISDIN K-Ox Eyes, 8
Ivabradine, 202

J

Jaw pain, 259
Journals (journaling), 88, 283
    for neuroticism, 26
    sleep, 86–87
Juicing, for dementia, 33

K

Kefir, 66, 171, 228
Kegel exercises, 6, 316
Keto (ketogenic) diet, 111, 112, 322
Keypad locks, 14
Kidney disease, 60, 62, 193, 321
Kidney stones, 15, 30, 129, 173, 211
Kimchi (kimchee), 66, 118, 228, 245,
  276
Knee arthritis, 264
Knee Raises, 290
Knee replacements, 3D technology for,
  273–75
Kombucha, 66, 276

L

Lactin-V, 296–97
Lactobacillus, 66, 67, 121, 123, 213, 228,
  276, 296
Lactulose Breath Test, 243–44
Lanoxin, 172, 202
Laser treatments, 18
Lasmiditan, 260–61
Lateral leg lifts, 148
Lateral pulldowns, 140, 258–59
Lateral raises, 133
Lawn care, 80
Laxatives, 169, 171, 219, 323–24
L-carnitine, 175
Lead shielding and X-rays, 161–62
Left ventricular-assist devices (LVADs),
  203, 204–5
Legionnaire's disease, 220
Leg lifts, 142
Legs Up the Wall, 10, 233–34
Leg swelling, 325–26
Legumes, 20, 112, 113, 171, 183
Lemon balm, 34, 225, 249
Lemon Dill Kraut, 120
Lentil Cassoulet with Lots of Vegetables,
  113–14
Leptin, 43
Leukemia
    CAR therapy for, 51–53
    combining cancer drugs, 56
    and perspiration pattern, 320–21

Lewy body dementia, 25
Lexapro, 26
Licorice tea, 312
LifeCoin, 138
Life transitions, coping with, 88–90
    acceptance of, 88
    finding creative outlets, 89
    publicly unveiling new self, 90
    rewriting the story, 90
    seeking support, 89
    shedding old mind-sets, routines,
      possessions, 89
    tributes or rituals to mark, 88–89
Lifting heavy objects, 283–84
Lipitor. *See* Statins
Lipoic acid, 106, 244
Lipoprotein (a), 193
Lockboxes, 14
Loneliness
    and aging well, 1, 2
    avoiding, 99
    caring for grandchildren, 97
    and dementia, 34
    and earwax, 16
"Love languages," 82–83
Low blood pressure, 198–99, 259
Low-calorie diets, 62
Low-dose estrogen therapy, 5–6, 45
Lower trapezius, 258
Low-fat diet, 112, 182–83
Low-protein diet, 231
Low-salt diet, 12
Lubricants, 6, 45
Lunesta, 2
Lung cancer, 77, 161
    new treatments for, 47
Lung emergencies, 305
Luvox, 218
Lye-cured olives, 117
Lying down bridges, 139–40
Lyme disease, 222–23
Lysine, 112, 224–25

M

Maastricht Acute Stress Test, 87
Macrophages, 229
Magic mushrooms. *See* Psilocybin
Magnesium, 34, 129, 191, 253
Male porn use, 318
Mammograms, 41–43
    earlier age for, 42–43
Marathon training, 200
Marijuana. *See* Cannabis
Marriage killers, 81–83
    feeling out of focus, 83
    giving love the way you want it,
      82–83
    long-ago missteps, 82
    seeking agreement, 83
Masked hypertension, 198
"Maskne," 323
Massage balls, 256–57
Massages, 178
    self-massage tools, 255–57
Massage sticks, 256
Matcha Cupcakes, 108
May-Thurner syndrome (MTS), 325–26
Meal prep, 105, 106
Measles and MMR vaccine, 219
Medical-alert pendants or bracelets,
  13–14
Medical care, 149–67
    asking right questions, 152–54
    health-care goals, 151–52
    health coaches, 154–56
    health-monitoring devices, 164–65

misdiagnosis, 160–61
    overcoming physician phobia,
      156–57
    patient priorities, 150–52
    surviving the hospital now, 158–60
    trusted health resources, 166
Medical errors, 160–61
Medical history, 158, 163–64
Medical phobias, 156–57
Medical research, sex-biased, 149–50
Medicare, 16, 38, 48, 175, 289
Medications. *See also specific medica-*
  tions
    after surgery, 159
    for alcohol use disorder, 29–30
    and dementia, 38
    dizziness vs. vertigo, 13
    and dry mouth, 15
    eye problems from, 171–73
    and gut microbiome, 170–71
    and low blood pressure, 199
    for menopause, 45–46
    for preventing diabetes, 58–59
    side effects, 168–70
    before surgery, 158, 159
    and tinnitus, 167
    website warning, 167–68
Meditation, 104, 265
    for autoimmune diseases, 276
    for brain health, 22–23, 31–32
    calming "monkey mind," 102
    for chronic inflammation, 239
    for eye floaters, 18
    for multiple sclerosis, 39
    stop-look-listen-smell (SLLS) protocol,
      26–27
    transcendental (TM), 31–32
Mediterranean diet, 49, 62, 182–83,
  238, 275
Melanoma, 50, 52, 55, 161
Melatonin, 2
    and COVID-19, 214, 217–18
Melittin, 46–47
Memory (memory loss), 21–24, 32
    aging and myths about, 3
    brain hacks for, 21–23
    breast cancer and PPIs, 53
    diagnosis of, 32
    and menopause, 23–24
    PPIs and breast cancer, 53
    remembering in the third person, 73
    remembering names, 27–28
    and saturated fats, 122
    and social anxiety, 73
    and testosterone, 317
    transcendental meditation for, 31
Ménière's disease, 11, 12
Meningitis, 161
Menopause
    alternative therapies for, 45
    and arthritis, 251–53
    and belly fat, 19–10
    and breast cancer, 43–46
    and diabetes, 57–58
    and headaches, 23–24
    and heart disease, 193
    link to man-made chemicals, 7–8
    medications for, 45–46
    resveratrol for symptoms of, 6–7
    safe treatment of, 45–46
    and sex, 317
    vaginal estrogen for, 5–6, 45, 212
"Menopause brain," 24
Mental fog, 35, 44, 66, 214, 235, 317
Metabolic equivalents (METs), 184–85
Metabolic stress test, 180

Metabolic syndrome, 61, 193
Metformin, 58–59, 170–71
Methylcobalamin, 130–31
Me Too Movement (#MeToo), 179
Metronidazole, 213, 296
Microbiome. *See* Gut microbiome
Microbiome therapy, 296–97
"Micro-moments" of connection, 86
Microtubule binding region (MTBR),
   38–39
Migraines, 259–61, 263
      CGRP drugs for, 260
      and dry eye, 263–64
      green light for, 263
      and menopause, 23–24
      non-drug options for, 261, 263
      preventive drugs, 259–61
      and strokes, 180
      vestibular, 12–13, 160
      yoga for, 261–62
Mild cognitive impairment (MCI), 17, 25
Milk
      acetyl-L-carnitine in, 33
      calcium in, 128–29
      expired, uses for, 122
Milk allergies, 312
Mindfulness meditation, 22, 39
"Mind over matter," 78–79. *See also*
   Cognitive behavioral therapy
Minor irritations, 79
MiraDry, 322
Misalignment problems, 9–10
Miscarriages, 110, 297
Misdiagnosis, 160–61
Miso, 66, 124–25, 228, 231, 276
MMR vaccines, 219
Mold, 223, 244, 304
"Mommy brain," 301
Money and adult child returning home,
   85
Money traps and happiness, 73–75
"Monkey mind," 102
Monounsaturated fatty acids (MUFAs),
   183
Mood and clothing, 70–72
Morning light, for mild concussions,
   235
Mosquitoes, 220–21
Mountain Brook, 234
Mouth lozenges, 16
Move-out date of adult child returning
   home, 85–86
MRSA (methicillin-resistant Staphylo-
   coccus aureus), 54–55
Mullein, 312
Multiple sclerosis (MS), 130, 171, 278
      autoimmune disease, 275, 276
      mindfulness meditation for, 39
Multivitamins, 215, 216, 239
Muscle contractions and calcium, 128
Muscle mass and vitamin C, 132
Mushrooms. *See* Psilocybin
Myalgic encephalomyelitis/chronic
   fatigue syndrome (ME/CFS), 214–15
Myasthenia gravis (MG), 328
Myers Cocktails, 231
MyWalgreens, 138

N

N-acetylcysteine (NAC), 215, 227
Naltrexone, 29
Naproxen, 24, 167, 203, 269, 301
Narcissistic personality disorder (NPD),
   68–70
      acceptance of partner with, 68–69
      avoiding confrontation, 69
      breaking the cycle, 69–70
      diagnosis of, 68
Nasacort, 172
Nasal congestion, 216
Nasal infections, 314
Nasal sprays, 171, 172
National Institutes of Health (NIH), 166
Natural births, 300
Natural healing, 175, 178, 227–50
      abnormal pap smear, 235–36
      acupuncture and surgery, 245
      after COVID-19 infection, 229–32
      charcoal, 241–42
      for chronic indigestion, 240
      for chronic tendonitis, 247–48
      colds and Pelargonium, 229
      face rash, 242–43
      "forest bathing," 237
      immune-boosters, 227–29
      for Parkinson's symptoms, 236–37
      restorative yoga, 232–35
      for SIBO, 243–45
      stopping inflammation, 238–39
      for ulcerative colitis, 240–41
      for varicose veins, 246
Natural killer (NK) cells, 52–53
Natural supplements. *See* Supplements
Nausea, 23, 29, 30, 50, 59, 159, 169, 173,
   181, 186, 198, 211, 243, 259, 324
Neck, "crick" or "kink" in, 284–85
Neck collars, 292–93
Neck pain, 9, 271, 327–28
      exercises for, 258–59
      stretches for, 266
      whiplash, 292–93
Negative Emotional Attractor (NEA), 94
Negative emotions, 25, 39
      and doomscrolling, 75–76
      finding meaning after death of
         loved one, 76–78
      getting through rough patches,
         88–90
      and imposter syndrome, 97–99
      using Instagram to lift spirits, 76
Nerivio, 261, 263
Neurofeedback, 282–83
Neurogenesis, 22
Neurontin, 45, 214
Neuropathy, 172, 186, 289
Neuroticism, 24–27
      overview of, 25
      strategies for, 25–27
Nexium, 60, 170
Night sweats
      and breast cancer, 44
      and diabetes, 57–58
      and heart attacks, 184
Nitrofurantoin, 212
Nocebo-effect, 195
Non-small cell lung cancer (NSCLC), 47
Nonsteroidal anti-inflammatory drugs
   (NSAIDs), 167, 170, 203, 218–19, 254
      and COVID-19, 175
      and late pregnancy, 301
Nonstick pans, 122–23
Noom, 156
Normal-weight obesity (NWO), 61–62
Nortriptyline, 259
"Numbing" behaviors, 94
Nutrition. *See* Diet
Nuts and seeds, 62, 112, 191

O

Obesity and overweight
      and belly fat, 20
      and diabetes, 61–62
      and folate deficiency, 131
      and glutathione, 228
      and heart disease, 181, 182, 186, 203
      and sleep disruptions, 2
      and sweating, 320
      and testosterone, 317
Obstructive sleep apnea (OSA), 304–5
Off-road running shoes, 141
Oleic acid, 117
Oleuropein, 117
Olive oil, 49, 117, 183, 191, 275
Olives, 117
Omega-3 fatty acids, 183–84, 215
      for colon cancer, 49
      for heart health, 183–84
      for inflammation, 238, 239, 293
      and insulin resistance, 191
Omega-6 fats, 191
Omega-9 fatty acids, 117
Omeprazole, 174
Ondansetron, 30
Online prescriptions, 167–68
Oophorectomies, 44
Ophthalmologists, 18, 172–73, 327
Oral steroids, 171, 287–88
Organic apples, 121
Orthostatic hypotension, 199, 293
Orthotics, 254
Oscillometric meters, 196–97
Osteoarthritis, 252–53, 264, 291
Osteopathic manipulative medicine, 178
Osteopenia, 128, 287
Osteoporosis, 144, 177, 287–88
      and anti-seizure drugs, 259
      bisphosphonate drugs for, 172
      and calcium, 127–28, 130
      chamomile tea for, 249
      and IVF, 295
      and oxytocin, 287
      and steroids, 287–88
Otoconia, 11, 291–92
Otolaryngologists, 11, 13, 54
Otoscopes, 165
Outpatient surgery, 162
Ovarian aging, 295–96
Ovarian cancer, 44, 46
Overweight. *See* Obesity and overweight
Oxalic acid, 129
Oxybutynin, 37
Oxytocin, 25–26, 123, 287

P

Pain, 251–80. *See also specific forms
   of pain*
      counting down for, 270
      learning to thrive with, 278–80
      living with, 280
      role of cannabis, 264
      self-massage tools, 255–57
      from sitting, 264–65
      3 easy ways to relieve, 285–86
Paint, volatile organic compounds in,
   311
Pancreatitis, 129, 324
Panic attacks, 181–82, 232
Pap smears, 235–36
Paraffin baths, 254
Parkinson's disease, 35–37
      coffee for, 110
      deep brain stimulation for, 35–36
      and medications, 37
      natural therapies for, 236–37
      and pupil size, 187
Paroxetine, 37, 45, 171, 298
Partners. *See* Relationships; Sex
Patient Priorities Care, 150–52

Paxil, 37, 298
Pelargonium, 229
Peloton, 146–48
Percussive therapy devices, 256, 257
Perfluorooctanoic acid (PFOA), 122–23
Perineural injection treatment, 272
Periodontal disease, 16, 50
Pessaries, 316
Pesticides, 118, 121, 228, 276
Petroleum jelly, 305
Pets
    and brain health, 22
    walking, 138
PET (positron emission tomography) scans, 38
PFAS (per-and polyfluoroalkyl substances), 7–8, 311
Phage therapy, 212–13
Phobias
    doctor, 156–57
    exposure therapy for, 157
    understanding, 157
Phonophoresis, 269–70
Phthalates, 276, 311
Physical injury, 281–86
    3 easy ways to relieve pain, 285–86
    4 common moves leading to, 283–85
Physical therapy (PT), 264, 269, 292–93
Physician phobias, 156–57
Phytic acid, 123, 129
Pickled vegetables, 118–20
    how to, 119–20
    recipes, 120
"Pins and needles," 30
Pioglitazone, 58–59
Piracetam, 32
Pizza boxes, 7
Plantar fasciitis, 267–69
Plant-based diet. *See* Vegetarian diet
Plaquenil, 172, 216, 217
Playing hard-to-get, 81
Pneumonia, 63, 161, 166, 174, 299, 305
Poison ivy, activated charcoal for, 242
Polysaccharides, 229
Pornography (porn use), 318
Portion sizes, 106
Positive attitude, 31, 208–9
Positive Emotional Attractor (PEA), 94
Postoperative delirium, 167
Postpartum depression (PPD), 299
Postsurgery depression, 76
Post-traumatic stress disorder (PTSD), 29, 230, 275–76, 281–83
Postural isometric lengthening (PIL), 285–86
Postural orthostatic tachycardia syndrome (POTS), 325
Potting mixes, 220
Powerade, 135
Power of attorney, 13
PPIs. *See* Proton-pump inhibitors
Prebiotics, 121
    for Baker's cyst, 247
Prediabetes, 58, 59, 63, 170
Prednisone, 130, 171, 328
Preeclampsia, 193, 300
Prefrontal cortex, 22, 31, 40
Pregnancy, 19
    and antidepressants, 298–99
    and bacterial vaginosis, 213
    and berberine, 50

and coffee, 110
drinking and miscarriages, 297
and family harmony, 300–301
flu and "vascular storm," 299–300
and heart disease, 180
IVF, 295–96
medication doses and IUGR, 297–98
"mommy brain," 301
natural births, 300
and NSAIDs, 301
and PFOA, 123
and strokes, 180
and thyroid dysfunction, 297
Premenstrual symptoms (PMS), 249, 252
Prilosec, 53, 60, 174
Probiotics, 48–49, 49, 66, 119, 227–28, 228
    for anxiety, 66–67
    for autoimmune diseases, 276
    in sourdough bread, 123
    for type 2 diabetes, 58
    for vaginal health, 213
Processed foods
    and anxiety, 66
    and cavities, 16
Procesed meats, 49, 191, 262
Procrastination, 79, 97
"Professional relatives," 15
Progressive muscle relaxation, 67
Prolozone therapy, 176, 272–73
Proning, 216
Propranolol, 259
Prostate cancer, 161, 318
Protein, aging and myth about, 111–12
Proton-pump inhibitors (PPIs), 169, 174
    breast cancer and cognitive issues, 53
    and diabetes, 60
    and gut microbiome, 170, 171
Prozac, 26, 171, 298
Psilocybin
    for cancer, 53
    for depression, 101–2
Psoriatic arthritis, 255
Psychotherapy, 29, 283. *See also* Cognitive behavioral therapy
Ptosis, 326–28
PTSD (post-traumatic stress disorder), 29, 230, 275–76, 281–83
Pulmonary rehabilitation, 307–8
Pulse oximeters, 163, 164, 165, 166
Pumpkin seeds, for diabetes, 62
Push-ups, 103, 142
Pyelonephritis, 211
Pyridostigmine, 328

Q

Quad exercises, 133, 139
Quercetin, 218, 231
Quinoa, 124, 125

R

Rear toners, 143
Receding gums and cavities, 16
Recipes
    Artichokes and Shell Beans Braised in White Wine, 114
    Avocado Sweet Potato "Toast" with Hummus, 108–9
    "Cheesy" Popcorn with Nutritional Yeast, 109

Chicken Almond Satay Wraps, 124–25
Choco-Banana "Nice Cream," 108
Creamy Curried Red Lentil Dip with Raw Veggies and Tortilla Chips, 109
Lemon Dill Kraut, 120
Lentil Cassoulet with Lots of Vegetables, 113–14
Matcha Cupcakes, 108
Roast Cod with Fennel and Tomatoes, 125–26
Roasted Sweet Potato & Kale Quinoa Bowl, 125
Spicy Carrot and Lime Salad, 120
Super Spinach Hummus, 126
Tamarind Tempeh Kebabs, 115
Zesty Papaya Salsa, 126
Recovery Factors, 215
Recumbent three-wheelers, 144
"Regulating" emotions, 94
Relationships. *See also* Sex
    annoying people, 95–96
    changing minds, 90–92
    death of loved one, finding meaning after, 76–78
    detoxing, 99–100
    doctor-patient, 152–54
    forgiveness, 97
    marriage killers, 81–83
    "micro-moments" of connection, 86
    partner with narcissistic personality disorder, 68–70
    playing hard to get, 81
    and porn use, 318
    preventing problems before they erupt, 79–81
    small talk, 94–95
Reproduction issues. *See* Pregnancy
Resistance band workouts, 138–40
    exercises, 139–40
    for neck pain, 258–59
    spot-train butt, 147
Resistance training. *See* Strength training
Respiratory conditions, xi, 303–14. *See also specific conditions*
    difficulty breathing (dyspnea), 303–5
    healthy home environment, 310–11
    lung emergencies, 305
    as post-COVID-19 symptom, 215
Resting heart rate (RHR), 199–200
Restless legs syndrome (RLS), 244
Restorative yoga, 232–35
Resveratrol, 6–7
Retail therapy, 72
Reticulospinal tract (RST), 27
Reverse lunges, 143
Reyvow, 260–61
Rheumatoid arthritis (RA), 193, 238, 247, 275, 278
    bee venom for, 46, 277
    and depression, 254–54
    and fever, 219
    hydroxychloroquine for, 172
Rhodiola, 232
Ribose, 215
Rifaximin, 244, 320
Rivastigmine tartrate, 37
Roast Cod with Fennel and Tomatoes, 125–26
Roasted Sweet Potato & Kale Quinoa Bowl, 125
Rock and Roll, 307
Rosemary oil, 34

Rotator cuff, 148, 284
Rotator cuff tear, 293–94
Rover, 138
"Rubber band" workouts, 138–40
    exercises, 139–40
    for neck pain, 258–59
    spot-train butt, 147
Running shoes, 141, 268
Ruts, eliminating, 71–72

S

Sacubitril, 202
Sadness. *See* Negative emotions
"Safety huddles," 80
St. John's wort, 171
Salad dressings, 107
Salt, 107, 119, 122
    and immune defenses, 221
Salt-cured olives, 117
SAMe (S-adenosyl methionine), 131, 232
SARS-CoV-2. *See* COVID-19
Saturated fats, 49, 116, 122
Sauerkraut, 66, 117, 118, 119, 228, 276
Sciatica, 269–70
Scurvy, 119
Sea salt, 122
Seated Hamstring Massage, 266–67
Seated Knee to Chest, 266
Seated Mountain Pose, 9
Seated Wrist Stretch, 267
Sea vegetables, 54–55, 122
Seaweed, 54–55
Second opinions, 152–53, 161
SECURE Act of 2019, 5
Selective norepinephrine reuptake
    inhibitors (SNRIs), 45
Selective serotonin reuptake inhibitors
    (SSRIs), 26, 45, 171, 298–99
Self-massage tools, 255–57
"Senior design," 4
Seniors. *See* Aging well
Sepsis, 161, 211, 212, 219
Serotonin, 30, 65, 67, 121
Sex
    after 70, 4
    and menopause, 317
    pain during, 5
    and porn use, 318
    and UTIs, 212
    women falling sleep after, 328
Sex-biased medical research, 149–50
    and heart disease, 179–80
Sex lubricants, 45
Sexually transmitted diseases (STDs),
    213, 296
Shampoo, 224
"Shinrin-yoku," 237
Shoes, 141, 221, 268
Shortness of breath, 52, 175, 181, 185, 186,
    195, 200, 202, 205, 214, 215, 259, 303, 305
Shoulder blade squeezes, 140
Shoulder pain, 266, 293–94
Shoulder Shrugs, 10
Shower benches, 14
Showers (showering), 224
    after exercising, 220
    medical-alert devices in, 13–14
"Sighing effect," 309
Sighs (sighing), 304, 308
Signature fashion style, 70
Silent heart attacks, 185–86
Single-arm rows, 133
Sinusitis, 216, 229
Sitting, 9–10
    and belly fat, 20
    "fidget-cisers" for, 142–43

and neck pain, 258–59
    pain from, 264–65
Skin cancer, seaweed for, 54–55
Skin elasticity, 8, 128, 248, 249
Skin rashes, 242–43, 244
Sleep. *See also* Insomnia
    for aging well, 2
    and atrial fibrillation, 206–7
    bedtime routine, 2, 105, 206, 214
    for belly fat, 20
    chamomile tea for, 214, 248–50
    for chronic inflammation, 239
    for colon health, 49
    for dementia, 34
    exercise and keeping cool, 135
    for eye floaters, 18
    for fascia, 273
    melatonin for, 2, 214, 217–18
    for menopause brain, 24
    and post-COVID-19, 214–15
    prebiotics for, 121
        ecommended amount, 2, 105,
        214, 239
Sleepiness, as medication side effect,
    169–70
Sleeping pills, 2, 149
Sleep journals, 86–87
Small-cell lung cancer (SCLC), 47
Small intestine bacterial overgrowth
    (SIBO), 174, 320
    natural relief for, 243–45
Small talk, 94–95
Smell (smelling)
    for chronic worry, 26–27
    loss of, as post-COVID-19 symptom,
        216, 218
    rotten egg, and SIBO, 320
    stop-look-listen-smell (SLLS) proto-
        col, 26–27
Smoking
    and COPD, 308
    and dementia, 33
    e-cigarettes, 311–12
    and glutathione, 228
    and heart health, 200, 203
    and lung cancer, 47
    thirdhand smoke, 314
Smoothies, for dementia, 33
Snacks, 107, 113
    exercise and keeping cool, 134
    guilt-free, 107–9
    planning ahead, 105, 106
    recipes, 108–9, 126–27
Sneakers, 141, 221, 268
Snowshoes, 136–37
Soccer Kicks, 290
Social anxiety
    and memory, 73
Social anxiety and memory, 73
Socialization, 1, 14, 34. *See also*
    Relationships
        caring for grandchildren, 97
        "micro-moments" of connection, 86
Social norms, 80
Social Security, 4–5
Socks, 137, 221, 233, 322
Sodium. *See* Salt
Sore throats, 46, 54, 224, 229
Sourdough bread, 123–24
Specialty massagers, 257
Speech therapy, after strokes, 210
Spices, 116
Spicy Carrot and Lime Salad, 120
Spicy foods, 45
Spider veins, 246
Spinal abscess, 160, 161

Spinal manipulation, 177, 178
Spinal mobilization, 177, 178
Splinters, activated charcoal for, 242
Splints, 254, 291
Sports drinks, 135
Squats, 133, 139, 142
Stain repellents, 7, 311
Stair climbing, 285
Statins, 189–91
    ASCVD Risk Score, 192–93
    CAC, 193–94
    and cholesterol myth, 189–90
    and diabetes risk, 64
    nocebo-effect, 195
    profit motive, 190
    side effects, 169
    3 questions to ask before taking,
        192–94
Stationary bikes, 145
Status quo, 91–92
Stem cells, for diabetes, 64
StepBet, 138
Steroid nasal sprays, 172
Steroids, 171, 287–88
Stevia, 127
Stop-look-listen-smell (SLLS) protocol,
    26–27
Strength training, 132–33
    for brain health, 27
    6 simple exercises, 133
Stress, 87–88
    and alcohol, 28
    and atrial fibrillation, 207–8
    and autoimmune diseases, 275–76
    calming "monkey mind," 102
    of caregiving, 72
    and chronic inflammation, 239
    and COVID-19, 230
    and heart health, 192, 200
    and increased gas, 265
    and menopause brain, 24
    natural healing of, 288
    and pain, 280
    prebiotics for, 121
    transcendental meditation for, 31
Stress incontinence, 315–17
Stress-induced cardiomyopathy, 195
Stretches (stretching), 10, 200, 265–67
    for fascia, 272–73
Strokes, 208–10
    and alcohol, 210
    and aspirin, 55
    and belly fat, 61
    dementia and calcium, 129
    and diabetes medications, 59
    heart monitors for, 201
    and menopause headaches, 23
    misdiagnosis of, 161
    and obesity, 61
    and positive thinking, 208–9
    preventive care, 180–81
    restoring mobility and sense of
        touch, 210
    speech therapy after, 210
    and unhealthy relationships, 99
    and vaginal estrogen, 5, 6
    and vitamin B12, 131
Successful aging. *See* Aging well
Sucrose, 107
Sudden cardiac arrest, 195
Sugar (sugar intake), 15, 66, 107, 191
    and belly fat, 19
    and chronic inflammation, 238
Sugary drinks and cavities, 16
Sumatriptan, 260, 261
Sunburn, 50, 135